01256644

HEALTH PSYCHOLOGY

HEALTH PSYCHOLOGY

A LIFESPAN PERSPECTIVE

Edited by

Gillian N. Penny

Nene College, Northampton, UK

Paul Bennett

*Gwent Psychology Services and University of Wales,
Cardiff, UK*

and

Mike Herbert

*International Medical College, Kuala Lumpur,
Malaysia*

harwood academic publishers
Switzerland • Australia • Belgium • France • Germany • Great Britain
India • Japan • Malaysia • Netherlands • Russia • Singapore • USA

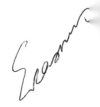
Copyright © 1994 by Harwood Academic Publishers GmbH, Poststrasse 22, 7000 Chur, Switzerland. All rights reserved.

Harwood Academic Publishers

Private Bag 8
Camberwell, Victoria 3124
Australia

3-14-9, Okubo
Shinjuku-ku, Tokyo 169
Japan

12, Cour Saint-Eloi
75012, Paris
France

Emmaplein 5
1075 A W Amsterdam
Netherlands

Glinkastrase 13–15
O-1086 Berlin
Germany

820 Town Center Drive
Langhorne, Pennsylvania 19047
United States of America

Post Office Box 90
Reading, Berkshire RG1 8JL
Great Britain

Library of Congress Cataloging-in-Publication Data
Health psychology: a lifespan perspective/edited by Gillian N. Penny, Paul Bennett & Michael Herbert.
   p. cm.
  Includes bibliographical references and index.
  ISBN 3-7186-5416-4. ISBN 3-7186-5415-6 (pbk).
  1. Clinical health psychology. I. Penny, Gillian N., 1947–
II. Bennett, Paul, 1942–   . III. Herbert, Michael, 1955–
R726.7.H43354 1994
613–dc20

93-17400
CIP

CONTENTS

CONTRIBUTORS

PAUL BENNETT
Community & Mental Health Unit, 12 Park Square, Newport, Gwent NP9 4EL, UK

ROGER BIBACE
Department of Psychology, Clark University, 950 Main Street, Worcester, MA 01610, USA

MICHAEL BOOTH
Department of Public Health, A27 Fisher Road, University of Sydney, NSW 2006, Australia

KEVIN J. CONNOLLY
Department of Psychiatry, University of Sheffield, Sheffield S10 2TN, UK

ROBERT J. EDELMAN
Department of Psychology, University of Surrey, Guildford, Surrey GU2 5XH, UK

SIOBHAN HART
1 Hicks Way, Crunch Croft, Sturmer Nr Haverhill, Suffolk CB9 7YU, UK

MIKE HERBERT
Department of Psychology, International Medical College, Kuala Lumpur, 21 Jalan Selangor, 46050 Petaling Jaya, Selangor, Darul Ehsan, Malaysia.

ROGER INGHAM
Department of Psychology, University of Southampton, Murray Building, Salisbury Road, Southampton SO9 5NH, UK

SUZANNE BENNETT JOHNSON
Department of Psychiatry, University of Florida, Box J-234, Gainesville, Florida 32610-0234, USA

MEGAN LEWIS
Institute of Behavioral Science, University of Colorado at Boulder, Boulder, Colorado 80309-0483, USA

SIMON MURPHY
Faculty of Health and Community Studies, University of the West of England, St Matthias Campus, Fishponds, Bristol, BS16 2JP, UK

DON NUTBEAM
Department of Public Health, A27 Fisher Road, University of Sydney, NSW 2006, Australia

GILLIAN N. PENNY
Department of Psychology, Nene College, Moulton Park, Northampton NN2 7AL, UK

KAREN S. ROOK
Program in Social Ecology, University of California, Irvine, CA 921717, USA

RALF SCHWARZER
Institut für Psychologie (WE7), Freie Universität Berlin, Habelschwerdter Allee 45, 1000 Berlin 33, Germany

LOTHAR R. SCHMIDT
Fachbereich 1 – Psychologie, Universität Trier, Postfach 3825, D-5500 Trier, Germany

M. SHELTON SMITH
School of Nursing, Vanderbilt University, Nashville, Tennessee 37240, USA

JANE M. USSHER
Department of Psychology, University College London, Gower Street, London WC1E 6BT, UK

KENNETH A. WALLSTON
School of Nursing, Vanderbilt University, Nashville, Tennessee 37240, USA

MARY E. WALSH
Department of Psychology, Boston College, McGurin 302, Chestnut Hill, MA 02167, USA

HEALTH PSYCHOLOGY:
A LIFESPAN PERSPECTIVE.
AN INTRODUCTION

GILLIAN N. PENNY, PAUL BENNETT AND MIKE HERBERT

The past twenty years have witnessed a rapid development of the field of health psychology. There has been increasing recognition of the links between medicine and psychology and the relevance of personal and psychosocial variables to health and illness. In turn, the theoretical basis, the concepts and constructs, used in health psychology is derived from social psychology. For example, it draws on attribution theory, social learning theory, and role theory to name but a few. Other fields of psychology which contribute significantly to health psychology include cognitive psychology, the psychology of individual differences, and learning theories. Throughout, there would seem to be some recognition of the differing influences on health and health behaviour which can be attributed to differences in personal, social, and cultural factors.

There has, however, been surprisingly little recognition within health psychology of the potential contribution of lifespan developmental psychology to inform our understanding of issues of health and illness. Yet it can be argued that health and illness are directly related to developmental processes, with morbidity and mortality showing distinct patterns across the lifespan. Ageing is directly linked to health status, and impacts on the demand for health care both in absolute terms and in the nature of the health care required. In addition, developmental and ageing processes may indirectly affect a variety of issues of interest to health psychologists such as illness prevention and health promotion, assessment and treatment of acute and chronic disease, health and illness behaviour and the experience of illness.

The main concern of lifespan developmental psychology is to understand the nature of change and stability which individuals experience through the life cycle from birth to death. Development is largely assumed to occur in an ordered sequence and with patterns of development common to groups of individuals. The developmental perspective focuses upon the biological, cognitive, social and personality processes which contribute to change throughout the lifespan. Such processes and patterns of development would, equally, seem relevant to understanding changes in health status and health and illness behaviour.

There has been some debate amongst developmental psychologists concerning the way in which change occurs during the life cycle. Traditional approaches [for example, Freud's classic theory of psycho-sexual development and Paiget's theory of cognitive development] emphasised the degree of change which occurred from birth to adolescence and assumed relative stability in adulthood. More recent approaches [for example, Baltes *et al.*, 1980] have recognised the degree of change that can occur in adulthood and an expanding elderly population has led to an increased focus upon late adult development and psychosocial processes in ageing. Thus, developmental periods through the life cycle are now commonly considered to comprise the prenatal, infancy, early childhood, middle and late childhood, adolescence, early adulthood, middle adulthood and late adulthood.

A number of theoretical models of lifespan development have been proposed to explain the patterns of change in individuals through the life cycle. They range from the classic theories of Buhler 1935, Jung 1960, Erikson 1958 and the more recent ones of Levinson 1978 and Gould 1972 which posit that development occurs through an ordered sequence of stages, to ones which emphasize stability and continuity throughout the lifespan such as that proposed by Costa and McCrae (1980). Of the first three, Erikson's theory (1958) is the more comprehensive and comprises eight stages, five emphasizing childhood development and three focussing upon adult development. Change follows a sequential pattern and the stages unfold in varying patterns of regularity. Each stage represents a struggle between two opposing tendencies and the way in which this tension is resolved has implications for future stages. Erikson argued that there is an optimal rate and sequence of development but that an individual's circumstances may alter the timing of this sequence. The theory suggests that the individual changes with age and that such changes are often experienced by different people at the same time.

Whilst Erikson's work derived from clinical experience, Levinson (1978) developed a model of adult development based on biographical interviews. His research revealed a series of developmental periods which were linked to specific chronological ages and comprised periods of transition which alternated with periods of stability. Each of the transitional periods has developmental tasks. The early adult transition, for example, provides a developmental bridge between adolescence and adulthood, whilst the phase from this bridge to the next transition is one of consolidation and the formation of a stable life structure. The mid-life transition comprises three tasks, but perhaps the most important is that of individuation or becoming one's own person. Here there are similarities to Erikson's last two psychosocial crises as well as to Neugarten's [1965] identification of increasing 'interiority' as a major process in mid-life. The re-appraisal which is associated with this phase may lead to significant changes from the previous life structure. Whilst Levinson proposes future transitions and tasks, moving through the age bands of 50 to 65 and beyond, as yet he has little empirical data to offer in support.

An alternative approach to development is the pluralistic one of Baltes and his colleagues (1980). They argue that not all developmental processes begin at birth, childhood or early adulthood, but that some may begin in old age. They also consider that some developmental processes may be curvilinear in that they may be important in childhood and in old age, but not in early or middle adulthood or vice versa. Individuals show considerable variation in development and this variability increases with age, particularly between adulthood and old age. The model is pluralistic in that three different types of influence on development can be identified: normative age graded influences such as biological development or typical events during adulthood focusing on, for example, the family; normative history-graded influences which comprise environmental, social and cataclysmic changes which affect the majority of a culture such as war or economic depression ànd which may have differential effects according to the age of the people who experience them; and non-normative influences which affect an individual but do not happen to most people.

Other theorists [for example, Neugarten, 1977] were also less satisfied with a life stage or crisis approach. They argued that to have a more coherent understanding of adult development one needs to study life events. Connections can be made between age or life stage and the probability of events taking place. The socio-historical context must also be considered. The same event, for example having a child at age 20 may have a very different impact on the woman compared to having it at age 40. Certain biological and social age-related events influence the individual's progression through the lifespan. Whilst development in childhood is largely regulated by biological factors, development in adulthood would seem to be regulated by social processes, so that the pattern of adult life would appear to follow a fairly regular course for most people.

Neugarten *et al.* [1965] found considerable consensus amongst representatives from various age groups about the appropriate ages for particular behaviours – such as the best ages for people to marry or to become grandparents. Similar studies in the 1980s indicate that the degree of consensus is declining, and Neugarten and Neugarten [1986] has consequently suggested that we may be moving towards an age-irrelevant society. Nevertheless, she argued, age norms still exert powerful influences on our behaviour. Neugarten posits the existence of an internal sense of the optimum time to reach certain social milestones – a social clock. She and her colleagues argue that off time events, that is those events which do not correspond to the appropriate age norms occurring either abnormally early or abnormally late, are more difficult to deal with. Socially expected events which do not occur at all, such as not getting married or not having children, may be particularly stressful.

The study of transitions focuses on the process of change in development. The concept of transition relates to a period of change or disequilibrium that may provide a bridge between one largely stable point in life and another relatively stable, but different, one. Normative and non-normative transitions correspond to Baltes' normative age graded and non-normative influences on development described earlier. Some transitions, such as the menopause and chronic disease, result from internal causes, while others, such as war or retirement from work, may be caused primarily by external forces. Theories about transitions tend to emphasize either internal changes or external events as the primary vehicle of change. Thus, Erikson's and Levinson's theories focus upon changes in adult development which result mainly from internal factors while Neugarten's and Baltes' work emphasizes external social factors as the main cause of transitions.

Both types of approaches are of interest. An emphasis on internal factors implies that there is a regular pattern of human development right through the life cycle, not only in the years of childhood. An emphasis on external social influences, such as that of Neugarten, points to the obvious role of social norms and expectations in creating stability and change and emphasises the individual in interaction with the environment.

These theories, thus, provide useful frameworks for understanding human development and indicate ways in which people may differ at different stages of their life cycle. They provide differing perspectives which enable us to account both for stability and for change, for commonality and for individuality along with a general developmental progression throughout the life cycle. Such approaches may also be of use to health psychology.

In particular, the following tenets of lifespan developmental psychology would seem to carry particular meaning for health psychology:

- the assumption of life long change.
- the assumption of progression; experiences at an early stage carry implications for future experiences.
- the biological, psychological and social developmental processes not only affect child development and the period of senescence, but also impact upon the adult years between.
- the concepts of life stages, crises or transitions imply that there are salient issues or problems at different points in the life cycles which are common to most people.
- the notion of normative or non-normative events suggest that an individual's experiences of an event may be affected by the timing of that event.

Such characteristics or assumptions of developmental psychology have considerable utility for enhancing our understanding of many of the concerns of health psychology. Issues pertaining to health status, health promotion and disease prevention, health and illness behaviour, individual differences and health, assessment and treatment of acute illness, and management of chronic disorders may be clarified through the application of concepts and theories of developmental psychology.

Any general underlying progression in the life cycle involving physical, psychological and social processes has implications for the individual's experience of health and illness, both physical and psychological. It suggests that there will be health issues common to particular life stages and that individuals may experience particular health concerns at specific points in the life cycle. The impact of a health problem may differ according to the stage of life in which it is experienced, both in terms of its meaning for the individual and their ability to cope with it. In addition, behaviours adopted to enable adjustment at one stage of the life cycle may have considerable implications for health in both current, and future, life stages.

Even when individuals from differing age groups experience a common disorder the implications of that health problem may differ considerably. As the psychological and social circumstances vary across the lifespan so health-related issues salient to children may be very different to those of adolescents, adults or the elderly. One can argue, therefore, that there is thus a need for a developmental approach to health which focusses upon each period of life and explores the problems and issues related to it.

Child health psychologists have been more aware of the influence of developmental processes on health issues than have health psychologists working with an adult population. Similarly, at the other end of the life cycle, the relationship between biological ageing and health has been examined. However, health psychologists have tended to study these age groups separately and there has been little attempt to consider health issues within an overall lifespan perspective.

This book represents a first attempt to remedy the current situation. Its aim is to explore aspects of health psychology from a lifespan perspective and to reflect the increasing awareness of a number of authors of the need to focus more directly upon developmental issues. The book does not attempt a comprehensive coverage of health and illness throughout the lifespan. Rather, the contributions have been chosen to represent dominant health issues at different stages of the life cycle and to illustrate the variety of ways in which developmental processes may be applicable to furthering our understanding of health and illness.

In selecting the life stages and health themes considered in the book the editors have drawn on the work of stage theorists such as Erikson, Gould, Levinson and Vaillant. We have chosen to focus upon five points in the life cycle; childhood, adolescence, early adulthood, middle adulthood and old age. Thus we have consciously emphasised the differing stages within the adult years, rather than taking the more traditional approach of focusing upon the differing stages of childhood, assuming a relatively stable period of adulthood and a decline into old age. This decision echoes recent moves within lifespan psychology itself and reflects the editors' perceptions of the need to introduce a more sequential approach to bring together the currently somewhat disparate fields of child health psychology, health psychology, and ageing and health, and to emphasise the progressive nature of people's experiences of health and illness.

In choosing the health issues within each of the stages we have considered the nature of developmental tasks postulated to be associated with these ages, the type of normative events commonly experienced within them (and the implications of non-normative ones), and the developmental processes operating at these times. We hope that the reader will perceive the variety of aspects of developmental issues from which our selection was made and that the chapters together form a compendium which illustrates the richness and diversity with which lifespan psychology can inform our understanding of health and illness.

Section I deals with health issues in childhood. The phenomenon of chronic illness is unusual at this time, being much more usual in the late adult and elderly phases of the life cycle. A basic assumption of childhood is that the dependency is limited and the main overall task is to develop independence, competence and mastery of the environment, and to begin the move out of the family into the wider social world. Chronic illness in childhood may disrupt this process of increasing autonomy. Suzanne Bennett-Johnson's chapter reviews these issues. In particular, she examines the inter-relationships between the children's illness and both patient and family functioning, and explores the implications of the differing age of the ill child on such functioning. The author also argues that the illness itself has an effect on children's development. In addition, she considers elements of disease specific functioning by examining children's responses to pain and discomfort, their knowledge about the illness and factors involved in adherence to the medical regimen. Her concluding remarks focus upon the question of measurement and the problem of correlation versus causation.

Bibace and colleagues focus upon children's perceptions of illness and review the various approaches which researchers have taken in attempting to understand them. The authors show how the four main approaches taken by researchers address rather different questions. The Health Belief Model, the cognitive developmental, script analysis and cognitive science approaches focus respectively upon the content of the child's health belief, the cognitive processes used by the child particularly that of causal reasoning, the sequence of events which children associate with illness and medical procedures and the biological bases of children's understanding of health related events. They argue for the utilisation of all four approaches, suggesting that the findings generated by such a multiplicity of approaches should be viewed as complementary rather than as exclusive. As well as being of interest in its own right, the way in which children construe health and illness has implications for health educators. An understanding of their concepts of health and illness, and the way in which they change as the children grow older, may lead to the development of more effective types of health educational approaches and materials. Accordingly the authors also draw attention to the potential implications of these models for health education, with particular reference to AIDS transmission.

One of the major tasks of adolescence is to develop a sense of identity and to take on a more adult role. This overall sense of identity encompasses more specific ones such as a sexual identity or an occupational identity. Erikson argues that the developmental crisis at this stage is resolved when the adolescent knows who and what he or she wishes to do and be. The search for, and the resolution of, that identity may have considerable implications for the health and well-being of the adolescent both in terms of their current and future potential health status.

The chapters in Section II address the theme of adolescence. Nutbeam and Booth's paper provides an overview of the various influences on health risk behaviour, whilst that of Ingham focuses more specifically upon sexuality in adolescence.

Nutbeam and Booth explore the physical, cognitive and social developments associated with adolescence and consider their influence on adolescent health and health behaviour. In particular, they draw attention to the model proposed by Irwin and Millstein which shows how a multiplicity of factors interact to predict risk-taking behaviour. The authors argue that adolescent health-compromising, risk-taking activities can only be understood within the context of their overall lifestyle. They suggest that such activities are not viewed by adolescents as directly relevant to health, but rather, they serve other functions such as integration into their peer group, and help to define the type of person they are. Thus, if one is to effect change in adolescent health risk behaviour, one has to understand the function that that behaviour serves.

By way of contrast Ingham, in the next chapter, examines a dominant theme in adolescence; that of emerging sexuality. He distinguishes between sexuality and the term 'sexual behaviour', arguing that the former permits a contemplation of wider ideas. In doing so, Ingham brings a European, 'new social psychological' perspective [Harre, 1985] to bear on issues of sexuality in people in this age group, particularly in connection with AIDS. He first establishes a rational for an ethnographic approach to research, presenting both his own data and those of other European workers and goes on to argue that there are two key ways in which psychology should develop. The first is by questioning current concepts of rationality assumed in many interpretations of behaviour. Secondly, he suggests that psychology should be more prepared to interact with, and adopt, the methodologies of other disciplines.

Once adolescence has been successfully negotiated and the sense of identity achieved, then Erikson argues that the individual is ready to share themselves with another and begin the development of intimate relationships. Thus, he argues that the main pre-occupation of early adulthood is the establishment of intimate relationships. Levinson too perceives the early adult phase as one of making choices and commitments, largely concerning occupations and marriage partners. With the development of a stable relationship comes the preparation for parenthood. Thus, a major feature of early to mid-adulthood is the establishment of a stable intimate relationship and successfully starting a family. Most societies place strong emphasis on the importance of having children. However, since infertility affects at least 1 in 10 couples, the potential for psychological morbidity is great. The chapter by Edelman and Connolly considers this issue of infertility. They argue that there is little evidence to support the notion of psychogenic infertility, but that there are stronger reasons to accept that at least some couples will react adversely to failure to conceive. In addition, they examine the claim that treatments for infertility themselves can carry a high psychological cost.

Early adulthood is a time of increasing commitment to work, family and community activities. It is also a time of increasing influence particularly when parenthood is achieved. The health behaviour of young adults is salient therefore not just for their own future well-being, but also because of the potential effect on the next generation. In their chapter, Murphy and Bennett take a broad perspective and attempt to identify social and individual determinants of health behaviour in young adults. They draw the readers attention to the problem that differences between age groups may reflect inter-generational differences, such as those that might arise from differences in education, rather than resulting from differing life cycle stages. Using an interactive model of health behaviour adopted by the World Health Organisation, they review the influences of genetic and/or individually acquired characteristics, micro-social, macro-social and physical environmental effects on health behaviour. The authors consider the implications of this interactive perspective to the methods of health promotion. They argue that there is a need for alternative health promotion programmes, which take cogniscence of the differing needs of different groups within society, and which target their audience more specifically in terms of their life cycle stages as well as their broader socio-economic circumstances and gender.

The boundaries of middle age vary from one theorist to another but the general consensus is that it comprises the period from 40 to 65 years of age. It is generally viewed as a time of maximal productivity with developmental tasks, comprising consolidating in a chosen career, raising children, and possibly caring for elderly parents. Theorists also touch upon issues of individuation and increasing interiority which occur at this stage. In their chapter, Wallston and Smith draw attention to the heightened sense of control which normally accompanies this life stage, proposing that individuals experience the greatest degree of control over their own lives and that of others during middle age than at any one stage in the life cycle. They acknowledge that peoples' desire for control may vary and that a gradual decline in health which is experienced during this stage may have implications for a person's perception of control over their health status. Wallston and Smith propose that control is a par-ticularly salient factor in any consideration of health issues, and they bring together a variety of studies which together illustrate the relevance of control beliefs to a number of illness factors including health status, psychological well-being, and length of survival in cancer patients. They argue convincingly for the need to examine inter-action effects between actual and perceived control when considering middle aged people with health difficulties.

Jane Ussher takes a narrower viewpoint of health-related issues in middle age and focuses upon aspects of the menopause; a biological phenomenon for women in mid-life to which the response may be socially mediated. In support of her contention,

Ussher examines attitudes to menstruation generally as well as the menopause specifically. She considers both society's and the medical profession's response to this biological process and examines the social and cultural context in which attitudes to reproductive processes are established. Ussher contends that any analysis of womens' health must include an understanding of the influence of menstruation and menopause. She continues by reviewing the evidence for the existence of reproductive syndromes and the types and efficacy of psychological responses to them.

In Section V the focus is upon the period of old age. The proportion of older people within Western societies is increasing, largely because of enhancements in life expectancy at older age. The most well established association with health has been that of ages and despite hopes that people would live longer morbidity-free lives, increased survival rates would seem to be accompanied by increased morbidity with greater numbers of health problems and more chronic illnesses. This pattern suggests an increasing demand on both formal and informal types of health care. The two chapters in the section on the elderly reflect obverse aspects of these issues covering both health related factors in the elderly themselves, and the health implications for those who provide social support to elderly people with low health status.

In their chapter Lewis, Rook and Schwarzer contend that there are two main issues in the health of the elderly which require consideration. The first relates to establishing those factors which might prevent or postpone the development of chronic illness and disability and the second involves clarification of those factors which enable the elderly to manage health problems. The authors focus upon the role of social relationships, notably social support and social control, in both the prevention or delay of chronic illness and its management once it has developed. They review research in both these areas and suggest questions which could usefully be addressed in future studies.

In the final chapter, Siobhan Hart focuses upon the costs of caring for older people by critically reviewing research which examines the psychological and physical health consequences of providing support to an ill relative. She draws attention to the need for studies which examine the effect on caregivers of the range of disorders which elderly people can experience, rather than the current situation in which the main emphasis is upon the carers of patients with dementia. Hart also reviews research which examines the coping strategies of carers and argues for more longitudinal studies if the effects of caring on health are to be more fully understood. In addition, she considers the evidence from intervention studies which explore the effectiveness of differing forms of carer support and proposes that there is a need to study what happens to carers following the death of the person cared for.

The editors hope that these ten chapters will provide the reader with a modest understanding of the way in which health psychology can benefit from a synthesis with lifespan psychology. It is hoped that the problems and themes presented by the various authors will stimulate further interest in the relationship between lifespan and health issues and encourage others to draw on the strengths of developmental psychology to provide a more comprehensive basis from which to explore the nature of health and illness within the field of health psychology.

REFERENCES

Baltes, P.B., Reese, H.W., Hayne, W. & Lipsitt, L.P. (1980). Life span developmental psychology. *Annual Review of Psychology*, **31**, 65–110.

Buhler, C. (1935). The curves of life as studied in biographies. *Journal of Applied Psychology*, **19**, 405–409.

Costa, P.T. & McCrae, R.R. (1980). Still stable after all these years: personality as a key to some issues in adulthood and old age. In P.B. Baltes and O.G. Brim, Jr. [eds] *Life Span Development and Behaviour*. Vol 3, 65–102. New York: Academic Press.

Erikson, E.H. (1980). *Identity and the Life Cycle: A Reissue*. New York: W.W. Norton.

Erikson, E.H. (1959). Identity and the Life Cycle. *Psychological Issues*, **1**(1), 1–171.

Gould, R.L. (1972). The phases of adult life: A study in developmental psychology. *American Journal of Psychiatry*, **129**, 521–531.

Gould, R.L. (1978). *Transformations: Growth and Change in Adult Life*. New York: Simon and Schuster.

Harre, R., Clarke, D. & DeCarlo, N. (1985). *Motives and Mechanisms*. London: Methuen.

Havighurst, R.J. (1972). *Developmental Tasks and Education*. 3rd edition (1st edition, 1948). New York: David McKay.

Jung, C.G. (1960). *The Stages of Life*. In *Collected Works*, vol 8. Princetown: Princetown University Press.

Levinson, D.J. (1978). *The Seasons of a Mans Life* (with C.N. Darrow, EE.B. Klein, M.H. Levinson & B. McKee). New York: Knopf.

Neugarten, B.L. (1965). A developmental view of adult personality. In Birren, J.E. [ed] *Relations of Development and Aging*. Springfield Illinois: C.C. Thomas.

Neugarten, B.L., Moore, J.W. & Lowe, J.C. (1965). Age norms, age constraints and adult socialization. *American Journal of Sociology*, **70**, 710–717.

Neugarten, B.L. (1977). Adaptation and the life cycle. In N.K. Schlossberg & A.D. Entine (eds) *Counseling Adults*. Monterey, California: Brooks/Cole.

Neugarten, B.L. & Neugarten, D.A. (1986). Age in an aging society. *Daedalus*, **115**(1), 31–49.

Vaillant, G.E. (1977). *Adaptation to Life*. Boston: Little, Brown.

SECTION I
Childhood

CHILDREN'S PERCEPTIONS OF ILLNESS*

ROGER BIBACE, LOTHAR R. SCHMIDT AND MARY E. WALSH

In the past decade, there have been at least four major reviews of the literature on children's perceptions of illness (Jordan and O'Grady, 1982; Eiser, 1985; Burbach and Peterson, 1986; Maddux *et al.*, 1986). It is interesting to note how studies related to children's conceptions of illness have been categorized in the past. There is considerable agreement among past reviewers (Jordan and O'Grady, 1982; Eiser, 1985) regarding two major types of studies in this area.

One diverse group of studies has been conducted within the framework of what is broadly interpreted as *developmental psychology*. Studies based on individual differences in knowledge are exemplified by cognitive-developmental psychologists. These have included studies which subscribe, in fairly strict fashion, to a Piagetian framework (e.g. Bibace and Walsh, 1980; Burbach and Peterson, 1986). Such studies use the concept of development as a "structural" or "organizing" principle for the creation of invariant sequences. Such sequences are exemplified in, but not limited to, normal ontogenesis. That is, since development is an "ideal," it can and has been applied to domains other than ontogenesis. Werner and Kaplan (1963), for instance, have applied their orthogenetic principle of development to psychopathology and to microgenesis. In contrast, other studies within the developmental framework equate development with changes associated with chronology in normal children (Campbell, 1975; Mechanic, 1964).

A second large group of studies focuses on "health beliefs." These studies are based on social psychological approaches contributing to children's beliefs regarding disease, in general, and to the articulation of a "health belief model" in particular. Within this tradition, Jordan and O'Grady (1982) group studies under three sub-headings: (a) preventive health behavior, (b) illness behavior, and (c) sick-role behavior. In all three areas, the attempt is to predict health behaviors from health beliefs. Even more

---

*Equality of contributions to this chapter is signified by alphabetical listing of authors.

broadly, this tradition has been labeled "the public health approach, exemplified by social psychologists and public health officials" (Jordan and O'Grady, 1982, p. 73). This approach has focused on "group differences in observable behaviors" (Jordan and O'Grady, 1982, p. 73).

In this review, we also wish to draw attention to two novel genres which are represented in children's perceptions of health and illness. These genres draw on theoretical frameworks which have, hitherto, not been heavily represented in research on children's perceptions of health and illness. Conversely, it is because of their increasing prominence in psychology generally, that we are now seeing applications of these theoretical frameworks to this area of study. One such framework is the analysis of scripts or broader psycholinguistic approaches. The other is that of cognitive science.

The perspective that is rarely, or no longer, represented in empirical studies is the psychoanalytic orientation. Though clinical case studies abound, there are few empirical group studies that rely on this perspective. This is interesting given that a primary metaphor for psychoanalysis is the body and the way it is fantasized (consciously and unconsciously) in healthy and diseased states.

It should be noted that children's health concepts are not examined in the literature as frequently as are concepts of illness. Gochman (1988) emphasized that because of contemporary overmedicalization, wellness should be the main target of investigation. However, health and illness are not necessarily related concepts. "Natapoff argues that at younger ages (e.g. up to 8 years) illness and health are seen as two separate concepts, not as interlinked or reversible ones. . . . However, there is a conceptual difficulty in treating health and illness as ends of the same continuum. There are not specific 'healthinesses' as there are specific illnesses, so there cannot be full reversibility between the two concepts" (Bird and Podmore, 1990, p. 176).

The analysis of health concepts and health behavior is important with regard to primary prevention and health education (Jordan and O'Grady, 1982; Maddux *et al.*, 1986). Gochman (1988) claims that we need basic research on "those personal attributes that relate to maintaining, restoring, and improving health" (p. 351). Therefore, ". . . assessments might be made of youngsters' beliefs about how well they generally cope with demands and challenges, including the challenge of remaining healthy and safe" (p. 352). On a practical level, children's knowledge of preventive behavior may be helpful for health education (Lohaus, 1990). However, preventive behavior is more likely to be shown if children learn it as a matter of course in daily living.

In his review, Lohaus (1990) shows that children provide definitions of health which are "negative," i.e. related to the absence of illness or of certain symptoms as well as definitions which are "positively" health oriented. In German studies (Poida, 1990; Huda, 1991) it was found that health was either defined as absence of illness or illness symptoms respectively, or as wellness, which also included the mood of the person. In addition, children often named behavioral aspects, such as healthy eating habits (especially eating fruits) or healthy activities, including diverse behaviors which one is able to engage in as a healthy individual. Children at a pre-operational level were, as expected, less specific (for example, one is healthy, one can play).

The dialectic among the four approaches to children's perceptions of illness is interpreted below as foci by investigators on different questions. Thus, the health belief model addresses questions related to "what," or the content of a child's health belief. The cognitive developmental approaches address questions related to "how," or the cognitive processes relied upon by a child. In the area of children's perceptions of illness, cognitive developmental psychologists have targeted the child's causal reasoning. A major issue for psychologists relying on the analysis of scripts has been linguistic analyses which focus on a child's perceived sequence of events regarding illness and medical procedures. The focal question from such a perspective is "What happens when?" Cognitive science in the area of health belief attempts to corroborate its commitment to neo-nativism generally, that is, to articulate the "biological givens" which enable the child to understand events in the "specific" domains of health. Thus, findings which demonstrate that children of a very young age, or a younger age than is ordinarily assumed by other approaches, can be interpreted as backing for the "hard-wiring" of the organism.

These four theoretical approaches to perceptions of illness have received unequal attention in the literature. The cognitive-developmental approaches has been the framework most frequently relied upon. This is probably due to the popularity of cognitive-developmental theorists in child psychology. The health belief model as a framework grows out of the domain of health educationists in preventive medicine. This framework has only much more recently been construed as part of health psychology. The last two frameworks are applications of relatively recent basic science orientations in psychology. Script analyses are derived from psycholinguistic frameworks; cognitive science, the most recent theoretical innovation, has had the fewest applications to children's perceptions of illness. In recent years a call for research proposals by a federal agency in America has demonstrated that the largest number have been in the area of cognitive-developmental psychology.

One of the appeals of the health belief framework is the ease with which it can be implemented. Studies aimed at determining *what* children believe about illness do not require learning novel frameworks and modes of interpretation. It is sufficient, within this framework, to administer questionnaires and to analyze the frequency with which certain contents or beliefs are held. Though "beliefs" and "attitudes" may be vague theoretical constructs, they still hold a considerable attraction for many psychologists as a basic psychological characteristic of a person.

An example which focuses on children's perceptions of cancer, may help to make this approach clearer. The health belief model, in its efforts to predict health behavior from health beliefs, would be likely to examine children's beliefs about a number of different aspects of cancer. Researchers within this framework would ask a number of children, in various age groups, a series of objective questions to determine their beliefs about such issues as the severity of cancer, the treatability of cancer and the perceived susceptibility of themselves or others to cancer. They would be particularly concerned about the way in which children perceive the benefit of health-related or illness-avoidant behavior and their reported intentions to take health actions, for example, "Do you think that you might ever try to smoke a cigarette?" In analyzing the data within the framework of the health belief model, sex and age group differences would likely be addressed. A study of children's health beliefs about cancer yielded some interesting information. For example, children perceived cancer, as opposed to other illnesses, as being more severe, less treatable, less understood and a disease people had a greater chance of getting (Michielutte and Diseker, 1982). Such findings could conceivably be useful to a health education program which was trying to change the content of children's illness beliefs.

The rationale for the cognitive/developmental approach, based on Piagetian and Wernerian frameworks, questions the exclusive reliance on the "product" or *what* is said or done by a person. This perspective addresses *how* that behavior comes about and relies primarily on an analysis of cognitive processes to answer the question "how." Thus, from this perspective, the interviewer must "probe" for the child's causal reasons for saying what s/he says about illness. That is, without probing, the interviewer runs the risk of not being able to determine the cognitive processes which purportedly are being relied upon by the child to say what s/he says. Another major complication in utilizing this framework is that there are no "ready-made" categories to bridge the theoretical abstractions of Piaget (1930) and Werner (1948) with the concrete examples of a child's response. Thus, the researcher is required to create categories that are both congruent with the theoretical framework and can be applied to the domain of illness. Bibace and Walsh (1981) have called such links between cognitive developmental theory and the conceptions of illness "categories of the middle range."

Consider once again the example of children's perception of cancer. Instead of considering what it is that children believe about cancer, (for example, that "cancer is more severe than other illnesses") the cognitive-developmental approach focuses on the developmentally-ordered ways of articulating how children understand the definition, cause and treatment of the illness (for example, "Young children believe that cancer is caused by touching a person with cancer, while older children believe that cancer is the consequence of physiological malfunctioning of body parts and systems and has both external and internal causes.") Researchers within this framework not only ask children what they think about various aspects of cancer (that is, the definition cause and treatment) but also ask them, through utilization of the "clinical method," to explain how the causes result in the illness (for example, "You just told me that cancer comes from smoking cigarettes. Can you tell me how smoking cigarettes brings about or treats the cancer?"). Through systematic exploration of the child's thinking, the cognitive-developmental approach focuses on the underlying processes that give shape to the content of a child's perceptions of illness.

Whereas cognitive-developmental studies focus on the child's conception of the cause of the illness, script researchers ask the child "what happens when?" type of questions. Consider once again the example of children's perceptions of cancer. Bearison and Pacifici's (1989) studies on children's event knowledge of cancer treatment required children to describe what happened when they went to the clinic for cancer treatment. The children were required to tell the experimenter "everything that happens to you when you come to the clinic from when you first arrive until you leave (e.g. what's the first thing that happens?)." These so-called events were coded into predetermined categories reflecting four levels of act generality.

Historians of science have argued that many technological advances (from telephones to computers) engender "metaphors" which are used by scientists to understand human behavior. The metaphor relied upon in this domain is that "the computational view of mind ... is central to cognitive science" (Newell, Rosenbloom and Laird, 1989, p. 93). Though there are various approaches within cognitive science, "disagreements between authors involve differences over the type of computation involved: for example, serial or massively parallel, symbol-based or connectionist" approaches (Anderson, 1991, p. 285). The importance of the metaphor is underscored in the assumption and strategies adhered to. Researchers in this tradition attempt to articulate the way in which the organism is "hard-wired" to solve problems in particular ways. As Fischer and Bidell (1991) point out cognitive scientists argue for "nativist inferences about cognitive capacities."

Siegal (1988), Keil (1989) and others attempt to demonstrate that even very young children are capable of making distinctions which cognitive developmental psychologists assume are characteristic of later stages of cognitive development.

The cognitive science approach is again illustrated in the example of children's perceptions of cancer. Its goal is to demonstrate that intuitive ideas occur at younger ages than previous research would suggest. With respect to children's perception of illness, the method for demonstrating these intuitive theories has been to present children with other children's ideas about illness, (for example, using puppets) in particular, the cause of the illness, and ask children whether these ideas are "right" or "wrong" (Siegal, 1988). Extrapolating from Siegal's research on illness, in the case of children's ideas about cancer, researchers within this framework might show children a video-tape of puppets telling each other that cancer comes from touching someone with cancer. The child subject is then asked if s/he thinks the puppet is "right" or "wrong." Further, children may be shown concrete demonstrations of how cancer could be caused (e.g. a doll next to a comb that had been used by someone with cancer) and asked "Will the doll get cancer if she now uses that comb?" The data from such studies would be used to demonstrate that children develop concepts of cancer or, more generally, concepts of illness, at much younger ages than previously thought. These studies argue that children have intuitive concepts of cancer and other diseases.

We will now articulate more fully these four approaches to children's perceptions of illness.

Cognitive-Developmental Approaches

The most common framework for examining children's concepts of illness has been provided by the cognitive-developmental perspective. A major assumption of this approach is that there are a limited number of categories which subsume the seemingly endless variety of ways in which people explain the meaning of an event to themselves and others. This approach further assumes that these forms of explanation can be ordered developmentally from least to most mature.

A number of recent reviews of studies of children's concepts of illness have examined the studies within this perspective (Jordan and O'Grady, 1982; Eiser, 1985; Burbach and Peterson, 1986; Maddux *et al.*, 1986). Some of the studies cited in these reviews, as well as other more recent studies, have measured the frequency of certain types of responses across the different age groups, for example, the number of references to the inside of the body. Others categorized responses according to some characteristics presumed to reflect the various developmental stages, for example, "confabulation" or "more sophisticated responses" (Perrin and Gerrity, 1981). Still others grouped responses into various categories of content themes, for example, "symptoms" or "diagnosis" (Campbell, 1975; Millstein, Adler and Irwin, 1981) and determined the age differences in the frequency of the various themes. Finally some of these approaches focused on the reasoning underlying children's various concepts of illness.

The initial study which utilized this latter approach (Bibace and Walsh, 1980) is now considered by some to be "the most detailed and well-defined system outlined thus far in the literature..." (Burbach and Peterson, 1986, p. 314). This research looks at the cognitive processes relied upon in various types of causal explanations for illness. These cognitive processes are categorized according to their developmental character-istics. The cardinal dimension for ordering these categories developmentally is the degree of differentiation between the self and the world (both animate and inanimate objects). In contrast to focusing on the content of a single response, or response-characteristic, this approach characterizes the form of reasoning, or organizational structure, used by the subject. In this approach, Bibace and Walsh specified six developmentally ordered explanations for the definition, cause and treatment of illness (see Table 1).

TABLE 1
Developmental Levels of Conception of Illness

Magical Level—Explanations Based on Association
1. Phenomenism. The child describes the illness in terms of any phenomenon s/he has experienced as associated with the illness, without clear differentiation of cause and effect. "A cold is from ... it's when your nose runs."
2. Contagion. The child describes the illness in terms of body experiences or symptoms. S/he associates a specific external cause with the illness, but cannot explain how the cause leads to the effect. "A cold is a runny nose and it's like from going outside in winter." (How?) "It's from being out in the winter time."

Concrete Level—Explanations Based on Sequence
3. Contamination. The child describes illness in terms of experienced symptoms and explains its cause as originating in external acts or situations. The child explains how a sequence of causal events leads to the illness by contacting or involving the body as a whole. "A cold is from when you're swimming in cold water or out in the snow. It stays in your body ... it goes up onto your chest."
4. Internalization. The child describes the illness and explains how a sequence of mechanical actions leads to changes in specific internal body parts. "A cold is when your nose gets stuffed up and you can't breathe. It's from the germs getting into your nose and lungs and clogging them up so you can't breathe. You sneeze to get the germs out."

Abstract Level—Explanations Based on Interaction
5. Physiological. The older child or adult describes an entire internal disease process involving the interaction of multiple causes and effects on multiple body parts. "A cold is a change within the body resulting in symptoms like coughing, sneezing, running nose, headaches and stuffed up sinuses. You catch the germs that are all around us. Coughing and running nose are the side effects of the body's fighting them off, it makes mucous to carry away the dead germs."
6. Psychophysiological. The older child or adult explains how multiple causes and effects interact by describing transformations at the cellular level. "A cold is the collection of symptoms that define the immune system's response to an invading virus. The white blood cells ... And this happens when the person is experiencing a lot of stress."

The forms of reasoning are general in nature and constitute the explanations for a wide range of illnesses. Indeed, the original research was based on children's responses to a number of illnesses (cold, heart attack, measles, cancer) but in the tradition of cognitive developmental psychology sought out the common forms of organization for such explanations. The original findings (see Table 2) have been confirmed in numerous studies over the past decade (Susman, Dorn and Fletcher, 1987; del Barrio, 1988).

While useful as "a model of developmental changes in children's health con-ceptualizations," this approach also has its limitations, some of which have been addressed over the years. For instance, Burbach and Peterson (1986) expressed concern regarding the statistical treatment of the data in the original study. Schmidt and

TABLE 2
Frequency of Response Categories
within Age Groups

Age	Category of developmental conception of illness					
	1	2	3	4	5	6
5–7	6	5	9			
8–10		2	12	6		
11–13			1	16	3	

Weishaupt (1990) have argued for the specification of the particular characteristics or attributes of various diseases, especially their concreteness. The methodological evaluation of Bird and Podmore (1990) was more negative: "There were several aspects of the present study which brought into doubt the usefulness of a Piagetian framework for interpretation of the findings" (p. 176). The authors abandoned an attempt to code children's responses using a Piagetian levels coding scheme, as reliability was unacceptably low. This was due to the brevity of statements given by the young children even after probing, which made the inference of causal connections between the various factors difficult to code.

However, over the years a number of studies have been done by others who have applied the Bibace and Walsh model to a variety of illnesses (e.g. Susman, Dorn and Fletcher, 1987; del Barrio, 1988; Young *et al.*, 1987). As the theory would predict, these studies have confirmed that the development of concepts of particular illnesses follow the same developmental trajectory as the development of the concept of illness more generally.

Recently, the growing concern about providing effective AIDS education has led Walsh and Bibace (1991) to examine the ways in which people understand this illness, particularly its causal mechanisms. Relying on the cognitive-developmental framework of our earlier work on conceptions of illness, this study examined conceptions of AIDS in a sample of school aged children. More specifically, this study examined children's causal reasoning about AIDS, which represents three major phases of cognitive development: pre-operational, concrete-operational and formal-operational thinking. Sixty subjects (age groups 5–7 years, 8–10 years and 11–13 years) were administered the Concepts of AIDS Protocol which addresses questions such as "What is AIDS?", "How do people get AIDS?", "Is there anything people can do so that they won't get AIDS?", etc. Responses were scored using the recently revised Concept of Illness Category System, which differs from the original scoring system insofar as it describes the criteria for each category in greater detail (Walsh, Crider and Bibace, 1989). The data confirm that, as a group, children's causal reasoning about AIDS parallels the way in which children think about illness in general. The same general category system encompasses children's explanations of a number of illnesses, including their explanation of AIDS. More specifically, the data could be organized in terms of three major categories or ways in which children conceptualize AIDS and its causes. Each of these three major categories could be broken down into two subcategories for a total of six categories (see Table 3).

The findings provide an initial empirical foundation for AIDS education curricula. The specific ways in which children of different ages explain AIDS and its causes can form the basis for preventive education programs (see Table 4). Young children, for

TABLE 3
Developmental Categories of Conceptions of AIDS

Explanations Based on Association
1. The child describes AIDS in terms of any phenomenon s/he has experienced as associated with any serious illness, without clear differentiation of cause and effect.
2. The child associates a specific cause with AIDS (e.g. winter weather) and describes specific symptoms/effects, but cannot explain how the cause leads to the illness.

Explanations Based on Sequence
3. The child describes AIDS in terms of common symptoms and explains its cause as originating in external activities or situations (e.g. "falling down and getting scratched"). S/He explains how a sequence of causal events leads to AIDS by contacting or involving the body as a whole (e.g. "scratches in your skin").
4. The child describes AIDS in terms of internal symptoms or organ malfunction (e.g. "your immune system falls apart"). S/He explains how specific causes lead, through a sequence of mechanical actions, to changes in specific internal body parts or processes (e.g. blood) and to some specific symptoms of the illness (e.g. "dirty needles put bad blood in you").

Explanations Based on Interaction
5. The child describes AIDS as a malfunction in a body organ or as an underlying condition that results in symptoms. S/He describes an entire internal disease process involving the interaction of multiple causes and effects on multiple body parts. (e.g. "They have weight loss, colds, no resistance to anything."; "It's a virus. It attacks white blood cells. They don't know how to react to it so they have no immune system. It's like they get other diseases. The immune system fights off any foreign bodies, germs; white blood cells fight off the germs, AIDS kills white blood cells, I think").
6. The older child or adult explains how multiple causes and effects interact by describing transformations at the cellular level. (e.g. "AIDS is a retrovirus—the human immunodeficiency virus. The genetic material of the retrovirus is RNA. The viral RNA serves as a template for making DNA which makes new virus particles. This virus ultimately impairs the functioning of the immune system rendering the person unable to fight other diseases.")

TABLE 4
Developmentally-Based AIDS Education

	Younger Children	Intermediate Children	Older Children
FEAR	vague fears; need reassurance from authority figures about their non-vulnerability	concrete fears; need strategies for excluding potential causes; need concrete information about non-causes	healthy fear; need specifics of biological mechanisms underlying causes and preventive behaviors
CAUSE	unconcerned with cause	preoccupied with discrete causes; need list of non-causes; not with details of mode of transmission	understand body systems; detailed biological explanations of various causes and mechanisms of transmission helpful
PREVENTION	unconcerned with prevention	beginning concept of prevention; introduce notion of prevention across many illnesses including AIDS; broad categories of preventive behaviors	understand prevention; need detailed biological explanations of preventive and the conditions under which they operate and which affect their use

example, will probably not profit from detailed explanations of the mechanisms of transmission of AIDS. For example, the precise nature of the drug use that results in AIDS (e.g. via the injection of the virus into the bloodstream and consequent damage to the immune system) will not be understood nor assimilated by children in the age range of 5 to 7 years. Children in this age range, however, are able to learn that two events are associated (e.g. drugs and AIDS). Thus, it is appropriate to instruct them that "dirty needles that people use to take drugs can make you very sick with AIDS." Children at the concrete level of understanding are able to comprehend in a concrete manner how a specific cause might lead to AIDS, but they are preoccupied at this age (8 to 10 years) with enumerating all manner of potential causes (e.g. touching, kissing, eating bad food, etc). The educational activity at this level can focus on distinguishing actual causes and what children labeled as "non-causes" of AIDS. The notion of prevention can be addressed with the most mature group whose understanding of cause is abstract and detailed enough for them to comprehend the mechanisms of prevention. They can understand at this level how a particular preventive measure works.

Bibace and Blinkoff (1991) have recognized the limitations of attempting to characterize an entire protocol (covering diverse illnesses) through a single method of scoring for stage of cognitive development. They studied the conceptions of illness of children ($8^{1}/_{2}$–9 years) and college students (19–21 years) using four different scoring criteria regarding cognitive processes. Thus, all subjects were scored according to four different criteria: (1) the traditional criterion used by Damon (1977) and Bibace and Walsh (1980), that is, the subject is assigned to a stage based on their two highest responses; (2) the subject is assigned to the stage represented by the most frequent responses, that is, the mode as representative of a stage (Strauss and Ephron-Wertheim, 1982); (3) the range of stages represented in the entire protocol as tapping "the stable or labile" levels of organization relied upon by the subject (Werner, 1948). Whereas the first three scoring methods are based on the subjects' spontaneous responses, which Fischer and Biddell (1991) label "functional level of development," the fourth method allows the subject to reflect upon and order hierarchically typical examples drawn from normative groups, from each of the six stages. This was labeled the subject's recognition response.

Children and college students replicated the usual developmental findings when relying on Damon's (1977) or the Strauss and Ephron-Wertheim (1982) criteria. Also as hypothesized, both children and college students' recognition responses were developmentally more mature than their spontaneous responses. This is particularly important for applications in educational and clinical settings.

Theoretically interesting is the contrast between the children and college students' range of responses regarding their conceptions of illness. The children clearly had an upper limit with regard to the level of cognitive development attained through any of the four scoring methods. That is, no child scored above stage four, i.e. their responses ranged from Phenomenism (Stage 1) to Internalization (Stage 4).

Unexpectedly, from a Piagetian, though not from a Wernerian, perspective was the range of responses in the college population across a variety of illnesses. Responses for the college group ranged from the lowest magical levels to the most abstract forms of thought. Indeed, eight of the 20 college students demonstrated this extreme range of cognitive processes. Another eight college students ranged from the cognitively immature stage of Contagion (Stage 2) to the most mature Psychophysiological stage (Stage 6). The presence of such "childish" or "immature" responses in college students needs to be taken into account by "stage" theories in developmental psychology. Psychoanalysis, with its emphasis on the co-existence of childish, irrational thoughts and feelings throughout life, would find such findings congruent with its theoretical expectations.

In Germany, Schmidt and Weishaupt (1990) have studied certain aspects of children's beliefs about illness from a developmental perspective. Scoring developmental dimensions of subjects' responses, Schmidt and Weishaupt's findings are consistent with Bibace and Walsh's (1980) findings insofar as the German samples demonstrate the expected developmental differences.

Poida (1990), working with an independent German sample, replicated the major findings of Schmidt and Weishaupt (1990). However, between the two studies there are significant differences with regard to the developmental levels of the answers. Most differences are to be found in the pre-operational as well as the concrete operational level with respect to causality and treatment. However, symptoms are rarely significantly different. The discrepancies reflect the fact that clinical interviews in the tradition of Piaget are, with regard to specific contents (characteristics and attributes of different illnesses), neither objective nor reliable (interviewing, scoring) nor independent of the sample characteristics (Burbach and Peterson, 1986).

The studies of German children are particularly interesting in that they allow for comparisons of children who live in orphanages and children who live with their families (Huda, 1991). Overall, Huda found that children in orphanages perform at lower levels of cognitive development, even though they knew more about the symptoms of pain. In general, it seems that the concepts of illness are relatively independent of the specific experiences of children who are not raised in a family. Some of the minor illnesses (e.g. colds, headaches) seem to be less focused upon and cared for in the orphanages. In contrast, measles and other diseases, which require children to be isolated, receive much more attention than in the usual family.

In contrast to the similarities between the American and German samples, Gökbas-Balzer (1991) compared Turkish children who live in Turkey and Turkish children who live in Germany. While 20–30% of the Turkish children living in Germany recognized AIDS as "the worst disease," none of the Turkish children living in Turkey considered AIDS as "the worst disease." Conversely, the latter sample regarded tuberculosis, jaundice and diptheria as very dangerous. These diseases were not regarded as dangerous by the Turkish children living in Germany. While differences with regard to cancer are not extreme, children in Turkey regard diseases as very dangerous which are not mentioned in Germany at all, especially tuberculosis, jaundice and diptheria, which seems to be a realistic evaluation in this region.

In the Turkish sample there was less knowledge about measles and heart infarction. Primary school children living in Germany knew much more about such "usual" diseases. Both groups mentioned some traditional treatments intrinsic to the culture, like reading the Koran, saying special prayers or consulting traditional healers sanctioned by that culture.

The literature on children's perception of illness and children's perceptions of anatomy and physiology (the insides of the body and how it works) remain isolated from one another. The findings from normal developmental psychology regarding the representation of the body (e.g. Goodenough Draw-a-Person) have not been integrated with children's perceptions of illness. For instance, Crider's (1981) work in North America and the work of Munari (1976) in Switzerland articulate the development of the insides of the body (anatomy & physiology). Munari asks the questions: As normal children grow older, which body parts are most frequently drawn? How do children reason with respect to referents (internal body parts and physiological transformations) which cannot be manipulated like physical objects? Munari finds that the heart is the body organ which appears first in children's drawings, followed by the brain and only much later by joints such as knees or the skeleton. Munari discusses these findings in terms of knowing, feeling, and perceiving. (For instance, the reliance on "concreteness" as the assumption relied upon by many authors in the perception of illness literature). Interestingly, as Munari points out, the heart is internal, can be felt or known, but is *not* perceived. In contrast, the knee, which is external, and can be perceived, felt, and known, only appears in children's drawing at a much later age than the heart. The brain, which can only be known (not perceived or felt) is most commonly drawn after the heart.

Developmental studies of the relationships between the representation of the body (anatomy and physiology) and illness (bodily dysfunctions, disabilities, or defects) have yet to be undertaken.

Health Belief Model

The health belief model (Maiman and Becker, 1974) provides another traditional theoretical framework for examining children's concepts of health. The most recent review of the major issues as well as some of the research studies in this area was completed by Gochman (1988). It should be noted that Gochman's review is not exhaustive, since he makes no mention of a number of studies considered significant by other reviewers such as Maddux *et al.* (1986) and Burbach and Peterson (1986). In fact, Gochman cites "the most current evaluations of children's health concepts" (p. 332) as Bruhn and Parcel (1982) and Gochman (1985).

The health belief model addresses the action component of a child's concept of illness. It is "an essentially cognitive paradigm for predicting the likelihood of persons taking health actions" (Gochman, 1988). The focus of this model is primarily the content of a person's beliefs about some or any specific aspect of health or illness. It does not attempt to look at the underlying structure of such beliefs, but instead addresses the action consequences or behaviors related to the various beliefs. The most common beliefs that the research examines are those related to perceived vulnerability to illness, perceived benefits of health-related or illness-avoiding behaviors, and intentions to take health actions. Most of the studies in this area have been carried out by Gochman and his associates (Gochman, 1988).

Working within this approach, Brown, Nassau, and Levy (1990) surveyed 441 fifth, seventh and tenth graders from one school district. "Students responded to one open-ended question, 'What upsets me most about AIDS is...' "(p. 296). Brown *et al.*'s analysis "revealed grade as a significant variable: fifth graders were most upset by AIDS lethality, while tenth graders felt helpless" (p. 296). Cognitive and emotional factors were posited to account for these differences. AIDS education strategies that consider grade-specific anxieties were suggested. The complementarity between "what upsets me about AIDS" (the health belief model) and the reasoning that underlies such beliefs (the cognitive-developmental approach) should be evident. Preventive interventions should consider relying on interventions which address both *what* is believed and the *kind of thinking* that results in a belief.

Cognitive Science Approaches

Recently, some new perspectives have been utilized in the study of children's concepts and experience of illness. Cognitive science (also referred to as structural constraint theory, rational constructivism, or neo-nativism) is relevant to children's perceptions of illness because of its focus on children's "intuitive theories" about biological phenomena (Carey, 1985). This perspective stresses innate biological factors (e.g. innate initial state; influence of maturation and the relation between evolution and cognition), constraints which limit the learner and structural issues, that is, the organization of the initial state. Cognitive science is the counterpoint to the health belief model which stresses environmental factors.

Fischer and Bidell (1991) provide an excellent review, appreciation and critique of this approach, focusing on the "theoretical claims and research methods of this new tradition," (p. 199) which "illuminate the relations between biological constraints and cognitive development" by drawing attention to "children's seemingly precious skills" (p. 199).

Siegal (1988) and F.C. Keil (personal communication, April, 1991) have studied children's conceptions of disease. Siegal, for instance, has criticized Bibace and Walsh's (1981) concept of "contagion" by relying on what Fischer and Bidell (1991) describe as "the argument from precocity." That is, Siegal claims that even very young children are able to make distinctions which negate the usefulness of the "contagion category." Contagion reflects a relative lack of differentiation between subject and object which leads to animism and immanent justice, which are characteristics of pre-operational thought in Piagetian developmental theory. The general counter-arguments, articulated by Fischer and Bidell (1991), are applicable to Siegal. That is, Siegal (1988) disregards the "principle of developmental variability" which is brought into play by the divergent "assessment conditions" relied on in his experiment in contrast to the replicated findings of Bibace and Walsh (1981).

Specifically, Siegal's experiments led him to conclude that "contrary to Bibace and Walsh (1981) and Kister and Patterson (1980), many preschoolers identify contagion and dismiss immanent justice as an explanation for colds . . . Immanent justice may be a factor in explanations for ailments . . . only if the illness is not easily within personal experience and another explanation is not salient." (p. 1358)

Keil agrees with Siegal's criticism of the immanent justice and magical aspects of "contagion" as articulated by Bibace and Walsh (1981) and cites the example of a kindergarten child who, when asked if "one can make another person sick by simply wanting it to be so" replied, "I know you can't get someone sick that way, because I've tried it and it doesn't work." This is an interesting example because in *all* cases of contagion noted by Bibace and Walsh (1981), in both normal children and in clinical encounters, the lack of differentiation between self and other results in the child's fears of being affected by the other person's disease brought about by close physical proximity, by breathing the same air as the sick person and so on.

In contrast to Keil's report of a normal subject, is the case drawn from Pollack's (1990) study of 21 children (age range 4 years to 12 years, 11 months). All children were HIV positive, eight of the children's mothers had already died of AIDS. All children were administered the Bibace and Walsh protocol (among other measures). Pollack describes one child (8 years, 9 months) from this group. This child is older than the children tested by Siegal or Keil. Further, this child had considerable personal experience with AIDS.

"For one child, entry into school had been a highly publicized and controversial issue. Now three years later when asked about AIDS she responded, 'AIDS is a virus. I got the virus . . . A virus means you got the disease and the cooties and the chicken pox and the measles. Everybody been teasing me about everything and I don't like it.' (How do people get AIDS?) 'They got it from me. I was born – they got AIDS from me . . . those kids in [names a school] got it from me because they been teasin' me . . . All I do is just give AIDS to them kids . . . I give AIDS to somebody if they don't like me.' (How?) 'All I have to do is call them names and they got AIDS' (15, age 8–9). Within the group who knew their diagnosis, this child's responses were lowest (Category 2). From a psychological perspective, these responses reflect magical thinking" (Pollack, 1990, p. 107).

What is particularly interesting in this response is how it illustrates the reciprocal influence of magical thinking. All normal subjects, children and adults, express irrational fears of contagion from others. Irrational influence and magical factors are assumed to endanger a person, for example, physical proximity, walking on the same side of the street, or breathing the same air.

The child in Pollack's study manifests the reciprocal of the normal child's fears. That is, she magically can exert power over other children who have been mean to her. The concept of retribution is explicit. The magical vehicle relied upon is that AIDS is brought about by calling people names: "All I have to do is call them names and they got AIDS."

Whether the person is expressing his/her fears of catching AIDS from others or believes s/he can communicate AIDS to others, responses characterized as "contagion" rely on insufficient differentiation between self and other and between words and actions. This inability to properly differentiate how interactions between oneself and others are regulated gives rise to irrational fears of contagion.

Eiser (1989) has proposed alternatives to the "stage" approach which "place greater emphasis to the role of experience" (p. 93). Eiser considers Nelson (1986) and Carey (1985) as "functionalists" in contrast to those espousing a stage-structural approach. The choice of Carey as an exemplar for such an experiential alternative is puzzling. Carey's work as a cognitive scientist is an expression of "neo-nativism." As Fischer and Bidell (1991) point out, this position assumes that concepts are hard-wired, requiring only minimal environmental stimulation.

The script analyses of Nelson (1986) rely on both general schemata for the representation of events and what Nelson calls "incidental learning." It is only the latter, from Nelson's perspective, that is experientially based.

Eiser, like other critics of Piaget, is sharply reminded by Fischer and Bidell (1991) that for Piaget "feedback from *actions on the world* (italics added) is considered to be the main source of knowledge about the world" (p. 205). It is, thus, inaccurate to portray Piaget as a "maturational determinist" who neglects experience. Fisher and Bidell, in a constructive fashion, attempt to reconcile the cognitive scientists and the cognitive-developmentalists through their analysis of the concepts of capacity and skill.

Similarly, Bearison (1991) has provided an excellent review and rebuttal of critiques aimed at Piaget, who has been misinterpreted as a "maturational determinist." Bearison reminds us that "For Piaget, the social foundations of knowing have been a consistent, if not always explicit, theme in all of his theoretical discussions" (p. 6). Indeed, Bearison quotes Piaget's statement that "There are many unnecessary problems arising from the fact that some have committed themselves from the outset to a dichotomy 'individual or society' while forgetting that there is a relational perspective according to which there exist only interactions" (Piaget, 1966, p. 249). This is an important reminder for those who stress solely or primarily the individual (e.g. the neo-nativism espoused by cognitive scientists) or society (e.g. experiential and environmental factors) espoused by the health belief model or by so-called "functionalists" such as Eiser.

Script Analytic Approaches

Bearison's (1991) work best exemplifies research with children's knowledge of illness based on script analyses. Bearison (1991) reminds us that a "script is a schematic representation of generalized and temporal sequence of socially contexted actions which enables one event to follow another toward the attainment of particular goals" (p. 471). Mandler (1983), Nelson (1986), and Schank and Abelson (1977) articulate this theoretical stance.

Nelson (1986), agreeing with Schank and Abelson (1977), describes a script as:

> ...an ordered sequence of actions appropriate to a particular spatial-temporal context and organized around a goal. Scripts specify the *actors*, *actions* and *props* used to carry out those goals within specified circumstances. The script is made up of *slots* and requirements on what can fill those slots. That is, the script specifies roles and props and defines obligatory and optional actions. For example, in a restaurant script a waiter or waitress is assumed, as are a menu, food, a bill, and a tip. Persons hearing a story about a restaurant can easily fill in these items from their general script knowledge.
>
> An important characteristic of scripts is that their format includes, and is in fact organized around, information about social goals and activities. Scripts are especially apt as initial representations for children, insofar as children depend on direction and guidance from adults in carrying through daily activities; thus the events they participate in inevitably include both types of information. (p. 15)

Bearison and Pacifici's (1989) studies on children aged 4 to 17 corroborated their hypothesis that "children possess well-organized knowledge about the events they experience in oncology clinics (compared to other common and recurring social events in their lives); that this knowledge is readily accessible to verbal recall; and that it reflects certain basic characteristics of the script model including the veridical and consistent sequencing of generalizable event representations over time" (p. 472). Bearison and Pacifici's findings included developmental factors. "Subjects in the youngest age group (4 to 6 years, 11 months), compared to the two older groups (7 to 9, 11 and 10 to 17.5) mentioned relatively fewer events, were less consistent and salient in their event representations and contained more sequence errors" (p. 484). For Bearison and Pacifici, the educational and clinical implications of such findings are that children would benefit from developmentally appropriate descriptions and explanations of the procedures they experienced during their visits to oncology clinics.

In contrast to the above theory-driven approaches is the choice of narratives based on attitudinal orientations. It is instructive to quote Bearison, who is a clinical/developmental psychologist whose studies of children seriously ill with cancer have been conducted within these divergent orientations. Bearison (1991) describes his research into children's event knowledge of cancer: "The children's responses (elicited by a research assistant) were recorded and transcribed on a computer, and every single event that they described was coded, numbered and statistically analyzed – what investigators refer to as number crunching" (page *xi*, 1991). However, at a certain point Bearison (1991) states, "I realized that we were losing the rich quality of what the children had been telling us. I remember talking about this to a clinical colleague, who compared it to plucking off the leaves of an artichoke but throwing away the heart" (p. *xii*). Bearison (1991) "undertook a *clinical and ethnographic* study of children's *experiences* of having cancer as opposed to the previous data-based number crunching kind of study. This time, instead of sending a research assistant to the field to collect data, I personally met with the children and listened to them tell me what it was like to have cancer. Their *stories, in their voices* are the focus of this book" (p. *xii–xiii*).

The issue of scientific and clinical perspectives raised by Bearison (1991) is extremely important. It has also been recognized by Bibace and Walsh (1981) in their insistence that approaches which glibly stress the complementarity of research and clinical approaches disregard important differences between an experimentalist's search for knowledge and a clinician's use of knowledge to help a person. This reversal of what constitutes the means and the ends should be acknowledged. Such an acknowledgement could lead to a more meaningful complementarity which, as in Bearison's examples, might lead to capturing both the leaves and the heart of the artichoke. A more holistic-developmental understanding of the child could emerge.

Another promising psycholinguistic approach to children's perception of illness has been initiated by Dent-Read (1991). Dent-Read focuses on communicating with hospitalized children by eliciting metaphors for body functioning and symptoms. Children were asked "what certain experiences felt like or reminded them of, such as their heart beating fast" (p. 3). The questions Dent-Read (1991) asked "were designed to elicit metaphors about body functions that pediatricians find difficult to assess, that is, exertion, abdominal pain, heart functioning and breathing hard" (p. 3). Metaphoric expressions were compared to literal descriptions. Children in three age groups (4–5, 6–7, 8–10 years) participated in individual interviews. Dent-Read found that "Children increased in the frequency with which they used metaphor as they increased in age" (p. 6). Further, "as expected, children used more metaphors about immediate body symptoms than about body states or general functioning (such as breathing hard or being tired)" (p. 6). Such findings, Dent-Read argues, are "useful to clinical psychologists ... because we can better understand children's experience and provide them with information and emotional support" (p. 6).

Dent-Read's (1991) study is interesting because it highlights the differences between this genre of study compared to those attempting to determine "the cognitive processes related to understanding the cause of the disease." Scientifically, such types of studies have little in common since they address different questions and issues. Dent-Read, for instance, focuses on the child's experience, both literal and metaphoric, and how that experience can be communicated to others through shared metaphoric similarities. In contrast, Bibace and Walsh (1980) focus on the child's conceptions or "how" the disease came about.

From the perspective of applied developmental psychology, scientific differences recede into the background. The convergence of these alternatives then emerge as clinically or educationally relevant to understanding both the individual child or groups of children.

Implications

It is clear from this review that children's perceptions of illness have been addressed from multiple theoretical and methodological perspectives. While some would argue that the findings reflective of these various perspectives are contradictory (Eiser, 1989), it would seem more useful to view them as complementary. These complementarities should address the objectives of scientists, educators, and clinicians.

REFERENCES

Anderson, J. (1991). Comments on foundations of cognitive science. *Psychological Science*, 2(5), 283–297.

Bearison, D.J. (1991). Interactional contexts of cognitive development: Piagetian approaches to sociogenesis. In L. Tolchinsky Landsman (Ed.), *Culture, schooling, and psychological development* (pp. 56–70). Worwood, NJ: Ablex Publishing.

Bearison, D.J. & Pacifici, C. (1989). Children's event knowledge of cancer treatment. *Journal of Applied Developmental Psychology*, 10, 469–486.

Bibace, R. & Blinkoff, R. (1991). *Assumptions in classifying children's conceptions of illness.* Manuscript in preparation.

Bibace, R. & Walsh, M.E. (1980). Development of children's concepts of illness. *Pediatrics*, 66, 912–917.

Bibace, R. & Walsh, M.E. (1981). Children's conceptions of illness. In R. Bibace & M.E. Walsh (Eds.), *New directions for child development: Children's conceptions of health, illness and bodily functions* (pp. 31–48). San Francisco: Jossey-Bass.

Bird, J.E. & Podmore, V.N. (1990). Children's understanding of health and illness. *Psychology and Health*, 4, 175–185.

Brown, L., Nassau, J.H. & Levy, V. (1990). What upsets me most about AIDS is ... A survey of children and adolescents. *AIDS Education and Prevention*, 2(4), 296–304.

Bruhn, J.G. & Parcel, G.S. (1982). Current knowledge about the health behavior of young children: A conference summary. *Health Education Quarterly*, 9, 238–262.

Burbach, D.J. & Peterson, L. (1986). Children's concepts of physical illness: A review and critique of the cognitive-developmental literature. *Health Psychology*, 5(3), 307–325.

Campbell, J.D. (1975). Illness is a point of view: The development of children's concepts of illness. *Child Development*, 46, 92–100.

Carey, S. (1985). *Conceptual changes in childhood.* Cambridge, MA: M.I.T. Press.

Crider, C. (1981). Children's conceptions of the body interior. In R. Bibace & M.E. Walsh (Eds.), *Children's conceptions of health, illness and bodily functions* (pp. 49–65). San Francisco: Jossey-Bass, Inc.

Damon, W. (1977). *The social world of the child.* San Francisco: Jossey-Bass.

del Barrio, C. (1988). The development of biological processes explanations: How children understand illness cause and cure. *Infancia y Appendizaia*, 42, 81–95.

Dent-Read, C.H. (1991, May). *Communicating with hospitalized children by eliciting metaphors for body functioning and symptoms.* Paper presented at the Midwestern Psychological Association, Chicago, IL.

Eiser, C. (1985). *The psychology of childhood illness.* New York, NY: Springer.

Eiser, C. (1989). Children's concepts of illness: Toward an alternative to the "stage" approach. *Psychology and Health*, 3, 93–101.

Fischer, K.W. & Biddell, T. (1991). Constraining nativist inferences about cognitive capacities. In S. Carey & R. Gelman (Eds.), *The epigenesis of mind: Essays on biology and cognition* (pp. 199–235). Hillsdale, NJ: Lawrence Erlbaum.

Gochman, D.S. (1985). Family determinants of children's concepts of health and illness. In

D.C. Turk & R.D. Kerns (Eds.), *Health, illness, and families: A life-span perspective.* New York: Wiley.

Gochman, D.S. (1988). Assessing children's health concepts. In P. Karoly (Ed.), *Handbook of child health assessment* (pp. 332–356). New York: Wiley.

Gökbas-Balzer, A. (1991). *Gesundheit und Krankheit: Konzepte von Turkischen Kindern.* Trier: Unpublished Thesis.

Huda, C. (1991). *Gesundheit und Krankheit: Konzepte von Heimkindern.* Trier: Unpublished Thesis.

Jordan, M.K. & O'Grady, D.J. (1982). Children's health beliefs and concepts: Implications for child health care. In P. Karoly, J.J. Steffen & D.J. O'Grady (Eds.), *Child health psychology* (pp. 58–76). New York: Pergamon.

Keil, F.C. (1989). *Concepts, kinds, and cognitive development.* Cambridge, MA: M.I.T. Press.

Kister, M.C. & Patterson, C.J. (1980). Children's conceptions of the causes of illness: Understanding of contagion and use of immanent justice. *Child Development*, 51, 839–849.

Lohaus, A. (1990). *Gesundheit und Krankheit aus der Sicht von Kindern.* Göttingen: Hogrefe.

Maddux, J.E., Roberts, M.C., Sledden, E.A. & Wright, L. (1986). Developmental issues in child health psychology. *American Psychologist*, 41(1), 25–34.

Maiman, L.A. & Becker, M.H. (1974). The Health Belief Model: Origins and correlates in psychological theory. *Health Education Monograph*, 2, 336–353.

Mandler, J. (1983). Representation. In P. Mussen (Ed.), *Manual of child psychology.* Vol 3. New York: Wiley, pp. 420–494.

Mechanic, D. (1964). The influence of mothers on children's health attitudes and behavior. *Pediatrics*, 33, 444.

Michielutte, R. & Diseker, R.A. (1982). Children's perceptions of cancer in comparison to other chronic illnesses. *Journal of Chronic Diseases*, 35, 843–852.

Millstein, S.G., Adler, N.E. & Irwin, C.E. (1981). Conceptions of illness in young adolescents. *Pediatrics*, 68, 834–839.

Munari, A. (1976). L'anatomie de l'enfants: l'etude genetique des conceptions anatomiques spontanees. *Archives de Psychologie*, 9, 5–34.

Nelson, K. (1986). Event Knowledge and Cognitive Development. In K. Nelson (Ed.), *Event knowledge: Structure and function in development* (pp. 1–20). Hillsdale, New Jersey: Lawrence Erlbaum Associates.

Newell, A., Rosenbloom, P. & Laird, J. (1989). Symbolic architecture for cognition. In M.I. Posner (Ed.), *Foundations of cognitive science* (pp. 93–131). Cambridge, MA: The MIT Press.

Perrin, E. & Gerrity, S. (1981). There's a demon in your belly: Children's understanding of illness. *Pediatrics*, 67, 841–849.

Piaget, J. (1930). *The child's conception of physical causality.* London: Kegan Paul.

Piaget, J. (1966). Le psychologie, les relations interdisciplinaires et le systeme des sciences. *Bulletin de Psychologie*, 254, 242–254.

Poida, E. (1990). *Kindliche Konzepte von Krankheit und Gesundheit*, Trier: Unpublished Thesis.

Pollack, S. (1990). Concepts of illness in HIV infected children. Unpublished doctoral dissertation, Seton Hall University.

Schank, R.C. & Abelson, R.R. (1977). *Script, plans, goals and understanding.* Hillsdale, NJ: Erlbaum.

Schmidt, L.R. & Weishaupt, I. (1990). Children's concepts of symptoms, causality, and the course of physical illness. In L.R. Schmidt, P. Schwenkmezger, J. Weinman & S. Maes (Eds.), *Theoretical and applied aspects of health psychology (pp. 255–265).* London: Harwood.

Siegal, M. (1988). Children's knowledge of contagion and contamination as causes of illness. *Child Development*, 59, 1353–1359.

Strauss, S. & Ephron-Wertheim, T. (1982). Structure and process: Developmental psychology as looking in the mirror. In I. Levin (Ed.), *Stage and structure: Reopening the debate* (pp. 59–76). New Jersey: Ablex Publishing Co.

Susman, E.J., Dorn, L.D. & Fletcher, J.C. (1987). Reasoning about illness in ill and healthy children and adolescents: Cognitive and emotional developmental aspects. *Developmental and Behavioral Pediatrics*, **8**(5), 266–273.

Walsh, M.E., Crider, C. & Bibace, R. (1989). *Developmental conceptions of illness: Revised scoring system*. Unpublished manuscript.

Walsh, M.E. & Bibace, R. (1991). Children's conceptions of AIDS: A developmental analysis. *Journal of Pediatric Psychology*, **16**(3), 273–285.

Werner, H. (1948). *Comparative psychology of mental development* (2nd ed.). New York: International Universities Press.

Werner, H. & Kaplan, B. (1963). *Symbol formation: An organismic-developmental approach to language and the expression of thought*. New York: John Wiley & Sons.

Young, M.H., McMurray, M.B., Rothery, S.A. & Emery, L.A. (1987). Use of the health and illness questionnaire with chronically ill and handicapped children. *Children's Health Care*, **16**(2), 97–104.

CHRONIC ILLNESS IN CHILDREN

SUZANNE BENNETT JOHNSON

Current estimates suggest that 10–20% of U.S. children have some type of chronic condition. Approximately half of these youngsters are victims of a chronic illness; the remaining suffer from visual or hearing impairments, or mental retardation (Gortmaker and Sappenfield, 1984). With the possible exception of asthma, most chronic diseases of childhood are relatively rare. However, in the aggregate, they constitute a significant minority that demand a disproportionate amount of health care services. For example, Smyth-Staruch et al. (1984) examined hospitalization and use of outpatient services during a 1-year period by a group of children suffering from some type of chronic medical condition. These children used 10 times more health care services than their "normal" peers.

This chapter will review recent psychological research relevant to childhood chronic disease. In keeping with current trends, both general and disease-specific functioning of children and their families will be addressed. Although only 10–15 years old, the available literature is quite extensive. Space limitations preclude a complete review of all relevant citations. Instead, primary themes and critical issues will be highlighted and examples provided.

GENERAL FUNCTIONING

Psychologists remain concerned with the chronically ill child's psychosocial adaptation. However, since the child lives within a family context, the impact of the child's disease on family members and the family's functioning has also been explored.

*Supported by grants RO1 HD13820 and PO1 DK39079 from the US National Institutes of Health. Correspondence should be addressed to: S.B. Johnson, Ph.D., PO Box 100234, University of Florida Health Science Center, Gainesville Fl 32610-0234, USA.

Patient Functioning

Current research on patient psychological adjustment contrasts sharply with similar studies conducted only 25 years ago. Rather than seeking to elucidate certain disease-related personality traits, factors that influence adaptation are now the subjects of inquiry. Further, the scope of study has been expanded to include school performance and peer relationships as well.

Psychological adjustment

Emotional disturbance is not the inevitable consequence of childhood chronic illness. In fact, most children with chronic disease cope remarkably well (Johnson, 1980; Drotar et al., 1981; Fielding et al., 1985; Hodges et al., 1985; Lemanek et al., 1986; Spaulding and Morgan, 1986). Longitudinal studies that have monitored youngsters' psychological adjustment from the time of diagnosis note some initial emotional upheaval that is usually resolved within six months to one year post-diagnosis (Kovacs et al., 1986; Wertlieb et al., 1986).

Nevertheless, there is some evidence that a minority of chronically ill children do have adjustment problems, and that the number of such children may be larger than would be expected in a physically healthy population (Pless, 1984; Wallander et al., 1988). Internalizing problems, such as anxiety, depression, or somatic complaints, may be disproportionately represented (Thompson et al., 1989). However, most standardized measures of psychological adjustment were developed for use with physically healthy children. In a healthy population, somatic symptoms such as loss of appetite, difficulty sleeping, and general fatigue, may be a valid sign of depression. In an ill population, they may be normal consequences of the child's disease rather than signs of a psychological disorder. For this reason there is some controversy as to whether internalizing problems are actually more prevalent than other types of problems among medically ill children (Wallander et al., 1988).

A number of investigators have examined disease-related factors as predictors of adjustment. Within a given disease, children who are in poorer health often exhibit more adjustment problems (Anderson et al., 1981; Steinhausen et al., 1983a, 1983b; Handford et al., 1986; Billings et al., 1987). Degree of impairment with activities of daily living also appears to correlate with psychosocial adjustment (Orr et al., 1984; Stein and Jessop, 1984). Physically handicapped children may exhibit poorer adaptation than ill, but less physically compromised children (Steinhausen, 1981; Wallander et al., 1989b). Disorders involving the brain seem to be particularly susceptible to behavioral and emotional difficulties (Hoare, 1984b; Breslau and Marshall, 1985; Spaulding and Morgan, 1986; Perrin et al., 1987; Kindlon et al., 1988; Walker et al., 1989; Wallander et al., 1989a).

Since the child lives within a family context, family factors have proved to be important predictors of psychosocial adjustment in ill and healthy populations alike. In a now classic study, Pless et al. (1972) studied the family functioning and adjustment of 209 chronically ill youngsters; 113 healthy children served as controls. Both family functioning and health status were associated with the children's adjustment. Chronically ill youngsters and those from more dysfunctional families had more adjustment problems. However, youngsters who were victims of a chronic illness and who lived in poorly functioning families had the highest incidence of psychological disturbance. This was particularly true of older youngsters, suggesting that there may be a cumulative effect over time of poor health and an unfavorable family situation.

Subsequent studies, conducted by different investigators with different groups of ill children, have consistently documented a link between parental adjustment or family functioning and the child's psychosocial adaptation (Hoare; 1984b; Margalit, 1986; Wertlieb *et al.*, 1986; Daniels *et al.*, 1987; Wells and Schwebel, 1987; Lavigne *et al.*, 1988; Varni *et al.*, 1989; Walker *et al.*, 1989; Wallander *et al.*, 1989c; Kronenberger and Thompson, 1990).

With the exception of longitudinal studies conducted by Kovacs *et al.* (1986) and Wertlieb *et al.* (1986), investigations of chronically ill children's psychosocial adaptation have been cross-sectional and correlational. Consequently, causal connections between study variables are sometimes difficult to verify. While poorer health may "cause" poorer adjustment, it is equally possible that poorer adjustment "causes" poorer health. Similarly, while poor family functioning may "cause" child maladjustment, behavior and emotional problems in the child could also "cause" family disruption. The available literature clearly documents important relationships between disease variables, family functioning, and child adjustment. However, the nature of these relationships should not be oversimplified.

As the research literature matures, there will be increasing attention to developmental issues. Children at different developmental stages cope with the demands of their illness in different ways (Worchel *et al.*, 1987; Band, 1990; Band and Weisz, 1990) which may, in turn, be related to the success of their adaptation. Certain developmental periods may be "at-risk" for certain types of adjustment problems. While clinical experience suggests that adolescence may be a particularly difficult developmental period, both Mrazek *et al.* (1987) and Wysocki *et al.* (1989) have documented the special problems exhibited by the chronically ill pre-school child. While we usually conceive of developmental issues in terms of physical maturity or the changing cognitive capacity of the child, diseases themselves may have a developmental course which may impact upon psychosocial adaptation. Some diseases get worse with increasing disease duration. Others are associated with periods of crisis followed by times of relative quiescence. The changing nature of chronic disease, in addition to the changing character of the child, will serve as important topics for future investigation.

Similarly, as we begin to understand what is wrong with chronically ill children, we will expand our inquiry to include what is right about their adaptation. It is certainly possible that the experience of having a chronic illness could have positive as well as negative repercussions. For example, Nelms (1989) found that chronically ill youngsters were more empathetic and emotionally responsive than "healthy" peers. We are likely to see more research of this type in years to come.

School performance
With the exception of central nervous system conditions, most chronic diseases of childhood are associated with normal intelligence. Nevertheless, academic under-achievement is common, a possible consequence of frequent school absences which seem to characterize this population (Weitzman, 1986). Recent studies suggest that certain diseases, such as recurrent otitis media, liver disease, or juvenile diabetes, may be associated with intellectual deficits (Feagans *et al.*, 1987; Ryan, 1989; Stewart *et al.*, 1991). Further, certain treatment procedures, such as cranial irradiation for acute lymphocytic leukemia, may have negative cognitive sequelae (Taylor *et al.*, 1987; Waber *et al.*, 1990). Currently, there is an increasing appreciation of possible

neuropsychological consequences associated with many chronic diseases or their treatment.

Peer relationships
In the past, peer relationships among chronically ill children have received relatively little attention (La Greca, 1990). However, this situation is rapidly changing. For example, a number of studies have examined nondisabled children's attitudes toward disabled peers. Attitudes seem to be influenced by type of disability, prior experience with children who have a particular handicap, the social context, and the age and gender of the child (Harper *et al.*, 1986; Newberry and Parish, 1986; Sigelman and Begleym, 1987; Royal and Roberts, 1987). Prior experience with children who have a disability, situations that do not place the handicapped child at a disadvantage, older age, and female gender all seem to be associated with more positive attitudes.

Family Functioning

A number of studies have examined the impact of a child's chronic condition on other family members. Most studies have examined maternal adaptation. Fewer studies have targeted father and sibling adjustment.

Parental adjustment
It is widely believed that the presence of a chronically ill child places increased stress on both the marital relationship and the family. However, divorce rates are comparable between parents who have or do not have a chronically ill child (Lansky *et al.*, 1978; Lavigne *et al.*, 1982; Sabbeth and Leventhal, 1984; Benson and Gross, 1989). It is possible that more subtle aspects of the marital relationship are affected; both positive (e.g. greater intimacy and communication) and negative (e.g. decreased support and increased marital friction) effects have been reported (Hauenstein *et al.*, 1988; Benson and Gross, 1989; Speltz *et al.*, 1990).

Mothers, in particular, appear to experience increased stress associated with parenting a chronically ill child (Wysocki *et al.*, 1989; Speltz *et al.*, 1990). Depression, anxiety, and somatic complaints have been noted (Fielding *et al.*, 1985; Hodges *et al.*, 1985; Walker and Greene, 1989; Wallander *et al.*, 1989b). Since mothers are the primary caretakers of chronically ill children, perhaps it is not surprising that mothers sometimes report more distress or adjustment problems than fathers (Borner and Steinhausen, 1977; Tavormina *et al.*, 1981; Walker and Greene, 1989). However, the small available literature is not consistent on this topic; some fathers report distress levels similar to or higher than that of mothers' (Gayton *et al.*, 1977; Fielding *et al.*, 1985).

Similar to trends found in the patient adjustment literature, there has been an increasing interest in factors associated with good or poor parental adjustment. Characteristics of the disease itself have been given some consideration. Breslau *et al.* (1982) reported that the impact of the disease on the child's ability to carry out activities of daily living may be one determinant of maternal distress. Mothers who were burdened with most of their child's daily care (e.g. eating, drinking, toileting), because the child was unable to carry out these functions, were more depressed, anxious, and distressed over their parenting role.

The changing nature of the disease may be an additional determinant of parental adjustment. In a rare longitudinal study, Kovacs *et al.* (1985) reported increased emotional strain at the time of the child's diagnosis, particularly in mothers. However, this initial emotional upheaval typically resolved within 6 months time. Other longitudinal studies have reported similar phenomena: an initial increase in anxiety associated with the diagnosis of some threat to the child's health, followed by a period of adaptation (McElroy *et al.*, 1986; Johnson *et al.*, 1990a). Although these studies focused on the point of disease diagnosis, one might expect changes in parental anxiety and distress at later points in the course of the disease, particularly for diseases associated with changing function or health status (Walker *et al.*, 1987).

Certain developmental periods may be associated with increased parental strain. The pre-school period may be a particularly difficult period due to the child's limited verbal ability (Walker *et al.*, 1987; Wysocki *et al.*, 1989; Spelz *et al.*, 1990). Of course, adolescence is always associated with a number of parental challenges that may become especially salient in a chronically ill child (Walker *et al.*, 1987).

Only recently have investigators begun to explore family factors that may be predictive of good or poor parental adjustment. As might be expected, spouse support or other forms of social support is one important determinant of maternal adjustment (McKinney and Peterson, 1987; Wallander *et al.*, 1989d). We can expect an increased number of studies of this type in the future. Hopefully, researchers will turn their attention to factors influencing paternal, as well as maternal, adaptation.

Sibling adjustment

As investigators sought to understand patient adaptation, and then maternal adjustment, the reactions of healthy siblings of the chronically ill child were given little attention. Fortunately, this situation is rapidly changing. However, as was characteristic of initial studies of patient and parental adjustment, studies of sibling adaptation have primarily focused on the detection of maladjustment, rather than predictors of good versus poor adaptation. Two reviews of this literature suggest that the presence of a chronically ill child within a family constellation is not consistently associated with emotional or behavioral problems in a physically healthy sibling (Drotar and Crawford, 1985; Lobato *et al.*, 1988). This conclusion should come as no surprise since chronic illness per se is not consistently associated with maladjustment in patients themselves or in their parents.

Investigators have begun to explore a variety of factors that might moderate the effect of a child's illness on sibling adjustment. Lavigne and Ryan (1979) provided evidence that the more visible the disease, the more likely the sibling will exhibit behavioral or emotional problems. Hoare (1984a) found disease duration to be predictive of sibling adjustment in an epileptic population; siblings who had lived with an epileptic brother or sister for a long time had more problems. However, in other diseases such as diabetes, living with the disease longer may be associated with better sibling adjustment (Lavigne *et. al.*, 1982). Wood *et al.* (1988) suggest both the type of illness and its severity may influence the extent and nature of adjustment reactions in healthy siblings. There are simply too few studies to draw firm conclusions. However, it is likely that the relationship between disease and sibling adjustment is complex, involving issues of visibility, impact on function, threat to life, and dynamic or static course.

Since family factors are important to patient and healthy child adjustment, they are important to sibling adjustment as well. Both patient and parental dysfunction are associated with poorer sibling adaptation (Daniels *et al.*, 1987). The relationship of the sibling's age and gender to that of the ill child's is an area of inquiry deserving increased attention. Lobato (1983) has pointed out that firstborn female children typically assume greater child care responsibilities than firstborn males or later-born children of either sex. Consequently, a female child older than the ill child might be particularly vulnerable. Lobato has provided supporting evidence from studies of older female siblings of mentally retarded children. Breslau *et al.* (1981) reported similar results in their analysis of the impact on siblings of cystic fibrosis, cerebral palsy, myelodysplasia, and other multiple handicaps.

Stein and Reissman (1980) have argued that the impact of a child's illness on a family need not be entirely negative. It is possible that the experience of living with an ill child could "set the stage" for the developmental of excellent communication skills, problem-solving ability, responsibility, and empathy. Unfortunately, the literature on both patient and family functioning has focused almost exclusively on maladaptive rather than adaptive behavior. An expanded focus on the positive as well as negative impact of childhood chronic illness would be a welcome change.

DISEASE-SPECIFIC FUNCTIONING

Chronic disease demands a long term, often a lifetime, commitment to disease management. While the physician provides recommendations for patient care, the child and family must manage the disease on a daily basis. The goal is to manage the disease successfully and to minimize functional disability. Often a great deal of information about the disease must be acquired. The child must be assisted in coping with the pain and distress associated with the disease or its management. Medical regimen adherence can be difficult, especially when the regimen demands numerous, complex or painful procedures to be carried out on a daily basis. Learning, distress, and adherence all involve human behavior and emotions. Hence, they are inherently psychological phenomena. Historically, psychologists were primarily concerned with the patient's or family's general adaptation to the disease. Today, there is greater interest in the child and family's disease-specific functioning. This exciting expansion, in both psychological service and research, has clear relevance to patient care.

Pain and Discomfort

Many chronic diseases of childhood are associated with painful symptomatology. For example, juvenile arthritis is a connective-tissue disease resulting in joint stiffness and pain. Chronic joint pain also occurs in patients with hemophilia due to internal hemorrhaging. Children with cancer may experience pain associated with tumor growth. Sickle cell anemia is associated with pain crises that occur when the patient's sickle-shaped cells block the flow of oxygen to the capillaries. Pain symptoms may be a sign of disease process or deterioration. When pain is an inherent aspect of the disease, helping the patient cope or manage pain may be a primary goal of psychological intervention.

Children sometimes experience pain as a consequence of medical interventions. In diabetes, for example, youngsters must take daily insulin injections and conduct finger sticks as many as four times a day to do blood glucose tests. Many pediatric cancer patients experience routine bone marrow aspirations and lumbar punctures which can be excruciating. Further, nausea and vomiting are common responses to many anticancer medications. Children with hemophilia are treated for internal hemorrhaging by intravenous infusion of medication to replace the children's missing clotting factor. Pain and discomfort associated with a medical procedure can interfere with its successful administration. In such cases, pain management is designed to increase patient cooperation and compliance.

Pain is not always associated with an identifiable organic cause. Headache, abdominal, or limb (growing) pain are some of the most common complaints of childhood. Oster (1972) reported prevalence rates of 20.6% for recurrent headache, 14.4% for recurrent abdominal pain, and 15.5% for recurrent limb pain; prevalence rates were higher for girls than for boys. In most cases, a specific disease or physical abnormality cannot be identified. Schecter (1984) estimates that less than 7% of abdominal pain, 4% of limb pain, and 5% of headache pain have an identifiable organic etiology. Although chronic pain has been traditionally classified as either organic or psychogenic, Levine and Rappaport (1984) have argued that pain is not necessarily an "either-or" phenomenon. Many somatic predispositions or dysfunctions cannot be identified or classified as true organic illness. However, somatic conditions, in combination with life style habits, environmental factors, and learned response patterns, can result in chronic pain. It is the psychologist's role to identify and modify the social, environmental, and behavioral determinants of the pain experience.

A variety of self-report, psychophysiological, and observational methods of assessing children's pain and distress have been developed (see Johnson, 1988, for a review). Further, both cognitive and behavioral interventions strategies have been used to help children successfully cope with pain (see Jay, 1988, for a review). Throughout the assessment and treatment literature, developmental issues repeatedly surface. Younger versus older children clearly display and cope with their distress differently (Jay *et al.*, 1983; Brown *et al.*, 1986; Wells and Schwebel, 1987; Worchel *et al.*, 1987; van Aken *et al.*, 1989; Jacobson *et al.*, 1990b). Other factors that seem to be predictive of children's pain and distress include gender (Katz *et al.*, 1987; van Aken *et al.*, 1989), prior experience (Wells and Schwebel, 1987; Jacobson *et al.*, 1990b), parental behavior (Osborne *et al.*, 1989; Jacobson *et al.*, 1990b), and health provider behavior (Weinstein *et al.*, 1982; Melamed *et al.*, 1983).

Knowledge About The Illness

Because many chronic diseases demand home care, the patient and parent must have an adequate understanding of the disease and its management. However, studies of disease knowledge have documented significant deficits. For example, children with diabetes often fail to inject insulin or glucose test properly (Epstein *et al.*, 1980; Johnson *et al.*, 1982). Parents treating children with hemophilia with factor replacement frequently use incorrect technique (Sergis-Deavenport and Varni, 1983). Children with asthma demonstrate poor knowledge of how to prevent or control attacks (Eiser *et al.*, 1988). Further, patients and parents seem to recall little of what the physician has told them immediately after a clinic visit (Page *et al.*, 1981). Clearly, patient and families know far less about a disease and its management than most health care providers realize.

Learning about a chronic illness can be an exceedingly complex task. Understanding the disease may mean more than knowing the "facts" about its etiology and treatment. Often the patient must learn to problem-solve, or apply the facts about the illness, in a variety of situations. More than cognitive knowledge is often required. Patients or parents must learn to give injections, conduct tests, administer intravenous medication, or carry out physical therapies. All of these tasks demand significant skill. Further, there may be little relationship, even within a disease, between various aspects of disease knowledge. For example, a patient may know the facts about diabetes but may not be able to apply those facts in different situations or may not be able to administer insulin or conduct a glucose test accurately (Johnson *et al.*, 1982; Harkavy *et al.*, 1983). This suggests that the health provider should assess *all* aspects of disease knowledge relevant to daily care.

As might be expected, cognitive developmental level is an important determinant of patient knowledge; older children typically know more about their condition than younger children (Etzwiler, 1962; Garner *et al.*, 1969; Partridge *et al.*, 1972; Johnson *et al.*, 1982). Further, cognitive development seems to be an important determinant of who benefits from educational programs designed to instruct children about their disease (Gilbert *et al.*, 1982; Harkavy *et al.*, 1983).

Since mothers are the primary caretakers of chronically ill children, it should come as no surprise that mothers are usually more knowledgeable than any other family member. However, adolescents are often as knowledgeable as their mothers and more knowledgeable than their fathers (Partridge *et al.*, 1972; Johnson *et al.*, 1982).

Knowledge about an illness is not consistently associated with either adherence or health status (Mazzuca, 1982; Johnson, 1984). However, it would be inappropriate to conclude that disease knowledge is unimportant. Rather, it is best to view both adherence and health as multi-determined. Adequate disease knowledge and skill provide the necessary but not sufficient conditions for good adherence and health to occur. Psychologists can contribute to improved patient care by developing adequate measures of patient knowledge and skill, by devising developmentally sensitive educational programs, and by evaluating the success of educational interventions.

Medical Regimen Adherence

Most chronic diseases require regular monitoring or intervention by the patient or family. The physician usually serves as a consultant rather than a direct service provider, offering recommendations to the family. During acute crises, the patient may be admitted to the hospital and cared for by the medical staff. However, the every day life of a child living with a chronic disease is characterized by patient or family, rather than physician, care. "Adherence" or "compliance" are terms we use to describe how well a patient or family follows the physician's disease management prescriptions.

Unfortunately, poor compliance is extremely common (Varni and Jay, 1984; Creer *et al.*, Johnson, 1989; Phipps and DeCuir-Whalley, 1990). Sometimes, noncompliance is inadvertent due to knowledge or skill deficits. The patient or parent may not understand or recall the provider's recommendations (Page *et al.*, 1981). Or, the patient may have insufficient knowledge or skill to carry out a regimen task accurately (Johnson *et al.*, 1982). In such cases, failure to comply with physician advice is not intentional. Nevertheless, the patient's health may be negatively affected.

Aspects of the regimen itself may influence compliance behaviors. Demands that are painful, labor-intensive, or incongruent with one's usual lifestyle may be complied with less. Treatments that are clearly life-sustaining or have immediate health consequences may be followed more consistently than procedures with more diffuse or distant connections to the patient's physical condition. For example, insulin injections are necessary for a child with diabetes to survive. Most children take their injections daily, but may fail to comply with other aspects of diabetes care (e.g. painful finger sticks for glucose tests, or dietary restrictions of favorite foods). For many chronic diseases, the treatment regimen is quite complex; patients may comply with one aspect of the regimen but not others (Johnson *et al.*, 1986; Johnson *et al.*, 1990b). For this reason, it is probably best to view patient adherence as a multifaceted phenomena rather than a unitary trait or characteristic of the patient. Not only should compliance with each regimen component be assessed, but determinants of compliance across regimen behaviors may differ.

Once again, developmental issues prove important. Although few investigators have monitored compliance over the course of the disease, there is some evidence that compliance is best at disease onset and may deteriorate thereafter (Litt and Cuskey, 1981; Hudson *et al.*, 1987; Jacobson *et al.*, 1987). We do not know yet whether compliance behaviors are modified by acute changes in a child's physical condition (e.g. patients may become more compliant in response to a medical crisis but exhibit a gradual decline in compliance thereafter). Similarly, we do not know whether compliance differs between patients who are living with a static, dynamic, or deteriorating pathological condition.

Far more frequently studied are compliance rates associated with the child's developmental level. Adherence appears to decline particularly during the adolescent years (Christensen *et al.*, 1983; Dolgin *et al.*, 1986; Johnson *et al.*, 1986; Tibbi *et al.*, 1986; Jacobson *et al.*, 1987, 1990a). Although adolescents frequently know more about their disease than younger children, they are often far less compliant. Nevertheless, adolescence is associated with increased patient responsibility for disease management (Kohler *et al.*, 1982; Anderson *et al.*, 1990). For example, in a study sample of youngsters with diabetes, Ingersoll *et al.* (1986) noted that parental participation in diabetes care had virtually ceased by the time the patient was 15 years of age. However, parental withdrawal was not always balanced by mature, responsible behavior on the part of the adolescent. Since the demands of adolescence are substantial, even for a physically healthy child, it may be unwise to place too much responsibility for disease management on the patient too quickly. Indeed, most successful behavioral intervention programs designed to improve patient adherence do so through increased parental participation (Weinstein and Cuskey, 1985).

Throughout childhood and adolescence, the family environment remains an important determinant of patient compliance. Low family conflict seems to be an especially salient correlate of good adherence; this finding has been reported in disease populations as varied as asthma (Christiaanse *et al.*, 1989), epilepsy (Friedman *et al.*, 1986), juvenile rheumatoid arthritis (Chaney and Peterson, 1989), and diabetes (Hauser *et al.*, 1990). Although it is usually assumed that family conflict causes poor adherence, it is certainly possible that poor patient adherence precipitates family conflict.

Good patient adherence is presumed to be critical to good patient health. However, for many diseases, the link between adherence and health is not as strong as might be expected. More complaint patients are not always in better health and interventions designed to improve patient compliance do not always result in improved health outcomes (Johnson, 1989). Yet, physicians frequently assume there is a one-to-one relationship between adherence and health. In fact, they often use health status measures as indices of patient compliance, labeling those patients in poor health as noncompliant. This approach is inappropriate for several reasons. First, it fails to recognize that both the effectiveness of the medical regimen prescription and patient compliance are critical to good or improved health. Indeed, no amount of patient adherence will make an ineffective treatment regimen effective! By focusing solely on the patient's behavior, the physician may fail to scrutinize his or her own medical recommendations. Further, using health status measures as indices of compliance, tells the provider nothing about what the patient did or did not do with regard to disease management. Consequently, the provider cannot give the patient any specific behavioral recommendations as to how the patient might better manage the disease. Finally, when the provider relies solely on indices of health status to assess patient compliance, there is a tendency to blame the patient whose health is poor or has deteriorated. This may interfere with the physician-patient relationship and may be particularly demoralizing to a patient who, in fact, has made every effort to adhere to the providers' recommendations. For these reasons, it is important to conduct independent assessments of both patient adherence and health status. Adherence should be assessed using behavioral methodologies so that specific recommendations for behavioral change can be provided to the patient.

Clearly, the psychologist can do far more than provide intervention programs to improve the adherence of selected, "problem" patients referred by the physician. Behavioral expertise is important to the everyday management of chronic disease. The physician must be educated to appreciate the difference between patient adherence and health and to assess both using independent and appropriate measurement strategies. Today, a physician would be considered remiss if he or she did not conduct laboratory assays or other assessments of the child's medical condition as part of a regularly scheduled clinic visit. Yet, behavioral assessment of the child's or family's disease management rarely occurs. In the future, behavioral assessment, like health status assessment, should become an integral part of standard pediatric practice.

Health Provider Behavior

While the patient's and family's adaptation and disease-specific functioning has been extensively explored, health provider behavior has been largely ignored. This is problematic because health provider behavior is critical to every aspect of managing a child's chronic medical condition. The provider informs and educates the child and family about the disease. The provider makes recommendations for everyday management of the child's medical condition. The provider intervenes with tests or treatments that may cause considerable patient pain or distress. Yet, we know little about which provider behaviors prove most helpful and which are detrimental to good patient care. This is an exceedingly important area of inquiry that is finally attracting increasing attention.

We do know that there are often large discrepancies between what the provider tells the patient and family and what the patient and family subsequently recall or understand (Page *et al.*, 1981). We are just beginning to elucidate factors that may underlie patient-provider miscommunication. These include the overuse of medical jargon (Korsch *et al.*, 1968; Gibbs *et al.*, 1987) and an apparent insensitivity to the changing cognitive capacity of the developing child (Perrin and Perrin, 1983). In some cases, providers appear to give too much responsibility for disease management to the child, before the child is cognitively or socially ready to accept it (Wysocki *et al.*, 1990). In other cases, large differences may exist between parents' and providers' treatment goals, impeding adherence with the provider's treatment recommendations (Marteau *et al.*, 1987).

Children as young as 4 or 5 years of age are very much aware of the different behaviors or roles exhibited by doctors versus patients. Doctors ask questions, perform therapeutic procedures, and prescribe treatments. Patients, on the other hand, are relatively passive participants in the doctor-physician interaction (Haight *et al.*, 1985). Interesting work done with adult populations suggests that patients can be taught to have a more active role, with positive consequences in terms of patient knowledge, satisfaction with care, adherence, and health outcomes (Anderson *et al.*, 1987; Greenfield *et al.*, 1988). Hopefully, this approach will be soon applied to childhood chronically ill populations as well.

Of course, provider-patient interactions involve more than the communication of medical information. An affective relationship is also established. Patient and parent feelings of satisfaction with medical care seems to be one predictor of patient adherence; more satisfied patients are more compliant (Litt and Cuskey, 1984; Hazzard *et al.*, 1990). We do not yet know the critical determinants of positive patient-provider rapport. However, interesting work by Stern and her colleagues (1989, 1991) suggests that many health professionals have stereotyped attitudes toward childhood victims of certain diseases, such as leukemia. These stereotypes appear to be quite negative; ill children are viewed as less sociable, less cognitively competent, less well-behaved, and less likely to be well adjusted in the future. Although these negative attitudes appear to be readily modified through the provision of appropriate information, current medical training often does not address the potential impact of provider perceptions on the doctor-patient relationship.

In addition to studying how providers communicate and relate, investigators are beginning to examine how health providers behave toward their patients, especially when carrying out tasks that may be painful or distressing to the child. Interesting work conducted in the dentist's office has shown that dentists' behavior can have important effects on children's anxiety and compliance (Weinstein *et al.*, 1982; Melamed *et al.*, 1983). This type of research needs to be expanded to a variety of medical settings.

CONCLUDING COMMENTS

Medicine's conquest of infectious disease sparked a revolution in health care. This, in turn, generated renewed interest in psychological aspects of medical conditions. Initially constrained by psychoanalytic theory, recent psychological research seems to have exploded into a wide variety of new and exciting directions. In previous sections, I have highlighted some of the more significant themes that characterize the current literature. Here, I would like to conclude with some methodological comments.

Measurement

As with most new areas of inquiry, investigators are frequently faced with the need to develop new measures of the constructs of interest. Since this can be a difficult and time-consuming enterprise, researchers often attempt to adapt available instruments for their purposes. Although this approach is sometimes successful, investigators should beware of acritical use of instruments developed with other (e.g. healthy) populations. For example, the Children's Depression Inventory includes items about the child's appetite, sleep habits, aches and pains, and feelings of tiredness (Kovacs, 1981). In a healthy child, these symptoms may represent signs of depression. However, in an ill child, the same symptoms may be a "normal" consequence of the child's medical condition. In other words, the same test items may mean something different in a chronically ill versus a healthy child. Unfortunately, higher scores achieved by chronically ill youngsters on such instruments, compared to their physically healthy peers, are sometimes misinterpreted as indicative of poorer adjustment in the chronically ill sample. Similar problems may arise when measures developed with adults are applied to pediatric populations.

When the focus is on disease-specific functioning, the development of disease-specific measures can hardly be avoided. Since different diseases require different regimen behaviors, measures of adherence and disease knowledge must be disease-specific. Even pain and distress may be exhibited differently across diseases. The situation is further complicated by the complexity of disease knowledge and adherence. For many chronic diseases, there are multiple skills and disease management behaviors required on a daily basis. In such cases, measures must be developed that are sensitive to the complexity of the patient's tasks. Fortunately, methodologies now exist that can be applied across diseases. For example, behavioral observation has been used to reliably assess skill in a variety of disease management tasks (Johnson *et al.*, 1982; Sergis-Deavenport and Varni, 1983). Similarly, behavioral observation has been used to assess pain and distress in children undergoing different kinds of medical procedures (Gilbert *et al.*, 1982; Elliot and Olson, 1983; Jay *et al.*, 1983; Kolko and Rickard-Figueroa, 1985). Once the investigator identifies a method of measurement, he or she may be able to successfully adapt a particular procedure for use with a specific illness group; in this way, an investigator may enter the realm of disease-specific measurement with a data-based approach.

In the past, investigators have emphasized measures that are sensitive to potential problems faced by children with chronic disease and their families: problems of poor adjustment to the disease, dysfunctional family reactions, pain and discomfort experienced as a result of the disease or its treatment, knowledge or skill deficits, poor adherence, or patient-provider miscommunication. These issues are clearly important and deserve our continued attention. However, measures also need to be developed that are sensitive to possible positive effects of learning to live with a chronic disease, permitting an expanded research focus on factors that encourage resilience, mastery, and pro-social behavior in the face of childhood chronic illness.

Developmental Issues

Throughout this chapter developmental issues have repeatedly surfaced. As children grow and mature, they change cognitively, emotionally, and socially. These developmental changes are central to our understanding of how chronic disease impacts on the child and family. Whether we are concerned with general psychological adaptation or disease-specific functioning, developmental issues remain paramount. However, in addition to changes associated with the child's growth and development, we must also be sensitive to changes associated with the disease process. The behaviors and reactions of newly diagnosed patients may be different from those who have learned to live with the disease. Diseases that are dynamic or associated with progressive deterioration may have different psychological sequelae than chronic conditions that are more static. An increased sensitivity to both child development and disease development should substantially enhance our understanding.

Correlation Versus Causation

In an area like childhood chronic disease, most psychological factors cannot be readily studied using experimental manipulation. Instead, research is typically characterized by a search for naturally-occurring associations. Hopefully, a causal hypothesis underlies the study of a possible link between observed variables. In the interest of economy, studies are initially cross-sectional; the relationship between study variables is examined in a sample at a single point in time. A significant association offers support for the study's hypothesis. Although correlational research is extremely important and should be guided by causal hypotheses, correlation does not confirm causation. Consequently, great care must be taken when we interpret our findings to consider alternative explanations. For example, we may hypothesize that a dysfunctional family environment may cause poorer medical regimen adherence. Indeed, we may be able to establish an empirical link between the two. Such an association supports our hypothesis but also suggests quite a different interpretation: poor adherence could lead to increased family dysfunction. Longitudinal studies may better address causal relationships between variables. However, longitudinal research is expensive, time-consuming, and practically difficult to conduct. Consequently, it is wise to base longitudinal research on a strong cross-sectional data-base. In developing that data-base, we need to be guided by causal hypotheses but not blinded by them.

REFERENCES

Anderson, B., Auslander, W., Jung, K., Miller, P. & Santiago, J. (1990). Assessing family sharing of diabetes responsibilities. *Journal of Pediatric Psychology*, **15**, 477–492.

Anderson, B., Miller, J., Auslander, W. & Santiago, J. (1981). Family characteristics of diabetic adolescents: Relationship to metabolic control. *Diabetes Care*, **4**, 586–594.

Anderson, L., Devellis, B. & Devellis, R. (1987). Effects of modeling on patient communication, satisfaction, and knowledge. *Medical Care*, **25**, 1044–1056.

Bakal, D. (1979). *Psychology and Medicine: Psychobiological Dimensions of Health and Illness*. New York: Springer.

Band, E. (1990). Children's coping with diabetes: Understanding the role of cognitive development. *Journal of Pediatric Psychology*, **15**, 27–41.

Band, E. & Weisz, J. (1990). Developmental differences in primary and secondary control coping and adjustment to juvenile diabetes. *Journal of Abnormal Child Psychology*, **19**, 150–158.

Benson, B. & Gross, A. (1989). The effect of a congenitally handicapped child upon the marital dyad: A review of the literature. *Clinical Psychology Review*, 9, 747–758.

Billings, A., Moos, R., Miller, J. & Gottlieb, J. (1987). Psychosocial adaptation in juvenile rheumatic disease: A controlled evaluation. *Health Psychology*, 6, 343–359.

Borner, S. & Steinhausen, H. (1977). A psychological study of family characteristics in juvenile diabetes. *Pediatric and Adolescent Endocrinology*, 3, 46–51.

Breslau, N. & Marshall, I. (1985). Psychological disturbances in children with physical disabilities: Continuity and change in a 5-year follow-up. *Journal of Abnormal Child Psychology*, 13, 199–216.

Breslau, N., Staruch, K. & Mortimer, E. (1982). Psychological distress in mothers of disabled children. *American Journal of Diseases of Children*, 136, 682–686.

Breslau, N., Weitzman, M. & Messenger, K. (1981). Psychologic functioning of siblings of disabled children. *Pediatrics*, 67, 344–353.

Brown, J., O'Leeffe, J., Sanders, S. & Baker, B. (1986). Developmental changes in children's cognition to stressful and painful situations. *Journal of Pediatric Psychology*, 11, 343–357.

Chaney, J. & Peterson, L. (1989). Family variables and disease management in juvenile rheumatoid arthritis. *Journal of Pediatric Psychology*, 14, 389–403.

Christensen, N., Terry, R., Wyatt, S., Pichert, J. & Lorenz, R. (1983). Quantitative assessment of dietary adherence in patients with insulin-dependent diabetes mellitus. *Diabetes Care*, 6, 245–250.

Christiaanse, M., Lavigne, J. & Lerner, C. (1989). Psychosocial aspects of compliance in children and adolescents with asthma. *Developmental and Behavioural Pediatrics*, 10, 75–80.

Creer, T., Harm, D. & Marion, R. (1988). Childhood asthma. In *Handbook of Pediatric Psychology*, edited by D. Routh, pp. 162–189. New York: Guilford Press.

Daniels, D., Moos, R., Billings, A. & Miller, J. (1987). Psychosocial risk and resistance factors among children with chronic illness, healthy siblings, and healthy controls. *Journal of Abnormal Child Psychology*, 15, 295–308.

Dolgin, M., Katz, E., Doctors, S. & Siegel, S. (1986). Caregivers' perceptions of medical compliance in adolescents with cancer. *Journal of Adolescent Health Care*, 7, 22–27.

Dronenberger, W. & Thompson, R. (1990). Dimensions of family functioning in families with chronically ill children: A higher order factor analysis of the family environment scale. *Journal of Clinical Child Psychology*, 19, 380–388.

Drotar, D. & Crawford, P. (1985). Psychological adaptation of siblings of chronically ill children: Research and practice implications. *Developmental and Behavioural Pediatrics*, 6, 355–362.

Drotar, D., Doershuk, C., Stern, R., Boat, T., Boyer, W. & Matthews, L. (1981). Psychosocial functioning of children with cystic fibrosis. *Pediatrics*, 67, 338–353.

Dunbar, F. (1955). *Emotions and Bodily Changes*. New York: Columbia University Press.

Eiser, C., Town, C. & Tripp, J. (1988). Illness experience and related knowledge amongst children with asthma. *Child: Care, Health and Development*, 14, 11–24.

Elliot, C. & Olson, R. (1983). The management of children's distress in response to painful medical treatment for burn injuries. *Behaviour Research and Therapy*, 21, 675–683.

Epstein, L., Coburn, P., Becker, D., Drash, A. & Siminerio, L. (1980). Measurement and modification of the accuracy of the determinants of urine glucose concentration. *Diabetes Care*, 3, 535–536.

Etzwiler, D. (1962). What the juvenile diabetic knows about his disease. *Pediatrics*, 29, 135–141.

Feagans, L., Sanyal, M., Henderson, F., Collier, A. & Appelbaum, M. (1987). Relationship of middle ear disease in early childhood to later narrative and attention skills. *Journal of Pediatric Psychology*, 12, 581–594.

Fielding, D., Moore, B., Dewey, M., Ashley, P., McKendrick, T. & Pinderton, P. (1985). Children with end-stage renal failure: Psychological effects on patients, siblings, and parents. *Journal of Psychosomatic Research*, 29, 457–465.

Friedman, I., Litt, I., King, D., Henson, R., Holtzmann, D., Halverson, D. & Kraemer, H. (1986). Compliance with anticonvulsant therapy by epileptic youth: Relationships to psychosocial aspects of adolescent development. *Journal of Adolescent Health Care, 7,* 12–17.

Gayton, W., Friedman, S., Tavormina, J. & Tucker, F. (1977). Children with cystic fibrosis: I. Psychological test findings of patients, siblings, and parents. *Pediatrics, 59,* 888–894.

Garner, A., Thompson, C. & Partridge, J. (1969). Who knows best? *Diabetes Bulletin, 45,* 3–4.

Gibbs, R., Gibbs, R. & Henrich, J. (1987). Patient understanding of commonly used medical vocabulary. *The Journal of Family Practice, 25,* 176–178.

Gilbert, B., Johnson, S., Spillar, R., McCallum, M., Silverstein, J. & Rosenbloom, A. (1982). The effects of a peer-modeling film on children learning to self-inject insulin. *Behaviour Therapy, 13,* 186–193.

Gortmaker, S.L. & Sappenfield, W. (1984). Chronic childhood disorders: prevalence and impact. *Pediatric Clinics of North America, 31,* 3–18.

Greenfield, S., Kaplan, S., Ware, J., Yano, E. & Harrison, F. (1988). Patients' participation in medical care: Effects on blood sugar control and quality of life in diabetes. *Journal of General Internal Medicine, 3,* 228–457.

Haggerty, R.J. (1984). Foreword: Symposium on chronic disease in children. *Pediatric Clinics of North America, 31,* 1–2.

Haight, W., Black, J. & DiMatteo, M. (1985). Young children's understanding of the social roles of physician and patient. *Journal of Pediatric Psychology, 10,* 31–43.

Handford, H., Mayes, S., Bixler, E. & Mattison, R. (1986). Personality traits of hemophiliac boys. *Developmental and Behavioural Pediatrics, 7,* 224–229.

Harkavy, J., Johnson, S., Silverstein, Spillar, R., McCallum, M. & Rosenbloom, A. (1983). Who learns what at diabetes summer camp. *Journal of Pediatric Psychology, 8,* 143–153.

Harper, D., Wacker, D. & Cobb, L. (1986). Children's social preferences toward peers with visible physical differences. *Journal of Pediatric Psychology, 11,* 323–342.

Hauenstein, E., Marnin, R., Snyder, A. & Clarke, W. (1988). Stress in parents of children with diabetes mellitus. *Diabetes Care, 12,* 18–23.

Hauser, S., Jacobson, A., Lavori, P., Wolfsdort, J., Herskowitz, R., Milley, J. & Bliss, R. (1990). Adherence among children and adolescents with insulin-dependent diabetes mellitus over a 4 year longitudinal follow-up: II. Immediate and long-term linkages with the family milieu. *Journal of Pediatric Psychology, 15,* 527–542.

Hawkins, D. (1982). Specificity revisited: Personality profiles and behavioral issues. *Psychotherapy and Psychosomatics, 38,* 54–63.

Hazzard, Hutchinson, S. & Krawiecki, N. (1990). Factors related to adherence to medication regimens in pediatric seizure patients. *Journal of Pediatric Psychology, 15,* 543–555.

Hoare, P. (1984a). Psychiatric disturbance in the families of epileptic children. *Developmental Medicine and Child Neurology, 26,* 14–19.

Hoare, P. (1984b). The development of psychiatric disorder among school children with epilepsy. *Developmental Medicine and Child Neurology, 26,* 3–13.

Hodges, D., Kline, J., Barbero, G. & Flannery, R. (1985). Depressive symptoms in children with recurrent abdominal pain and their families. *Journal of Pediatrics, 107,* 622–626.

Hudson, J., Fielding, D., Jones, S. & McKendrick, R. (1987). Adherence to medical regime and related factors in youngsters in dialysis. (1987) *British Journal of Clinical Psychology, 26,* 61–62.

Ingersoll, G., Orr, D., Herrold, A. & Golden, M. (1986). Cognitive maturity and self-management among adolescents with insulin-dependent diabetes mellitus. *Journal of Pediatrics, 108,* 620–623.

Jacobson, A., Hauser, S., Lavori, P., Wolfsdor, J., Herskowitz, R., Milley, J., Bliss, R., Gelfand, E., Wertlieb, D. & Stein, J. (1990a). Adherence among children and adolescents with insulin-dependent diabetes mellitus over a four-year longitudinal follow-up: I. The influence of patient coping and adjustment. *Journal of Pediatric Psychology*, **15**, 511–526.

Jacobson, A., Hauser, S., Wolfsdorf, J., Houlihan, J., Milley, J., Herskowitz, R., Wertlieb, D. & Watt, E. (1987). Psychologic predictors of compliance in children with recent onset of diabetes mellitus. *Journal of Pediatrics*, **110**, 805–811.

Jacobson, P., Manne, S., Gorfinkle, K., Schorr, O., Rapkin, B. & Redd, W. (1990b). Analysis of child and parent behavior during painful medical procedures. *Health Psychology*, **9**, 559–576.

Jay, S. (1988). Invasive medical procedures: Psychological intervention and assessment. In *Handbook of Pediatric Psychology*, edited by D. Routh, pp. 401–425. New York: Guilford Press.

Jay, S., Ozolins, M., Elliott, C. & Caldwell, S. (1983). Assessment of children's distress during painful medical procedures. *Health Psychology*, **2**, 133–147.

Johnson, S.B. (1989). Adherence behaviors and health status in childhood diabetes. In *Neuropsychological and Behavioral Aspects of Diabetes*, edited by C. Holmes, pp. 30–57. New York: Guilford Press.

Johnson, S.B. (1988). Chronic illness and pain. In *Behavioral Assessment of Childhood Disorders*, 2nd edition, edited by E. Marsh and L. Terdal, pp. 491–527. New York: Guilford Press.

Johnson, S.B. (1984). Knowledge, attitudes, and behavior: Correlates of health in childhood diabetes. *Clinical Psychology Review*, **4**, 503–524.

Johnson, S.B. (1980). Psychosocial factors in juvenile diabetes: A review. *Journal of Behavioral Medicine*, **3**, 95–116.

Johnson, S.B., Pollack, T., Silverstein, J., Rosenbloom, A., Spillar, R., McCallum, M. & Harkavy, J. (1982). Cognitive and behavioral knowledge about insulin dependent diabetes among children and parents. *Pediatrics*, **69**, 708–713.

Johnson, S.B., Riley, W., Hansen, C. & Nurick, M. (1990a). Psychological impact of islet cell antibody screening: Preliminary results. *Diabetes Care*, **13**, 93–95.

Johnson, S.B., Silverstein, J., Rosenbloom, A., Carter, R. & Cunningham, W. (1986). Assessing daily management of childhood diabetes. *Health Psychology*, **5**, 545–564.

Johnson, S.B. Tomer, A., Cunningham, W. & Henretta, J. (1990b). Adherence in childhood diabetes: Results of a confirmatory factor analysis. *Health Psychology*, **9**, 493–501.

Katz, E., Kellerman, J. & Ellenberg, L. (1987). Hypnosis in the reduction of acute pain and distress in children with cancer. *Journal of Pediatric Psychology*, **12**, 379–394.

Kindlon, D., Solee, N. & Yando, R. (1988). Specificity of behavior problems among children with neurological dysfunctions. *Journal of Pediatric Psychology*, **13**, 39–47.

Kohler, E., Hurwitz, L. & Milan, D. (1982). A developmentally staged curriculum for teaching self-care to the child with insulin-dependent diabetes mellitus. *Diabetes Care*, **5**, 300–304.

Kolko, D. & Rickard-Figueroa, J. (1985). Effects of video games on the adverse corollaries of chemotherapy in pediatric oncology patients: A single-case analysis. *Journal of Consulting and Clinical Psychology*, **53**, 223–228.

Korsch, B., Gozzi, E. & Francis, V. (1968). Gaps in doctor-patient communication: I. Doctor-patient interaction and patient satisfaction. *Pediatrics*, **42**, 855–871.

Kovacs, M. (1981). Rating scales to assess depression in school aged children. *Acta Paedopsychiatrica*, **46**, 305–315.

Kovacs, M., Brent, D., Steinberg, T., Paulauskas, S. & Reid, J. (1986). Children's self-reports of psychologic adjustment and coping strategies during the first year of insulin-dependent diabetes mellitus. *Diabetes Care*, **9**, 472–479.

Kovacs, M., Finkelstein, R., Feinberg, T., Crouse-Novak, M., Paulauskas, S. & Pollock, M. (1985). Initial psychologic responses of parents to the diagnosis of insulin-dependent diabetes mellitus in their children. *Diabetes Care*, **8**, 568–575.

Kronenberger, W.G. & Thompson, R.J. (1990). Dimensions of family functioning in families with chronically ill children: A higher order factor analysis of the Family Environment Scale. *Journal of Clinical Child Psychology*, **19**, 380–388.

La Greca, A. (1990). Social consequences of pediatric conditions: Fertile area for future investigation and intervention? *Journal of Pediatric Psychology*, **15**, 285–308.

Lansky, S., Cairns, N., Hassenein, R., Wehr, J. & Lowman, J. (1978). Childhood cancer: Parental discord and divorce. *Pediatrics*, **62**, 184–188.

Latimer, P. (1978). Psychophysiologic disorders: A critical appraisal of concept and theory illustrated with reference to the irritable bowel syndrome (IBS). *Psychological Medicine*, **9**, 71–80.

Lavigne, J., Nolan, D. & McLone, D. (1988). Temperament, coping, and psychological adjustment in young children with myelomeningocele. *Journal of Pediatric Psychology*, **13**, 363–378.

Lavigne, J. & Ryan, M. (1979). Psychologic adjustment of siblings of children with chronic illness. *Pediatrics*, **63**, 616–627.

Lavigne, J., Traisman, H., Marr, T. & Chasnoff, I. (1982). Parental perceptions of the psychological adjustment of children with diabetes and their siblings. *Diabetes Care*, **5**, 420–426.

Lemanek, K., Moore, S., Gresham, F., Williamson, D. & Kelley, M. (1986). Psychological adjustment of children with sickle cell anemia. *Journal of Pediatric Psychology*, **11**, 397–410.

Levine, M. & Rappaport, L. (1984). Recurrent abdominal pain in school children: The loneliness of the long-distance physician. *Pediatric Clinics of North America*, **31**, 969–991.

Litt, I. & Cuskey, W. (1981). Compliance with salicylate therapy in adolescents with juvenile rheumatoid arthritis. *American Journal of Diseases of Children*, **135**, 434–436.

Litt, I. & Cuskey, W. (1984). Satisfaction with health care: a predictor of adolescents' appointment keeping. *Journal of Adolescent Health Care*, **5**, 196–200.

Lobato, D. (1983). Siblings of handicapped children: A review. *Journal of Autism and Developmental Disorders*, **13**, 347–363.

Lobato, D., Faust, D. & Spirito, A. (1988). Examining the effects of chronic disease and disability on children's sibling relationships. *Journal of Pediatric Psychology*, **13**, 389–407.

Margalit, M. (1986). Mother's perceptions of anxiety of their diabetic children. *Developmental and Behavioral Pediatrics*, **7**, 27–30.

Marteau, T., Johnston, M., Baum, J. & Bloch, S. (1987). Goals of treatment in diabetes: A comparison of doctors and parents of children with diabetes. *Journal of Behavioral Medicine*, **10**, 33–48.

Mazzuca, S. (1982). Does patient education in chronic disease have therapeutic value? *Journal of Chronic Diseases*, **35**, 521–529.

McElroy, E., Steinschneider, A. & Weinstein, S. (1986). Emotional and health impact of home monitoring on mothers: A controlled prospective study. *Pediatrics*, **78**, 780–786.

McKinney, B. & Peterson, R. (1987). Predictors of stress in parents of developmentally disabled children. *Journal of Pediatric Psychology*, **12**, 133–150.

Melamed, B., Bennett, C., Jerrell, G., Ross, S., Bush, J., Hill, C., Courts, F. & Ronk, S. (1983). Dentists' behavior management as it affects compliance and fear in pediatric patients. *Journal of the American Dental Association*, **106**, 324–330.

Mrazek, D., Casey, B. & Anderson, I. (1987). Insecure attachment in severely asthmatic preschool children: Is it a risk factor? *Journal of the American Academy of Child and Adolescent Psychiatry*, **26**, 516–520.

Nelms, B. (1989). Emotional behaviors in chronically ill children. *Journal of Abnormal Child Psychology*, **17**, 657–668.

Newberry, M. & Parish, T. (1986). Enhancement of attitudes toward handicapped children through social interactions. *Journal of Social Psychology*, **127**, 59–62.

Orr, D., Weller, S., Satterwhite, B. & Pless, I. (1984). Psychosocial implications of chronic illness in adolescence. *Journal of Pediatrics*, **194**, 152–157.

Osborne, R., Hatcher, J. & Richtsmeier, A. (1989). The role of social modeling in unexplained pediatric pain. *Journal of Pediatric Psychology*, **14**, 43–61.

Oster, J. (1972). Recurrent abdominal pain, headache and limb pains in children and adolescents. *Pediatrics*, **50**, 429–436.

Page, P., Verstrete, D., Robb, R. & Etzwiler, D. (1981). Patient recall of self-care recommendations in diabetes. *Diabetes Care*, **4**, 96–98.

Partridge, J., Garner, A., Thompson, C. & Cherry, T. (1972). Attitudes of adolescents toward their diabetes. *American Journal of Diseases of Children*, **124**, 226–229.

Perrin, E. & Perrin, J. (1983). Clinicians' assessments of children's understanding of illness. *American Journal of Diseases of Children*, **137**, 874–878.

Perrin, E., Ramsey, B. & Sandler, H. (1987). Competent kids: Children and adolescents with a chronic illness. *Child: Health, Care and Development*, **13**, 13–32.

Phipps, S. & DeCuir-Whalley, S. (1990). Adherence issues in pediatric bone marrow transplantation. *Journal of Pediatric Psychology*, **15**, 459–475.

Pless, I. (1984). Clinical assessment: Physical and psychological functioning. *Pediatric Clinics of North America*, **31**, 33–45.

Pless, I., Roghmann, K. & Haggerty, R. (1972). Chronic illness, family functioning, and psychosocial adjustment: A model for the allocation of preventive mental health services. *International Journal of Epidemiology*, **1**, 271–277.

Royal, G. & Roberts, M. (1987). Students' perceptions of and attitudes toward disabilities: A comparison of twenty conditions. *Journal of Clinical Child Psychology*, **16**, 122–132.

Ryan, C. (1989). Neuropsychological consequences and correlates of diabetes in childhood. In *Neuropsychological and Behavioral Aspects of Diabetes*, edited by C. Holmes, pp. 58–84. New York: Springer-Verlag.

Sabbath, B. & Leventhal, J. (1984). Marital adjustment to chronic childhood disease: A critique of the literature. *Pediatrics*, **73**, 762–768.

Schechter, N. (1984). Recurrent pains in children: An overview and an approach. *Pediatric Clinics of North America*, **31**, 949–968.

Sergis-Deavenport, D. & Varni, J. (1983). Behavioral assessment and management of adherence to factor replacement therapy in hemophilia. *Journal of Pediatric Psychology*, **8**, 367–377.

Shapiro, A. (1978). Placebo effects in medical and psychological therapies. In *Handbook of Psychotherapy and Behavioral Change: An Empirical Analysis*, edited by S. Garfield and E. Bergen, pp. 369–410. New York: Wiley.

Sigelman, C. & Begleym, N. (1987). The early development of reactions to peers with controllable and uncontrollable problems. *Journal of Pediatric Psychology*, **12**, 99–115.

Smyth-Staruch, K., Breslau, N., Weitzman, M. & Gortmaker, S. (1984). Use of health services by chronically ill and disabled children. *Medical Care*, **22**, 310–328.

Spaulding, B. & Morgan, S. (1986). Spina bifida children and their parents: A population prone to family dysfunction? *Journal of Pediatric Psychology*, **11**, 359–374.

Speltz, M., Armsden, G. & Clarren, S. (1990). Effects of craniofacial birth defects on maternal functioning postinfancy. *Journal of Pediatric Psychology*, **15**, 177–196.

Stein, R. & Jessop, D. (1984). Relationship between health status and psychological adjustment among children with chronic conditions. *Pediatrics*, **73**, 169–174.

Stein, R. & Reissman, C. (1980). The development of the impact-on-family scale: Preliminary findings. *Medical Care*, **18**, 465–472.

Steinhausen, H. (1981). Chronically ill and handicapped children and adolescents: Personality studies in relation to disease. *Journal of Abnormal Child Psychology*, **9**, 291–297.

Steinhausen, H., Schindler, H. & Stephan, H. (1983a). Comparative psychiatric studies on children and adolescents suffering from cystic fibrosis and bronchial asthma. *Child Psychiatry and Human Development*, **14**, 249–458.

Steinhausen, H., Schindler, H. & Stephan, H. (1983b). Correlates of psychopathology in sick children: An empirical model. *Journal of the American Academy of Child Psychiatry*, **22**, 559–564.

Stern, M. & Arenson, E. (1989). Childhood cancer stereotype: impact on adult perceptions of children. *Journal of Pediatric Psychology*, **14**, 593–605.

Stern, M., Ross, S. & Bieglass, M. (1991). Medical students' perceptions of children: modifying a childhood cancer stereotype. *Journal of Pediatric Psychology*, **16**, 27–38.

Stewart, S., Silver, C., Nici, J., Walker, D., Campbell, R., Uauy, R. & Andrews, W. (1991). Neuropsychological function of young children who have undergone liver transplantation. *Journal of Pediatric Psychology*, **16**, 569–583.

Tavormina, J., Boll, T., Dunn, N., Luscomb, R. & Taylor, J. (1981). Psychosocial effects on parents of raising a physically handicapped child. *Journal of Abnormal Child Psychology*, **9**, 121–131.

Tavormina, J., Kastner, L., Slater, P. & Watt, S. (1976). Chronically ill children: A psychologically and emotionally deviant population? *Journal of Abnormal Child Psychology*, **4**, 99–100.

Taylor, H., Albo, V., Phebus, C., Sachs, B. & Bierl, P. (1987). Postirradiation treatment outcomes for children with acute lymphocytic leukemia: Clarification of risks. *Journal of Pediatric Psychology*, **12**, 395–411.

Thompson, R., Kronenberger, W. & Curry, F. (1989). Behavior classification system for children with developmental, psychiatric, and chronic medical problems. *Journal of Pediatric Psychology*, **14**, 559–575.

Tibbi, C., Cummings, K., Zevon, M., Smith, L., Richards, M. & Mallon, J. (1986). Compliance of pediatric and adolescent cancer patients. *Cancer*, **58**, 1179–1184.

van Aken, M., van Lieshout, C. & Katz, E. (1989). Development of behavioral distress in reaction to acute pain in two cultures. *Journal of Pediatric Psychology*, **14**, 421–432.

Varni, J. & Jay, S. (1984). Biobehavioral factors in juvenile rheumatoid arthritis: Implications for research and practice. *Clinical Psychology Review*, **4**, 543–560.

Varni, J., Wilcox, K. & Hanson, V. (1989). Mediating effects of family social support on child psychological adjustment in juvenile rheumatoid arthritis. *Health Psychology*, **8**, 421–431.

Waber, D., Gioia, G., Paccia, J., Sherman, B., Dinklage, D., Sollee, N., Urion, D., Tarbell, N. & Sallan, S. (1990). Sex difference in cognitive processing in children treated with CNS prophylaxis for acute lymphoblastic leukemia. *Journal of Pediatric Psychology*, **15**, 105–122.

Walker, L., Ford, M. & Donald, W. (1987). Cystic fibrosis and family stress: Effects of age and severity of illness. *Pediatrics*, **79**, 239–246.

Walker, L. & Greene, J. (1989). Children with recurrent abdominal pain and their parents: More somatic complaints, anxiety, and depression than other patient families? *Journal of Pediatric Psychology*, **14**, 231–243.

Walker, L., Ortiz-Valdles, J. & Newbrough, J. (1989). The role of maternal employment and depression in the psychological adjustment of chronically ill, mentally retarded, and well children. *Journal of Pediatric Psychology*, **14**, 357–370.

Wallander, J., Feldman, W. & Varni, J. (1989a). Physical status and psychosocial adjustment in children with spina bifida. *Journal of Pediatric Psychology*, **14**, 89–102.

Wallander, J., Varni, J., Babani, L., Banis, H., DeHaan, C. & Wilcox, K. (1989b). Disability parameters, chronic strain, and adaptation of physically handicapped children and their mothers. *Journal of Pediatric Psychology*, **14**, 23–42.

Wallander, J., Varni, J., Babani, L., Banis, H. & Wilcox, K. (1988). Children with chronic physical disorders: Maternal reports of their psychological adjustment. *Journal of Pediatric Psychology*, **13**, 197–212.

Wallander, J., Varni, J., Babani, L., Banis, H. & Wilcox, K. (1989c). Family resources as resistance factors for psychological maladjustment in chronically ill and handicapped children. *Journal of Pediatric Psychology*, **14**, 157–173.

Wallander, J., Varni, J., Babani, L., DeHanne, C., Wilcox, K. & Banis, H. (1989d). The social environment and the adaptation of mothers of physically handicapped children. *Journal of Pediatric Psychology*, **14**, 371–387.

Weinstein, A. & Cuskey, W. (1986). Theophylline compliance in asthmatic children. *Annals of Allergy*, **54**, 19–24.

Weinstein, P., Getz, T., Ratener, P. & Domoto, P. (1982). The effect of dentists' behaviors on fear-related behaviors in children. *Journal of the American Dental Association*, **104**, 32–38.

Weitzman, M. (1986). School absence rates as outcome measures in studies of children with chronic illness. *Journal of Chronic Diseases*, **39**, 799–808.

Wells, R. & Schwebel, A. (1987). Chronically ill children and their mothers: Predictors of resilience and vulnerability to hospitalization and surgical stress. *Journal of Developmental and Behavioral Pediatrics*, **8**, 83–89.

Wertlieb, D., Hauser, S. & Jacobson, A. (1986). Adaptation to diabetes: Behavior symptoms and family context. *Journal of Pediatric Psychology*, **11**, 463–479.

Wood, B., Boyle, J., Watkins, J., Nogueira, J., Zimand, E. & Carroll, L. (1988). Sibling psychological status and style as related to the disease of their chronically ill brothers and sisters: Implications for models of biopsychosocial interaction. *Developmental and Behavioral Pediatrics*, **9**, 66–72.

Worchel, F., Copeland, D. & Barker, D. (1987). Control-related coping strategies in pediatric oncology patients. *Journal of Pediatric Psychology*, **12**, 25–38.

Wysocki, T., Huxtable, K., Linscheid, T. & Wayne, W. (1989). Adjustment to diabetes mellitus in preschoolers and their mothers. *Diabetes Care*, **12**, 524–529.

Wysocki, R., Meinhold, P., Cox, D. & Clarke, W. (1990). Survey of diabetes professionals regarding developmental changes in diabetes self-care. *Diabetes Care*, **13**, 65–68.

SECTION II
Adolescence

HEALTH BEHAVIOUR IN ADOLESCENCE: RISKS AND REASONS

DON NUTBEAM AND MICHAEL L. BOOTH

INTRODUCTION

Adolescence is both a period of transition from childhood to adulthood and an important period in the life span in itself. It is characterized by major physical and intellectual development which is associated with important changes in social relationships, as young people struggle to meet external expectations of them to behave as adults, and their own perceptions and reactions to what this means. The period of adolescence has particular importance for health throughout the rest of the life span. For example, most adult smokers initiate their habit during adolescence (Marsh and Matheson, 1983) and involvement in sports as an adolescent is a strong predictor of participation in regular physical activity as an adult (Dishman, Sallis and Orenstein, 1985). It is a period during which patterns of behaviour are initially tried out and eventually become established. These include behaviours which may have immediate consequences affecting health status (drug and alcohol misuse), those which substantially influence future health status (tobacco use) and those which may have life-long consequences (high-risk behaviours which lead to disability).

This chapter outlines the nature and timing of the important developmental changes (physical, cognitive and social) which characterise adolescence. The concept of "risk-taking" is then discussed as a central approach to understanding the associations between the various aspects of developmental change and health behaviour. Finally, recent empirical evidence which has examined the inter-relatedness of health behaviours (or "lifestyle") and their associated determinants is discussed. Ultimately, the study of adolescent health behaviour is a complex and expanding field. The main aim of this chapter is to introduce the key issues and to provide references for the further information of interested readers.

DEFINING ADOLESCENCE

Although chronological age is not always an appropriate marker for developmental changes it is certainly the most convenient and is widely used. There is some disagreement as to the ages that should be used to identify the boundaries of adolescence (particularly the upper age limit), but the onset of puberty is widely accepted as marking the beginning of adolescence. Although, the onset of puberty may vary considerably between individuals and typically occurs earlier in females than in males, the age of ten years is used by many authorities (including the World Health Organisation; WHO, 1980) because it includes the onset of puberty in both sexes and in most individuals. Unfortunately, no such phenomenon suggests an appropriate upper age limit to adolescence. In most Western cultures the end of adolescence is identified by the development of the ability to live independently of parents and the commencement of a vocation (or, at least, vocational education). The age of 19 years is therefore commonly used to mark the beginning of adulthood. In more traditional cultures adolescence may be a relatively brief period, commencing with puberty and ending shortly after with certain rites of passage which deliver the individual into "instant" adulthood. Consequently, the upper age limit of adolescence must remain flexible and responsive to the cultural context in which it is being used. A useful guide is the age at which the mainstream culture expects adult roles to be adopted. The extended period from 10 to 19 years of age will be used as the definition of adolescence in this chapter.

PHYSICAL DEVELOPMENT AND ADOLESCENT SEXUALITY

Pubescence is generally considered the most important marker of the beginning of adolescence. It is a rapid change to physical maturity and involves a spurt of physical growth, the appearance of secondary sexual characteristics and the attainment of reproductive maturity.

Rapid increases in height and weight commence at about $10\frac{1}{2}$ years of age in girls and at about $12\frac{1}{2}$ years of age in boys and last about 2 years in both sexes. However, the rate of increase in both height and weight is generally greater in boys than girls, leaving boys, on average, heavier and taller than girls. Sexual development accompanies the height and weight growth spurts in both sexes.

This spurt in growth combined with sexual and reproductive maturity has enormous implications for the ways in which adolescents behave and the consequences of their behaviour for health. Sexual curiosity is associated with sexual maturity, and experimentation with sexual behaviour is an unsurprising consequence of such curiosity. Although the study of adolescent sexual behaviour is severely constrained by practical, methodological problems (Nielson, 1987), it is clear that knowledge, beliefs, attitudes and behaviour vary substantially as a function of gender, age, socio-economic status and cultural or ethnic background. There are clear differences between girls and boys in their attitude to sex, with girls more likely to associate sex with love and personal commitment and boys generally doing the opposite, dissociating sex from love (Hamburg and Trudeau, 1981; Miller and Simon, 1980). Differences in the desired level of sexual activity was well summarized by McCabe and Collins (1990): "males want more than they get sexually and females get more than they want".

The consequences of unprotected sexual intercourse among adolescents are substantial. Unwanted pregnancy is one obvious outcome which leads to an unenviable choice for most teenagers of either giving birth and compromising the mother's own social, educational and economic development (and consequently disadvantaging their child), or seeking an abortion – which, if available, will frequently be sought in the later stages of pregnancy with greater risks to health and future fertility (UN, 1988). In addition, unplanned and/or unprotected sexual intercourse also carries with it the risk of sexually transmitted infection. The incidence of sexually transmitted diseases among adolescents has increased markedly in both developed and developing countries in the past twenty years (Silber and Woodward, 1985). Among the major diseases are gonorrhoea and chlamydia infections, herpes, and in the past decade HIV infection leading to AIDS. The impact of these diseases on adolescents is greatly compounded by a failure to seek advice either because of ignorance of the symptoms, or because of the reluctance of some young people to seek help because of their expectations that they will meet with hostility and rejection.

Studies conducted in the United States and Australia indicate that most adolescents are sexually experienced by the age of 18 years (McCabe and Collins, 1990; Zelnick and Shah, 1983). Because adolescent sexuality is a taboo subject in many societies, many young people have vague or distorted ideas about sexual behaviour. They may fail to recognize the risk of pregnancy or contracting a sexually transmitted disease through sexual intercourse, are naturally impulsive and less likely to plan ahead than an adult, and are less likely to make the best use of available health care services (Collins and Robinson, 1986; Friedman, 1989; Silber, 1985).

Several studies have identified that the older the adolescent at first intercourse the more likely they are to be better informed about the relative risks of their behaviour, and to use contraception consistently and effectively (Faulkenberry, Vincent, James and Johnson, 1987; Freeman, Rickels, Huggins, Mudd, Garcia and Dickens, 1980; Reichelt and Werley, 1981; Zelnick, Kanter and Ford, 1981). Such findings would tempt a conclusion that prevention efforts might be best directed towards achieving a delay in the first sexual experiences. But this would be ignoring the reality of life for many teenagers of both sexes who are constantly bombarded with apparently conflicting messages about sexual behaviour from adults, peers and the media. Efforts to break down taboos about adolescent sexuality, to improve communication between adults (particularly parents) and adolescents, and to improve access to information and relevant services would all help substantially to avoid the unwanted and frequently health-compromising consequences of adolescent sexual behaviours.

COGNITIVE DEVELOPMENT

As well as the fundamental physical changes which occur during adolescence, a great many of the psycho-social attributes which shape and regulate the occurrence of health behaviours are either acquired or consolidated during adolescence. Young people's attitudes and beliefs, their motivations and personal control, and their self image and self esteem are subject to considerable development and reform during adolescence. This development is substantially determined by important changes in cognitive abilities which shape adolescents capacity to understand their world and where they fit into it.

The writings of Piaget remain very influential in understanding the cognitive development of children and adolescents (Inhelder and Piaget, 1958; Piaget, 1972). He asserted that children through to adolescence go though four stages of cognitive development: sensorimotor, preoperational, concrete operational and formal operational thought. (The last stage is of greatest relevance to adolescent cognitive development). He suggested that the operations and the way they are organized within any of the four stages imply shifts in the underlying structure which results from interaction with the physical and social world. Piaget also argued that the progression through the four stages of development is universal and invariant.

During the early years of adolescence the first stage of formal operational thought enables young people to think abstractly and to engage in hypothetical-deductive reasoning – generating different solutions to problems and testing them in a planned way until a workable solution is found. During the middle years of adolescence, the new ideas and speculations are increasingly tested against the realities of experience and formal operational thought becomes more consolidated. Such new ideas are further developed as young people test out their personal tolerance limits, and the social acceptability of various actions and behaviours. This experimentation with, and testing out of new ideas and behaviours has great relevance to the development of health behaviours such as smoking, drug and alcohol use, and has contributed significantly to an understanding of risk-taking behaviour among young people.

Although Piaget's theory remains influential, it has been the subject of substantial criticism (Keating, 1988). Perhaps of greatest importance is the suggestion that only 40–60% of late adolescents and adults appear to use formal operational thought in the way described by Piaget (Keating, 1980; Neimark, 1979). For the rest of the adolescent population, far less progression is made between concrete and formal operational thought. Such a view has important implications for understanding and predicting adolescent health behaviour, and has obvious consequences for developing health promotion messages and programmes for young people.

Beyond this basic work on cognitive development theory, research in the field of social cognition has assisted our understanding of how people conceptualize and reason about their social world, how they interact with other individuals and groups, and how they reason about themselves. Key aspects of social cognition have been described by Elkind in his theory of adolescent egocentrism (Elkind, 1967; Shantz, 1983). This theory has been a durable and rich source of hypotheses on adolescent behaviour. Elkind suggested that adolescent egocentrism is a direct result of the emergence of formal operational thought and is represented by two complementary types of thinking; the imaginary audience and the personal fable. The imaginary audience is the belief that others are as preoccupied with their behaviour as are the adolescents. The personal fable reflects the development of a sense of personal uniqueness (so no-one can understand how they feel) and a sense of omnipotence and indestructibility.

An understanding of cognitive development is of great importance in understanding the evolution of behaviours relevant to health. Cognitive development in adolescence is characterized by an increased interest and capacity for experimentation, and a narrowly focussed and self-centred view of the world, combined with feelings of indestructibility. Such characteristics make for a complex melting pot from which emerge behaviour patterns that are both resistant to change and of immense importance to health.

THE SOCIAL CONTEXT OF ADOLESCENT
HEALTH BEHAVIOURS

The period of adolescence is not only marked by physical and intellectual development. These developments are also accompanied by significant changes in social relationships, which in turn substantially influence behaviours – particularly those which are largely socially defined such as sexual behaviour, smoking and alcohol use.

The popular perception of parent-adolescent relationships being characterized by conflict and stress has not been borne out by empirical studies (e.g. Kandel and Lesser, 1972; Youniss and Smolar, 1985). Only a relatively small proportion of families experience a dramatic decline in the quality of relationships (Rutter, Graham, Chadwick and Yule, 1976) and those that do are more likely to be single-parent families or stepfamilies (Montemayor, 1986). This is not to say that relationships do not change and that some conflict does not occur. Most research highlights a transformation in parent-child relationships often accompanied by an increase in minor arguments (e.g. Steinberg, 1988), usually centred on issues of greater autonomy. Associated with this changing parental relationship is an increase in the time spent and intimacy shared with peers, but most adolescents do so within an atmosphere of a continued positive relationship with their parents (Montemayor and Flannery, 1991).

A strengthened relationship with peers may serve important functions in the transition from childhood to adulthood. For example, it is been suggested that peers may provide emotional support (Blos, 1979), that peer groups provide the opportunity for learning about relationship development (Sullivan, 1953), and that associating with peers facilitates the development of an identity separate from the family role (Youniss, 1980).

This changing pattern of social relationships has important implications for health related behaviours, particularly where such behaviours are socially defined. Parents obviously shape the physical and social environment in which young people live. They will often define in explicit terms the level of tolerance and social acceptability of a range of behaviours. Family functioning, parental family management techniques, and parental behaviour and example have all been associated with adolescent health behaviours, particularly with 'anti-social' behaviours including smoking, alcohol misuse, and the use of illicit drugs (Baumrind, 1987; Loeber & Dishion, 1983).

Peer influence can be exerted through explicit pressures, but is more often manifested through more subtle forms of social reinforcement, or isolation. Association with peers who use illicit drugs, smoke or use alcohol is one of the strongest predictors of these behaviours among adolescents (e.g. Kaplan, Martin and Robbins, 1982). Peer relationships are not all negative in their impact on health behaviour, however. Research conducted in Europe has indicated a clear and positive relationship between patterns of regular physical activity and peer support for such activity (Wold, 1989). Social, emotional and other forms of practical support may also be provided by peers (Foster-Clark & Blyth, 1991). The relative strength of parental and peer influence varies by issue. Peer influence tends to be greater in lifestyle choices including fashion, drug use and anti-social behaviours, whereas parental influence tends to be greater on more substantial and future-oriented issues such as education and vocation (e.g. Kandel and Andrews, 1987).

Although the family and peers are the primary social influence on health-related behaviour, they are by no means the only significant social factors. Important secondary social influences on behaviour include both the school and the mass media. Again, the extent of this influence varies considerably from individual to individual, and from issue to issue.

In the case of the media, television and newspapers are recognized as important sources of health information for adolescents and adults alike (e.g. Freimouth, Greenburg, Dewitt and Romano, 1984). More specifically, media exposure has been associated with uptake and brand choice among adolescent smokers (Chapman and Fitzgerald, 1982), greater consumption of non-nutritious snacks and incorrect perceptions of the nutritional values of foods high in salt, sugar and fat (Atkin, 1976, 1980), and alcohol consumption (Atkin, Hocking and Block, 1984). Against this the mass media influence health behaviour in more positive ways, either incidently (as part of "normal" news and entertainment) or more deliberately as part of a planned media campaign (Flay and Burton, 1990; Montgomery, 1990).

In the case of the school, there is clear evidence of a relationship between school experience and social behaviours. In summary, the more positive the experience, the more positive the health behaviours (Nutbeam, Aaro and Catford, 1989). The reverse is also true in that dislike of school, and/or under-achievement are closely associated with health compromising behaviours including substance misuse and unsafe sex (Jessor and Jessor, 1977). As with the media, the school is also used as a vehicle for promoting positive health behaviours – an approach which has met with varying levels of success over the past two decades (e.g. Botvin, 1983; Thompson, 1978; Perry, 1991). In general, this research has identified that the actual influence of both school and media are more limited than might be expected, and probably a good deal less important than family and friends. The school and the media act most powerfully to reinforce or undermine existing adolescent beliefs and behaviours, rather than actually determining them.

The study of the social context of adolescent health behaviour has been considerably influenced by social learning theory. This theory, most substantially articulated by Bandura (1977, 1986), emphasizes the notion that behaviours are gradually acquired and shaped as a response to the positive and negative consequences of those behaviours. Parents, teachers, peers, siblings and "significant others" (such as pop stars and sports heroes) provide the reinforcing or negative feedback necessary to shape and maintain a behaviour. These individuals also serve as role models, providing examples of appropriate and inappropriate behaviours, and their consequences. Eventually, as the adolescent matures, these rewards and punishments may become internalized.

Social learning theory also highlights the importance of the environment in which behaviour occurs as the *source* of cues, rewards and punishments. This distinguishes social learning theory from cognitive theories which focus much more on an adolescent's *construction or perception* of their environment. However, more recent discussion of social learning theory recognizes that young people are capable of imagining or anticipating the response of parents, peers and significant others towards a behaviour, and of placing a value on the behaviour and/or its consequences (Bush and Iannotti, 1985).

RISK-TAKING BEHAVIOUR IN ADOLESCENCE

Adolescents are no longer afforded the tolerance that children receive, but neither have they had the opportunity to acquire the skills, knowledge and experience that generally temper adult behaviour. They are faced with the opportunity to engage in adult behaviours such as sexual activity, alcohol consumption and motor vehicle use without necessarily recognising the possible negative consequences of their actions. Even if the possibility of some negative outcome is acknowledged, the sense of invulnerability that attends adolescence often precludes an appropriate change in behaviour. Adolescents are frequently confronted by behavioural choices which require varying levels of personal experience for an appropriate response. How much alcohol is too much? How fast is too fast to drive? At face value adolescents often appear to be taking unnecessary risks which are likely to impact on their health and well-being. Understanding the functions served by risk taking and their relationships with the physical, social and cognitive changes that take place during adolescence is crucial in determining how to reduce risk taking or to minimise harm associated with particular behaviours.

Most people engage in various forms of risk-taking behaviour. That is, behaviour where there is the potential for a harmless outcome but also a variable risk (compared with many other behaviours) of an injurious or other negative outcome. Risk-taking behaviour is a commonly identified feature of adolescence as young people gain greater independence and develop new social relationships, experiment with new forms of behaviour, and test out the limits of their tolerance (both physical and social). Risk-taking behaviour can have negative outcomes that are directly related to the behaviour (e.g. alcohol use leading to motor vehicle accidents), or more remote to the behaviour (e.g. cigarette smoking) or which may have both immediate and long-term consequences (e.g. unprotected sexual intercourse). However, defining a particular behaviour as a risk behaviour is not as simple as might be imagined (Irwin, 1987). The personal, social and physical resources an adolescent has available to cope with the potential outcomes may substantially determine the real level of risk being encountered. Alcohol and illicit drug use are two examples where health effects are dependent upon the individuals access to these resources. As such, the same behaviour may represent a serious risk for one individual and a relatively minor risk for another. Not all risk-taking behaviour is negative and taking risks in a controlled, positive environment may contribute to the healthy development of adolescents (Baumrind, 1987; Damon, 1984). Despite these variables in definition some behaviours are clearly associated with a much higher likelihood of a negative health outcome and it is these behaviours that have been given closest attention in the literature on adolescent health.

Irwin and Millstein (1991) suggested a classification of negative risk-taking behaviours based on their aetiological factors; (1) behaviours that are inherently pathogenic, e.g. suicide, (2) behaviours that are primarily the result of environmental forces, e.g., violent 15 behaviours, and (3) behaviours that result from an interaction between the biopsychosocial processes of adolescence and the environment and which include vehicle use, sexual activity and substance use. Most discussions of risk-taking behaviour in the literature are restricted to the third category as these are considered most amenable to adaptation.

The pioneering work of Jessor and Jessor (1977) and subsequent studies have identified that risk taking behaviour by adolescents is far from a random, anti-social action. Such risk behaviours are a means to an end, and they often fulfil an important personal or social function. These functions include:

(1) a means of expressing opposition to adult authority and the conventional society whose values and norms are not shared by the younger generation, e.g. unconventional music and drug taking,
(2) a way of identifying with and being accepted into the peer group, e.g. smoking is a well-established mark of peer-group membership,
(3) an expression and confirmation of valued attributes of personal identity. Drinking and driving, for example, is a way of showing that one is "cool" or "experienced",
(4) as a sign that one has gone from a less mature to a more mature status,
(5) a coping mechanism for dealing with anxiety, frustration, inadequacy, and failure or with the anticipation that failure is likely, and
(6) simply for the fun or pleasure or release from an otherwise boring routine.

The development of a theoretical model to represent risk-taking behaviours is a necessary prerequisite for the design and implementation of effective interventions aimed at reducing the prevalence of these behaviours. Jessor and Jessor (1977) were the first investigators to attempt to develop a fairly comprehensive model of what they called "problem behaviour", that is, delinquency, precocious sexual activity, alcohol abuse and use of illicit drugs. The Jessors' early work stimulated a great deal of interest and more recent research has allowed the development of more refined models of risk-taking behaviours. Several models have been developed (Daitzman and Zuckerman, 1989; Irwin and Millstein, 1991; Slovic, 1987; Udry, 1988; Zuckerman, 1986) and have placed emphasis on different factors. Irwin and Millstein (1991) have presented a model which was based on the Jessors' earlier work and which has attempted to incorporate the results of more recent research, particularly the effects of biological factors such as hormone levels and the timing of puberty in relation to peers (see Irwin and Millstein, 1986, for a more detailed discussion of the model).

The model identifies two, interacting sets of primary (predisposing) factors termed biopsychosocial factors and environmental factors. Biopsychosocial factors are described as endogenous to the individual and include affective states, sensation-seeking, attitudes, beliefs, knowledge, intentions, the value placed on independence and expectation for academic performance. Environmental factors are those external to the individual and include factors such as the quality of family life, peers, school and the broader society. The two sets of predisposing factors may place the adolescent in a position of increased vulnerability when precipitating factors for risk behaviours are encountered. Again, precipitating factors are divided into biopsychosocial and environmental factors and include the effects of the school environment, peer and social pressures and a poor ability to resist those pressures, a lack of experience and/or knowledge and substance availability and use. The relative influence of each of these many factors and the ways in which they may interact are yet to be determined and will require a substantial research effort. At the very least, Irwin and Millstein's model clearly illustrates the complexity of the problem and the multitude of factors that must be considered.

Although most of the research to date has focussed on behaviours with more immediate health consequences (e.g., substance abuse and unprotected sexual activity) Donovan, Jessor and Costa (1991) have attempted to apply problem behaviour theory to other health behaviours (physical activity, hours of sleep, seat belt use and diet). Although the strength of the relationships between the model's explanatory variables and the health behaviours studied was only modest, the results were consistent across behaviours, gender and age. Although reasonably confident prediction of adolescent health behaviour is not within our grasp, the findings of Donovan *et al.* certainly represent a promising start.

HEALTH BEHAVIOURS AND LIFESTYLES

Risk-taking behaviours are frequently examined in isolation from other behaviours, and sometimes in isolation from the physical/social environment which contributes to them. Hence there are numerous studies of adolescent smoking behaviour, alcohol use, patterns of physical activity and dietary choices. While there are merits in examining these problems individually (it may be more practical and manageable and such individual behaviours are often directly associated with defined health outcomes) this approach to studying adolescent health behaviours misses the important relationships between behaviours which become apparent in the examination of a range of health behaviours. Their health behaviours do not exist in isolation but are associated with each other in clusters (Irwin and Millstein, 1986; Jessor and Jessor, 1977; Jessor, 1984; Udry, 1988). For example, there is considerable evidence of relationships between the inappropriate use of licit drugs (alcohol, cigarettes and prescription drugs) and illicit substances (Jessor and Jessor, 1977; Newcomb and Bentler, 1986; Yamaguchi and Kandel, 1984) and between substance use and early (often unprotected) sexual activity (Kegeles, Millstein, Adler, Irwin, Cohn and Dolcini, 1987; Mott and Haurin, 1987; Zabin, 1984).

The work of Jessor (1984) in examining clusters of "problem behaviours" has been instrumental in highlighting these important relationships between behaviours and he has drawn attention to the important theoretical and practical implications of such findings. Firstly, Jessor has shown that these risk behaviours are, in some way, associated within the adolescent's social context – as one behaviour is associated with another it suggests that there are socially organized opportunities to learn and practice them together. Secondly, he has indicated that different risk behaviours may share an underlying psychological and/or social meaning so they each serve a similar function for the adolescent. Thirdly, and most importantly he indicated that interventions aimed at reducing the incidence or magnitude of risk behaviours may be more effective if they are directed toward the cluster of risk behaviours (and their common underlying causes) rather than at isolated behaviours. Finally, it suggests that adolescent health behaviours may best be conceived as constituting a "lifestyle" rather than as isolated behaviours.

As well as the findings of Jessor who demonstrated the clear links between so-called "problem behaviours", more recent studies have identified clusters of positive health behaviours such as physical activity, healthy food choices and seat-belt use (Nutbeam, Aaro and Catford, 1989; Nutbeam, Aaro and Wold, 1991). These latter analyses were based on data available from a WHO co-ordinated study of health behaviour among adolescents (aged 11–15) from 11 countries in Europe (Aaro and Wold, 1989). The group of health-enhancing behaviours (healthy food choices, regular physical activity, good oral hygiene and the use of seatbelts) clustered consistently between age groups and between the eleven countries included in the study (Austria, Belgium, Finland, Hungary, Israel, Norway, Spain, Sweden, Switzerland and the UK (Scotland and Wales)). Similarly, the group of health-damaging behaviours (alcohol misuse, smoking, unhealthy food choices) appear to cluster in individuals. Although the size of the effects observed in these analyses were modest and variable in strength between countries, they were consistent in their relationships with a range of psychosocial predictors. For example, clusters of health-damaging behaviours were consistently associated with lower parental socio-economic status, negative attitudes to school and future education, negative relationships with parents and regular use of free time with friends away from home. Alternatively, the cluster of health-enhancing behaviours was consistently associated with higher socio-economic status, positive attitudes to school, and good parental relationships.

The consistency in the inter-relatedness of individual behaviours led the investigators to use terms such as "health-promoting" or "health-compromising" lifestyles as more meaningful descriptions of the clusters of health behaviours. However, this research has been based in a traditional, and narrowly focussed definition of "lifestyle", based on a collection of individual behaviours. The concept of lifestyle is now generally regarded as representing a wider set of social and behavioural characteristics including, for example, young people's membership of social groups, their exposure to the media, and their choice of leisure-time activities. For these reasons studies of adolescent lifestyles should not be limited to behaviours which are mainly important in predicting mortality and morbidity. Findings from studies such as the WHO cross national survey indicate the need for further investigation of the lifestyle concept as a means to better understand individual health behaviours. They also point to the need to further refine the construction of research instruments to describe adolescent lifestyles in a more sophisticated way than is presently the case.

CONCLUDING REMARKS

Adolescence, as a period in the lifespan, is second only to infancy in the rapidity of physical, cognitive and social change. Those who wish to understand and influence adolescent health behaviours must constantly bear this in mind. Attempts to understand health behaviours must take into account an adolescent's physical development, cognitive abilities (and limitations) and the social context of health behaviour.

Physical development and sexual maturity have a direct impact on adolescent behaviour in a range of ways which impact on health. The consequences of unprotected sexual intercourse were highlighted earlier, as too were the difficulties of identifying an appropriate preventive response. Recognition of the importance of cognitive development and the social context of health behaviour is crucial to determining a workable response. It is also important to recognize the fact that behaviours which adults may perceive as representing unacceptable risks to health may fulfil an important function for young people – and are unlikely to be conceived of as relevant to health at all.

The key to a better understanding, and to the construction of a workable health promotion response, may lie in an understanding of individual health behaviours within this wider frame of reference. Research in the past fifteen years has indicated how health behaviours cluster, and how these clusters of behaviours are related to psycho-social and environmental variables, as well as a range of other behaviours which may not be health related. Attempts to influence individual health-compromising behaviours will be greatly enhanced through a recognition of their perceived benefits to young people, and of their position in this more complex lifestyle framework.

ACKNOWLEDGMENTS

The authors wish to express their gratitude to Professor John Collins and Dr. David Bennett for their helpful comments on earlier versions of this chapter.

REFERENCES

Aaro, L. E. & Wold, B. (1989). Health behaviour in schoolchildren. A WHO cross-national survey. Research protocol for the 1989–90 study. Department of Social Psychology, University of Bergen and WHO-EURO, Copenhagen.

Atkin, C.K. (1976). Children's social learning from television advertising: Research evidence from observational modelling of product consumption. *Advances in Consumer Research*, 3, 513–519.

Atkin, C.K. (1980). Effects of television on children. In E.L. Palmer & A. Dorr (Eds.), *Children and the Faces of Television: Teaching, Violence and Selling* (pp. 287–306). New York: Academic Press.

Atkin, C.K., Hocking, J. & Block, M. (1984). Teenage drinking: Does advertising make a difference? *Journal of Communication*, 34, 157–167.

Bandura, A. (1977). *Social Learning Theory*. Englewood Cliffs, NJ: Prentice Hall.

Bandura, A. (1986). *Social Foundations of Thought and Action*. Englewood Cliffs, NJ: Prentice Hall.

Baumrind, D. (1987). A developmental perspective on adolescent risk-taking in contemporary America. In C.E. Irwin Jr., (Ed.), *New Directions for Child Development 37: Adolescent Social Behavior and Health* (pp. 93–125). San Francisco: Josey-Bass Inc.

Blos, P. (1979). *The Adolescent Passage: Developmental Issues*. New York: International Universities Press.

Botvin, G.J. (1983). Prevention of adolescent substance abuse through the development of personal and social competence. In T.J. Glynn & C.G. Leukefeld (Eds.), NIDA Research Monograph 47. *Preventing Adolescent Drug Abuse: Intervention Stragegies* (pp. 115–140). Rockville, ML: National Institute on Drug Abuse.

Bush, P.J. & Ianotti, R. (1985). The development of children's health orientations and behaviors: Lessons for substance use prevention. In C.R. Jones & R.J. Battjes (Eds.), NIDA Research Monograph 56. *Etiology of Drug Abuse: Implications for Prevention* (pp. 45–74). Rockville, ML: National Institute on Drug Abuse.

Chapman, S. & Fitzgerald, B. (1982). Brand preference and recall in adolescent smokers: Some implications for health promotion. *American Journal of Public Health*, 75, 491–494.

Collins, J.K. & Robinson, L. (1986). The contraceptive knowledge, attitudes and practice of unmarried adolescents. *Australian Journal of Sex, Marriage and Family*, 7, 132–152.

Daitzman, R. & Zuckerman, M. (1989). Disinhibitory sensation seeking, personality, and gonadal hormones. *Personality and Individual Differences*, 1, 103–110.

Damon, W. (1984). Peer education: The untapped potential. *Journal of Applied Developmental Psychology*, 5, 331–343.

Dishman, R.K., Sallis, J.F. & Orenstein, D.R. (1985). The determinants of physical activity and exercise. *Public Health Reports*, 100, 158–171.

Donovan, J.E., Jessor, R. & Costa, F.M. (1991). Adolescent health behavior and conventionality-unconventionality: An extension of problem-behaviour theory. *Health Psychology*, **10**, 52–61.

Elkind, D. (1967). Egocentrism in adolescence. *Child Development*, **38**, 1025–1034.

Faulkenberry, R.J., Vincent, M., James, A. & Johnson, W. (1987). Coital behaviours, attitudes, and knowledge of students who experience early coitus. *Adolescence*, **22**, 321–332.

Flay, B.R. & Burton, D. (1990). Effective mass communication strategies for health campaigns. In C. Atkin & L. Wallack (Eds.), *Mass Communication and Public Health: Complexities and Conflicts* (pp. 129–146). London: Sage Publications.

Foster-Clark, F.S. & Blyth, D.A. (1991). Peer relations and influences. In R.M. Lerner, A.C. Peterson & J. Brooks-Gunn (Eds.), *Encyclopedia of Adolescence* (Vol. 2, pp. 767–771). New York: Garland Publishing Inc.

Freeman, E.W., Rickels, K., Huggins, G.R., Mudd, E.H., Garcia, C.R. & Dickens, H.O. (1980). Adolescent contraceptive use: Comparisons of male and female attitudes and information. *American Journal of Public Health*, **70**, 790–797.

Freimouth, V.S., Greenburg, R.H., DeWitt, J. & Romano, R.M. (1984). Covering cancer: Newspapers and the public interest. *Journal of Communication*, **34**, 62–73.

Friedman, H.L. (1989). The health of adolescents: Beliefs and behaviour. *Social Science and Medicine*, **29**, 309–315.

Hamburg, D. & Trudeau, M. (1981). *Biobehavioral Aspects of Aggression*. New York: Alan Liss, Inc.

Inhelder, B. & Piaget, J. (1958). *The Growth of Logical Thinking from Childhood to Adolescence*. New York: Basic Books.

Irwin, C.E. (1987). Editor's Notes. In C.E. Irwin Jr., (Ed.), *New Directions for Child Development 37: Adolescent Social Behavior and Health* (pp. 1–12). San Francisco: Josey-Bass Inc.

Irwin, C.E. & Millstein, S.G. (1986). Biopsychosocial correlates of risk-taking behaviours during adolescence: Can the physician intervene? *Journal of Adolescent Health Care*, **7** (suppl.), 82S–96S.

Irwin, C.E. & Millstein, S.G. (1991). Risk-taking behaviours during adolescence. In R.M. Lerner, A.C. Petersen & J. Brooks-Gunn (Eds.), *Encyclopedia of Adolescence* (Vol. 2, pp. 934–943). New York: Garland Publishing Inc.

Jessor, R. (1984). Adolescent development and behavioral health. In J.D. Matarazzo, S.M. Weiss, J.A. Herd, N.E. Miller & S.M. Weiss (Eds.), *Behavioral Health: A Handbook for Health Enhancement and Disease Prevention* (pp. 69–90). New York: Wiley.

Jessor, R. & Jessor, S.L. (1977). *Problem Behavior and Psychosocial Development: A Longitudinal Study of Youth*. New York: Academic Press.

Kandel, D. & Andrews, K. (1987). Processes of adolescent socialization by parents and peers. *International Journal of the Addictions*, **22**, 319–342.

Kandel, D. & Lesser, G. (1972). *Youth in Two Worlds*. San Francisco: Jossey-Bass.

Kaplan, H.B., Martin, S.S. & Robbins, C. (1982). Applications of a general theory of deviant behavior: Self-derogation and adolescent drug use. *Journal of Health and Social Behavior*, **23**, 274–294.

Keating, D.P. (1980). Thinking processes in adolescence. In J. Adelson (Ed.), *Handbook of Adolescent Psychology*, (pp. 211–246). New York: Wiley.

Keating, D.P. (1988). *Adolescent's Ability to Engage in Critical Thinking*. Madison, WI: National Centre for Effective Secondary Education.

Kegeles, S., Millstein, S.G., Adler, N.E., Irwin, C.E., Jnr., Cohn, L. & Dolcini, P. (1987). The transition to sexual activity and its relation to other risk behaviours. *Journal of Adolescent Health*, **8**, 303.

Loeber, R. & Dishion, T. (1983). Early predictors of male delinquincy: A review. *Psychology Bulletin*, **93**, 68–99.

Marsh, A. & Matheson, J. (1983). Smoking attitudes and behaviour among adults. Office of Population and Census Statistics, HMSO, London.

McCabe, M.P. & Collins, J.K. (1990). *Dating, Relating and Sex*. Sydney: Horwitz-Grahame.

Miller, P. & Simon, W. (1980). The development of sexuality in adolescence. In J. Adelson (Ed.), *Handbook of Adolescent Psychology* (pp. 383-408). New York: Wiley Interscience.

Montemayor, R. (1986). Family variation in adolescent storm and stress. *Journal of Adolescent Research*, 1, 15-31.

Montemayor, R. & Flannery, D.J. (1991). Parent-adolescent relations in middle and late adolescence. In R.M. Lerner, A.C. Petersen & J. Brooks-Gunn (Eds.), *The Encyclopedia of Adolescence*, (Vol. 2, pp. 729-734). New York: Garland Publishing Inc.

Montgomery, K.C. (1990). Promoting health through entertainment television. In C. Atkin & L. Wallack (Eds.), *Mass Communication and Public Health: Complexities and Conflicts*. London: Sage Publications.

Mott, F.L. & Haurin, R.J. (1987, April/May). The inter-relatedness of age at first intercourse, early pregnancy, and drug use among American adolescents: Preliminary results from the National Londitudinal Survey of Youth Labor Market Experience. Paper presented at Annual Meeting of the Population Association of America, Chicago, Illinois.

Neilson, L. (1987). *Adolescent Psychology: A Contemporary View*. New York: Holt, Reinhart and Winston.

Neimark, E.D. (1979). Current status of formal operations research. *Human Development*, 22, 60-67.

Newcomb, M.D. & Bentler, P.M. (1986). Cocaine use among adolescents: Longitudinal associates with social context, psychopathology, and use of other substances. *Additive Behaviours*, 11, 263-273.

Nutbeam, D., Aaro, L. & Catford, J. (1989). Understanding children's health behaviour: The implications for health promotion for young people. *Social Science and Medicine*, 29, 317-325.

Nutbeam, D., Aaro, L. & Wold, B. (1991). The lifestyle concept and health education with young people. *World Health Statistics*, 44, 55-61.

Perry, C.L. (1991). Conceptualizing community-wide youth health programs. In D. Nutbeam, B. Haglund, P. Farley & P. Tillgren (Eds.), *Youth Health Promotion* (pp. 1-21). London: Forbes Publications.

Piaget, J. (1972). Intellectual evolution from adolescence to adulthood. *Human Development*, 15, 1-12.

Reichelt, P. & Werley, H. (1981). Contraception, abortion and venereal disease: Teenagers knowledge and the effect of education. In F. Furstenburg, R. Lincoln & J. Menken (Eds.), *Teenage Sexuality, Pregnancy and Childbearing* (pp. 305-317). Philadelphia: University of Pennsylvania Press.

Rutter, M., Graham, P., Chadwick, F. & Yule, W. (1976). Adolescent turmoil: Fact or fiction. *Journal of Child Psychology and Psychiatry*, 17, 35-56.

Shantz, C.U. (1983). Social Cognition. In J.H. Flavell & E.M. Markmann (Eds.), *Handbook of Child Psychology* (Vol. 3, pp. 495-555). New York: Wiley.

Silber, T.J. (1985). Adolescent sexuality: Developmental and ethical issues: In *Health of Adolescents and Youths in the Americas* (pp. 87-94). Washington D.C.: Pan American Health Organisation.

Silber, T.J. & Woodward, K. (1985). Sexually transmitted diseases in adolescence. In *Health of Adolescents and Youths in the Americas* (pp. 129-141). Washington D.C.: Pan American Health Organisation.

Slovic, P. (1987). Perceptions of risk. *Science*, 236, 280-285.

Steinberg, L. (1988). Pubertal maturation and parent-adolescent distance: An evolutionary perspective. In G. Adams, R. Montemayor & T. Gullotta (Eds.), *Advances in Adolescent Development* (Vol. 1, pp. 71-97). Beverly Hills, CA: Sage.

Sullivan, H.S. (1953). *The Interpersonal Theory of Psychiatry*. New York: Norton.

Thompson, E.L. (1978). Smoking education programs 1960–1976. *American Journal of Public Health*, **68**, 250–257.

Udry, J.R. (1988). Biological predispositions and social control in adolescent sexual behavior. *American Sociological Review*, **52**, 841–855.

U.N. (1988). *Adolescent Reproductive Behavior: Evidence from Developed Countries* (Vol. 1). New York: United Nations.

Wold, B. (1989). *Lifestyles and Physical Activity: A Theoretical and Empirical Analysis of Socialization among Children and Adolescents*. PhD Thesis: University of Bergen, Faculty of Psychology.

World Health Organisation (1980). *Final Report, Regional Working Group on Health Needs of Adolescents*, Manilla, Philippines.

Yamaguchi, K. & Kandel, D.B. (1984). Patterns of drug use from adolescence to young adulthood: 3. Predictors of progression. *American Journal of Public Health*, 74, 673–681.

Youniss, J. (1980). *Parents and Peers in Social Development: A Sullivan-Piaget Perspective*. Chicago: University of Chicago Press.

Youniss, J. & Smolar, J. (1985). *Adolescent Relations with Mothers, Fathers, and Friends*. Chicago: University of Chicago Press.

Zabin, L.S. (1984). The association between smoking and sexual behavior among teens in US contraceptive clinics. *American Journal of Public Health*, 74, 261–263.

Zelnick, M., Kanter, J.F. & Ford, K. (1981). *Sex and Pregnancy in Adolescence*. Beverly Hills, CA: Sage Publications.

Zelnick, M. & Shah, F.K. (1983). First intercourse among young Americans. *Family Planning Perspectives*, 15, 64–70.

Zuckerman, M. (1986). Sensation seeking and the endogenous deficit theory of drug abuse. In S.I. Szara (Ed.), *Neurobiology of Behavioral Control in Drug Abuse*. NIDA Research Monograph 74 (DHHS Publication No. ADM 87-1506). Washington DC: U.S. Government Printing Office.

SEXUALITY AND HEALTH IN YOUNG PEOPLE:
Perceptions and behaviour related to the threat of HIV-infection

ROGER INGHAM

Until some twenty years ago, there had been relatively little work in the field of sexual behaviour by psychologists. Quite why this should have been so is not altogether clear, although the private nature of much of sexual behaviour raises many methodological and ethical problems which are not easy to overcome. Further, many areas of social psychology develop from the need to solve practical and applied problems, and sexual activity has not, generally, been seen as an area in which solutions have been required. This may have not only led to a reluctance by psychologists to enter the field in the light of possible 'surprise' by colleagues (and sometimes more extreme reactions – see, for example, Kinsey *et al.*'s (1948) description of the hostility experienced, and Allgeier (1984) on Masters and Johnson), but also to possible difficulties in funding. Further, it is not clear why potential respondents to studies would be motivated to participate.

Recently, however, two factors have arisen which have altered the context in which such studies take place. In the first place, the rapid growth in the numbers of unplanned teenage pregnancies in the United States (with over one million per year at present) has created a massive public health problem, and led to the establishment of research programmes intended to explain (and 'correct') the apparent widespread lack of appropriate contraceptive behaviour amongst young people. Secondly, the 'discovery' of the Human Immunodeficiency Virus and its transmission character-istics have placed the understanding of sexual behaviour near the top of the priority list of problems needing solutions. The context of this concern is, of course, virtually world-wide, with very high rates of infection being reported in some developing countries. Since at present the progress towards finding either a vaccine or a cure appears to be depressingly slow, it is generally recognised that behaviour change represents the most hopeful avenue by which the spread of the virus can be contained.

The required behaviour changes include those that prevent the exchange of certain body fluids known to act as transmitters, including blood, semen and vaginal fluids. In particular, widespread alterations to medical practice now ensure that blood used for transfusion is screened, and, wherever possible, sterile needles are used for injections, and rubber gloves are used for surgical procedures. These changes depend on adequate training of medical staff, as well as on the availability of finance to ensure adequate supplies, a condition that can not be fully met in some developing countries.

Thus, to the extent that behaviour change amongst medical staff has been achieved so cases of transmission via medical procedures have been drastically reduced in number. However, the behaviour of the general population still causes serious concern. Exchange of blood through, for example, the sharing of syringes by intravenous drug users remains a major route of transmission of HIV, and the exchange of semen, vaginal fluids and blood during sexual intercourse constitutes another. Thus, a great deal of research attention has been paid to aspects of these behaviours, how they can be explained and, in particular, how they can be altered in order to reduce the risk of transmission. Greatest attention has been focussed on those people who engage (or who are thought to engage) more frequently in the behaviours which carry the highest risk of transmission, including intravenous drug users, men who have sex with other men, and individuals who have sex with 'multiple' partners, whether or not involving commercial transactions.

It is important to stress that it is preferred not to talk in terms of 'risk-groups' as such, since transmission occurs via specific behaviours rather than via group membership or individual group identity. Thus, for example, a prostitute (or 'commercial sex-worker') who insists on condom use with all clients may well be at lower risk of infection than someone who has sex with many different partners but does not regularly adopt safer sex procedures (see, for example, Day, 1988, 1990). Nevertheless, on the grounds that risk behaviours are thought to be more likely amongst certain sectors of the population, research efforts have tended to focus on these particular sectors. Since a higher proportion of young people are more likely to engage in drug use and sexual activity, they have emerged as a particular target for research attention. The relative lack of previous work in this area has added to the urgency of this endeavour.

DEFINITIONS AND RANGE OF ATTENTION

The term *sexuality* is preferred to 'sexual behaviour' since attention is thereby focussed on considerably wider issues than simple frequency counts and scores on questionnaires. *Sexuality* incorporates aspects of individual and group identity, as well as knowledge, attitudes and emotions regarding sexual expression and experience. Individual meanings and understandings are seen as being embedded within a system of societal discourses. As such, it could be argued that there are few, if any, areas of human experience which are not related in some way to sexualities. However, as will be seen later, few psychologists engaged in this area of work have fully adopted this wider definition.

Given the very wide range of issues which could be encompassed under the term 'sexuality', as well as interpretations of the term 'health' which incorporate both physical and psychological dimensions, one chapter could clearly not aim to cover all the relevant material and issues. Rather, this chapter reviews some of the research carried out in the area of sexual activity in young people, with a particular focus on the issues raised by the threats associated with HIV infection. In this sense, the emphasis is on health behaviours, as well as the alternative interpretations and understandings of relevant issues and contexts. The intention is critically to examine the dominant approaches currently in use, and to propose that an expansion of current methods and theoretical approaches is required.

Finally, the term *young people* is preferred to the more commonly used 'adolescence' since it is rather more neutral in meaning. The latter term carries implications of homogeneity amongst people within certain age brackets, which may lead to certain assumptions and associations regarding their behaviour and attitudes. As Warwick and Aggleton (1990) have argued it is important to investigate the variation *within* particular age groups, particularly how this variation may be related to socio-economic status, gender, ethnicity, sexual orientation and other aspects (although there is little work as yet which has adequately explored these variations).

For the purposes of this chapter no specific age range is selected, although it is probably true to say that the majority of studies conducted on 'young people' have restricted themselves to ages ranging from sixteen to early or mid-twenties (with many studies in the United States being conducted on college students). The lower age band is generally determined by problems of accessing people below this age, given the legal position in most countries. However, as will be pointed out later, a reasonable proportion of young people have commenced their sexual careers by this age, so some of the data collected rely on retrospective accounts going back a number of years in some cases.

METHODOLOGICAL ISSUES

Since the majority of reported studies in the psychological literature have adopted questionnaire or survey methods, and since there are strong reasons to argue that data collected through these means present only a partial picture, some brief consideration needs to be given to the alternative methodologies available, and their relative advantages and drawbacks.

Questionnaire studies clearly have advantages in allowing relatively large-scale data to be obtained at relatively low cost, and statistical analyses of the data permit the testing of formal theoretical models. Self-completion questionnaires may encourage honesty since they are normally completed under conditions of anonymity; alternatively, the very lack of involvement due to the anonymity may lead to spurious responses. Validity checks are, of course difficult to design. The reported frequencies of certain activities can be measured, as well as scores on psychological variables which might be expected to have some predictive utility with regard to behaviour, such as knowledge, attitudes, beliefs, perceived risk levels, and so on.

However, such approaches are not without problems. A major problem arises (as with any self-completion questionnaire study) in relation to the understanding of the language used in the items and response formats. These issues are of particular importance in the field of sexual behaviour and experience precisely because the terminology used in this area is open to ambiguity and misunderstanding. Consider the following few examples:

Sexual partner
Coxon's (1988) work with gay men (under the umbrella of Project SIGMA) identified a number of serious methodological problems in the study of sexual activity. Amongst these was the lack of agreement on the meaning of 'sexual partner'. In other words, what does one have to do to someone, or have done to one, in order to qualify as a 'sexual partner'? As Coxon points out, in terms of considering risk-reduction, considerable detail is required in order to assess the probability of transmission of HIV. Thus, for example, a couple who engage in mutual masturbation might well consider themselves to be in a sexual relationship, and to be 'sexual partners'. However, a questionnaire that simply asked for information on, for example, numbers of sexual partners during the previous year (as many questionnaires in this area do) would clearly miss the subtlety required, and could well lead to over-estimation of levels of risk behaviour.

Sexual activity
The publications emanating from a current study in the United Kingdom (the Women's Risk and AIDS Project) identify further problems concerning the meaning of some key terms. For example, many questionnaire studies ask respondents to note the number of 'sexual partners' (or people 'with whom they have engaged in sexual intercourse', or somesuch phrase). Responses are often correlated with some other measure in attempts to improve predictability. However, such acceptance at face value of the answers given often ignores, or makes invisible, the actual *contexts* in which such sexual activity takes place. Thus, for example, '... there is no language for women's ambivalence about male sexuality, or for the concepts which fall between 'sex' and 'rape' for identifying pressures to have sexual intercourse, or women's ambivalence in situations where they are reluctant to have sexual intercourse, but are also reluctant to refuse it' (Holland *et al.*, 1991). Clearly, treating answers to such simple items on questionnaires implies a sense of volition which will, in some cases, be completely inappropriate.

Medical terminology
Some studies assume a level of knowledge of bio-medical phenomena which is inappropriate. A pertinent example of the dangers involved was provided by one of the early studies on lay perceptions of HIV-infection carried out in the United Kingdom, Warwick and his colleagues (Warwick *et al.*, 1988) found wide variation in the understanding of the nature of transmission of the virus itself. The authors categorised the range of responses obtained from discussions with young people into three groups, which they labelled the *miasmatic*, the *serendipitous* and the *endogenous*. None of these matched bio-medical explanations regarding transmission. Whilst the authors stress the relevance of these lay understandings in the context of health education and promotion, it is equally important to stress their implications with regard to questionnaire items concerning knowledge of transmission routes. It can not be assumed that respondents to questionnaires share understandings of the meanings of terms with those constructing such questionnaires.

Accurate questionnaire data are vitally important for certain purposes. These include the description of the prevalence of certain activities (always assuming that the problematic issues of terminology have been overcome as far as possible), how these are affected by demographic and other indices, the construction of models for predicting the likely spread of infection (for example, see Anderson and May, 1988; Solomon *et al.*, 1989), and similar aims. They are also, of course, useful for investigating aspects of knowledge, beliefs, attitudes, and other similar traditional social psychological variables. However, for the purposes of exploring the more complex and subtle aspects of individuals' sexualities, motivations, meanings, and so on, they are severely limited and limiting.

The major alternative approach being used at present involves the collection of data through accounts from young people. Although such interviews are extremely time-consuming, and do, of necessity, involve much smaller samples, they provide the opportunity for much more detailed exploration of important aspects of the experiences and behaviour of the people concerned. Ambiguities in terminology can, to a large extent, be identified and overcome, issues can be returned to in order to provide internal reliability checks, a relaxed and conversational style by the interviewer can help to produce an honest and thoughtful account, and so on. A number of studies are currently under way in the United Kingdom using such methods; these include the Women's Risk and AIDS Project (WRAP) (see Holland *et al.*, 1990, 1991) and the Social Aspects of Risk-reduction Project (see Ingham *et al.*, 1991, 1992; Woodcock *et al.*, 1992a). This chapter draws primarily on these approaches, given the limitations of purely questionnaire based studies outlined earlier. There appears to be considerably less work using qualitative approaches being conducted in the United States (Gagnon's work (Gagnon, 1977; Gagon and Simon, 1973) being a major exception) and elsewhere.

The major method used in the projects mentioned above involves loosely structured interviews with young people which can last anything from one hour to three and a half hours (depending on how loquacious the interviewee is, and how much they have to tell). In addition to obtaining specific details regarding relationships and sexual activities, analysis of the ways in which the respondents talk about, and make sense of (to the extent that they are able), their experiences reveals a great deal of important contextual and background information. The data obtained through these means are considerably more complex than those obtained through questionnaire surveys (and take considerably longer to analyse), but the richness provides an important complement to the more superficial data from survey studies. It is difficult to argue that one method is in any sense superior to another; rather, that in such an important area as this, a multi-method approach is to be recommended. It should be added that qualitative data can be analysed in a quantitative manner – the difference lies in the fact that the categories derived emanate from the respondents' own interpretations and meanings, rather than through imposition by the researchers.

MAIN THEORETICAL APPROACHES USED

In addition to studies designed to simply measure some basic frequencies (of, for example, age at first intercourse, contraceptive use, numbers of partners) most studies conducted by psychologists have used one of three theoretical approaches. These are (a) the individual differences approach, (b) the 'rational' health behaviour approach and (c) the 'sexual scripts' approach.

(a) Individual Differences

A number of the early studies in the United States attempted to search for correlates of particular aspects of sexual behaviour. Thus, for example, Zuckerman *et al.* (1972) report that sexual experience in undergraduates was correlated with the Disinhibition scale of his Sensation-seeking questionnaire. Some of the various sub-scales correlated with particular activities or experiences; for example, Endurance correlated negatively with numbers of partners but positively with orgasmic frequency for females but not for males (clearly, the effect of Endurance is gender specific!). Zuckerman *et al.*'s later conclusion regarding sexual permissiveness and 'health' is straightforward – 'Sexual permissiveness in college students seems to be an expression of a healthy capacity for warm interpersonal relationships rather than a neurotic search for security and reassurance of self-worth or a narcissistic need for ego gratification' (Zuckerman *et al.*, 1976, p. 18).

An alternative approach to the study of individual differences in sexual activity has been developed by Mosher and colleagues (Mosher and Cross, 1971; Mosher and Vonderheide, 1985). They introduced the 'sex-guilt' questionnaire, which measured general expectations of punishment for violating perceived sexual standards. Similarly, Byrne and colleagues (Byrne and Fisher, 1983; Fisher *et al.*, 1988) introduced the notions of erotophilia and erotophobia – expressing positive and negative sexual attitudes respectively. These measures have been correlated with various sexual behaviours and associated activities (such as contraceptive use). In general, it has been found that those with greater sex-guilt and a more erotophobic attitude are *less* likely to use appropriate contraception and therefore *more* likely to put themselves at risk of disease and/or unwanted pregnancy. The argument is that those with more positive attitudes towards sexual activity are more likely to acknowledge the possibility and to prepare themselves appropriately.

Using these scales, Daugherty and Burger (1984) investigated the relative importance of a number of possible sources of influence over sexual activity and attitudes. They report (in common with a number of other studies) that males have lower sex-guilt, higher erotophilia and more sexual partners than females. There were various differences in the reported sources of influence between the sexes, although for both actual sexual behaviour was related to perceived attitudes of peers.

Although studies of this type have drawn attention to some possibly important variables, their limitations must be recognised. For example, the last study reported above fails to distinguish in any sense the different meanings that sexual activity might have for males and females, or the different contexts in which such activity takes place. Thus, to point to differences between males and females in relative influences assumes that what is in fact being influenced is similar for both sexes. More recent evidence demonstrates that this is far from the case, as will be discussed later.

(b) Health Beliefs

An alternative approach to that involving individual differences in sexual activity has stemmed from work in the field of health psychology. There are a number of models available to guide thinking and research; probably the most widely used are the Health Belief Model (Rosenstock, 1974; Rosenstock *et al.*, 1988) and the Theory of Reasoned Action (Ajzen and Fishbein, 1980). Given that sexual behaviour carries with it certain levels of risk (and that this has been the major reason for the recent interest), it is not surprising that models used to try to understand other risk-related behaviours have been applied to the field. More specifically, Byrne and his colleagues (Byrne and Fisher, 1983; Fisher, 1990) have developed a specific model to predict sexual behaviour and contraceptive use.

There are some problems inherent in these general social cognitive approaches, however. Firstly, the level of precision required in the measurement of the variables makes it necessary to adopt highly structured questionnaires. Apart from the issues identified earlier relating to terminology and restrictions of response format, there is a tendency to attempt to reduce the numbers of items relating to particular variables to as small a number as possible. Thus, for example the outcome measure for 'intention to use condoms' is often a single item, which reduces the range of variation possible and possibly serves to exaggerate the meaning of, say, a one point difference on a seven-point scale.

Similarly, the wording and response formats of items assessing beliefs, attitudes and subjective norms are highly precise (in that slight alterations to the wording can produce quite significant changes in responses made) and again, just one or two items are normally used to produce the relevant scale scores. The items are 'transparent', in that individuals who wish to portray consistent (and apparently 'rational') answers can do so readily. Indeed, given some of the questionnaires used in these studies, the authors should be asked to account for the failure to reach 100 percent of the variance explained!

Assessing the subjective norm component of the Theory of Reasoned Action (or Planned Behaviour) poses particular issues. One problem arises in selecting the 'significant others' for studies of sexual behaviour. One recent study (Schmidt, 1991) used an interesting example – 'current partner' was used as a 'significant other'. The problem arises when the respondents are asked about their behavioural intentions regarding condom use with a *new* partner. Thus, the relevant item was 'do you think that your partner expects you to use a condom with a new partner?'. It is debatable whether respondents would be able to estimate what their current partner would think of them even having a new partner, let alone whether or not they would use a condom with them!

A further point worth making about the Theories of Reasoned Action and Planned Behaviour is that they deal primarily with the issue of intentions. Although the authors claim that intentions are the best predictors of behaviour, the empirical evidence for such an assertion is not strong. Very few studies have been performed which relate intentions at Time One to actual behaviour at Time Two.

At a more theoretical level, the use of such models as these raises questions concerning the concept of 'rationality'. Thus, it is implicitly assumed that people actually wish to behave in a health-preserving and risk-reducing way; the outcome measures are inevitably a 'sensible' course of action (as defined by those who know what is indeed 'sensible') and that falling short of this behaviour reflects some form of 'deficit', be it in the individual's knowledge, perceived risk, perceived vulnerability, or whatever. This issue will be returned to, when some alternative ways of considering the notion of 'rationality' will be discussed.

(c) Sexual Scripts

The third approach to the study of sexual behaviour in young people involves a more socially grounded approach. Gagnon and his colleagues (Gagnon and Simon, 1973; Gagnon, 1977) have developed a theoretical framework based on the notion of sexual scripts, which were originally regarded as "... heuristic devices to be used by observers to better interpret sexual conduct at three levels: cultural scenarios, interpersonal interactions and intrapsychic processes' (Gagnon, 1986). More recently, however, it has become accepted that "... many everyday actors ... self-consciously 'script' or near 'script' their own interactions as they negotiate their lives" (Gagnon, op. cit.). They propose that individuals engaged in sexual activities can frequently be regarded as following prescribed and rehearsed scripts; these are not only intended to encourage self-control, but also to 'manage' the other person(s) involved. Such scripts are learned, or acquired, from a variety of sources, including peers, parents, teachers, the media, and others. Of course, the scripts acquired from these various sources may well not be consistent with each other!

Gagnon's analysis includes discussion of the ways in which such sexual scripts alter as people grow older and enter different forms of relationships. Thus, young people at the early stages of their sexual careers will have less well formed scripts than when they are older and more experienced. The effects of the absence of well formed and practised scripts leads, it is argued, to a greater likelihood of 'inefficient' sexual behaviour, lower consistency of contraceptive use, and other effects. Further, inappropriate scripts may be adopted in particular situations, as in, for example, Maticka-Tyndale's suggestion that condoms are scripted as purely contraceptive devices (rather than infection-control devices) with young adults "... relying on their believed ability to avoid coitus with infected partners as their major preventive mechanism" (1991, p. 45).

REVIEW OF RECENT RESEARCH

Much of the work outlined above relates primarily to work carried out in what might be termed the 'pre-AIDs era'. The primary aim of the work was not only to explore sexual behaviour in its own right, but, in many cases, specifically to further the understanding of contraceptive behaviour in the context of pregnancy avoidance.

The threat posed by HIV infection has not only added urgency to this endeavour, but has also altered the nature of the enquiry. The emphasis has shifted from the use of any form of contraceptive to the specific use of condoms, since only barrier methods prevent (or at least reduce) the possibility of transmission of the virus. In this section, some of the recent work in the area is reviewed, and an attempt is made to highlight some of the important themes which are emerging. Particular attention is paid to results from qualitative approaches in view of the restrictions imposed by purely questionnaire based approaches.

The key issue to be addressed is the extent to which young people take the threat of HIV infection seriously to the extent of either altering their current behaviour towards more regular use of safer sexual activity, or, for those not yet sexually active, adopting safer activities from the outset (which may include delaying the start of their sexual careers). There is little doubt at present that the vast majority of young people (at least in the UK and other developed countries) are aware of AIDS, of the major routes of transmission and at least the basics of what they ought to do to avoid infection (Ingham, 1990; Abrams *et al.*, 1990; Clift *et al.*, 1989), and yet there is little evidence of change towards 'safer' behaviour. In the attempts to address these issues, a number of other important aspects have been identified which help to provide a wider contextual framework for understanding and explanation than that used in much of the earlier research.

(a) Perceived personal invulnerability

One of the most consistent findings to emerge from recent work has been very clear evidence that, even though young people are well informed regarding the major routes of transmission of the HIV virus, and that infection has severe consequences, they do not believe themselves to be at risk. Abrams *et al.* (1990), based on their survey of young people in and around Dundee, report that, whilst the respondents estimated that 50 percent of their age group would die of AIDS related illnesses within five years, their estimates of their own chances of becoming infected were very low.

Woodcock *et al.* (1992a) explored this area in some detail through their qualitative accounts from young people. During discussion of their own reactions to, and perceived threat of, HIV infection respondents were asked to justify (where appropriate) their own perceptions of invulnerability. A few simply dismissed the risk as being exaggerated by the media or the Government or some other agency. Of the majority who recognised the inherent risk, however, various arguments were put forward. These were grouped under the following categories:

(i) *"Life is a gamble anyway"*. Although not strictly speaking a justification of perceived invulnerability, this category includes those individuals who did not take the threat of HIV infection any more seriously than other risks in life.

(ii) *"My partners are safe"*. These respondents had their own ways of assessing risk which related to perceived properties of their sexual partners. Included in these were the belief that their partners were 'not promiscuous' (although a definition of 'promiscuous' was rarely forthcoming!). Some respondents argued that because their partners had previously only had one partner at a time ('serial monogamy') they were unlikely to be at risk due to their earlier behaviour.

Assessments of partners' riskiness were often made on the bases of some completely irrelevant criteria, including their occupation, their parents' occupation(s) and/or where they lived. This latter criterion could either be based on parts of particular towns or cities, or on the basis of towns or cities themselves.

(iii) *"I am safe"*. Many respondents regarded their own lifestyle and behaviour as being sufficient to discount them from risk. Because of the high level of publicity given to the so-called 'risk groups', people who do not see themselves as belonging to one or more of these could reason that they are therefore 'safe'. A perception of personal invulnerability was in many cases not based on an objective assessment of their own past or present behaviour but on a sense of personal identity in relation to these 'risk groups'.

(b) Barriers to effective action regarding risk reduction

Whether or not individuals feel themselves to be vulnerable to HIV-infection, there appear to be a number of barriers to taking effective action in order to reduce risk.

(i) Misunderstanding of advice

Various pieces of advice have been given in government sponsored campaigns in the UK and elsewhere over the past few years. The language in which these campaigns are couched can create problems in interpretation – it has already been demonstrated how some terms appear to be understood in different ways by people. Sometimes, official medical language is simply not understood in the manner intended (cf Warwick *et al.*, 1988; Sherr, 1987; Coxon, 1988), although it must be acknowledged that more colloquial 'street' language would cause offence to some readers and viewers of media campaigns.

Specific advice has also been shown to be misunderstood. For example, in 1990, the then Chief Medical Officer for the United Kingdom received massive publicity for his advice to 'use a condom if you don't know your partner'. Ingham *et al.* (1991) explored the meaning of 'knowing' in this context amongst a sample of young people. They report that most of the young people interviewed did indeed believe that they 'knew' their sexual partners; what they understood by 'knowing', however, was not what the Chief Medical Officer had in mind. In many cases, the respondents reported that they had 'known' their partners through being at the same school, living in the same street, going to the same youth club, or whatever. What they didn't know, in the majority of cases (and what the Chief Medical Officer presumably meant by his advice), was anything about the sexual histories of their partners which would have enabled them (at least in theory) to make some form of risk-assessment. Since these respondents felt that they had 'known' their partners, then the second part of the advice – to use condoms – did not seem relevant.

Ingham *et al.* (1991) considered various aspects of first intercourse, including the length of time between becoming 'a couple' and intercourse, what the respondents did actually 'know' about their partner's sexual histories, how these related to condom-use, and other factors. The authors conclude that advice which contains such ambiguous terminology can actually be counter-productive, in that people appear to believe that they are following the advice when they are clearly not doing so in the manner intended.

(ii) Positive reasons for not following advice received

A further feature of national campaigns in the UK was the suggestion that young people should 'get to know their partner' before engaging in sexual relations with them. This advice was presumably intended not only to enable open and frank discussion between the couple on matters relating to safer sex, contraception, and other relevant matters, but also to enable some form of 'risk assessment' to be made of potential partners. People were encouraged to find out about their partner's sexual history as part of this 'getting to know you' stage of the relationship.

Ingham *et al.* (1992) draw attention to some of the very real and practical difficulties involved in following such advice. For example, during the early stages of relationships, feelings of jealousy and resentment were reported by their respondens whenever partners mentioned earlier partners. In other cases, respondents who had had little prior sexual experience did not want to reveal this to their new partners; conversely, those with extensive prior experience did not want to reveal this fact either. A further issue related to trust; some respondents reported that to discuss with their current partners about previous partners and sexual experiences implied that, in due course, when the current relationship was over, their own behaviour and activities would become the subject of discussion with new partners.

Thus, in addition to the difficulties of talking about sexual and relationship issues (see below), there are some quite 'rational' and understandable reasons for not following the advice to share sexual histories with new partners.

(iii) Difficulties of talking about sexual matters

Many young people report great difficulty in discussing sexual matters, whether with a new partner or with others in their social worlds, such as parents, teachers, and so on. Thus, even in cases where people are persuaded of the need to take the threats seriously and where they are motivated to act appropriately, difficulties are still reported. These relate to a lack of confidence regarding their own knowledge, as well as not having a suitable language with which to communicate.

This is not surprising, given the ways in which young people become acquainted with sexual activities and the issues surrounding sexuality. Research into, for example, the sex education received from either school or home reveals some serious shortcomings (Farrell, 1978; Allen, 1987; Thomson and Scott, 1991). Woodcock *et al.* (1992b) report that many respondents in their research felt that their sex education lessons were of little value, being either too early or too late, being too biological or too vague, and often conducted by teachers who were perceived to be very embarrassed by the whole area and who clearly (or so it appeared to the young people) would rather not have been there. Under these circumstances, it is perhaps not at all surprising that talking about sex comes to be seen as problematic.

The situation at home appears to be equally difficult. Fathers were generally reported as avoiding the subject whenever it was raised, or to treat the area in a 'jokey' manner. Ingham *et al.* (in prep.) considered not only the levels of information acquired from parents, but also the 'atmosphere' that the young people reported with regard to sexual issues. Mothers were more likely than fathers to discuss matters with their children, but often adopted one of a number of rather limited approaches – these varied, for example, from a moral appeal ("don't do it until you're married") to a *laissez-faire* attitude ("do what you want but be careful"), with some appearing not to mention the areas involved at all. Very few cases of parents discussing health risks were described, the majority of cases in which 'warnings' were given related to pregnancy. The females in the sample reported more discussion with their mothers on sexual matters than did the males.

Thus, the two main potential sources of talking about (and, by implication, developing the skills and vocabulary to discuss) sex would appear to be under-used. In addition to this apparent lack, other less direct sources of knowledge of sex tend to encourage enigmatic associations. Thus, young people learn from an early age that it is a topic to be joked about surreptitiously, and that *double entendres* and other evasive styles are often used.

Studies in which young people have been asked directly about their main sources of knowledge about sex support the data obtained through the qualitative analyses reported by Woodcock *et al.* (1992b). Thus, for example, 'friends' are often cited as the major source of information, as are older siblings. The media are cited frequently, although most studies do not specify in detail as to whether 'fact' or fictional programmes are being referred to. In any event, considering what is known about some of the misconceptions regarding young people's knowledge, as well as some of the sensationalist treatment in certain sections of the media, it is a matter of concern that these sources are often cited as the major means through which many young people acquire their 'knowledge' regarding sexual issues.

There is some evidence that many young people are themselves not happy with this state of affairs. In a survey of 600 school and college students (aged 12 to 18) carried out by Ingham (1990) for the World Health Organisation, not only was an item on current main sources of information asked, an item asking for where they would *prefer* to obtain information was also included. Whilst the most frequently reported current sources for males were friends and television, the preferred sources stated were teachers and both parents. For females, the most frequently cited sources were mothers and friends, with preferred sources being both parents. These results were country specific, in that similar studies carried out in Cyprus and Croatia obtained different patterns of results.

(c) Social processes

Whilst much of the research conducted in the United States during the 1970s and 1980s tended to adopt a primarily individual approach to the study of sexual activity, more recent work (especially in European countries) has drawn attention to some of the wider social processes which affect the area. From a methodological viewpoint, it is only when more attention was given to the use of more qualitative approaches in this field that some of these social processes became apparent. Although this type of work is still (relative to other approaches) in its infancy, some of the issues to emerge are briefly described below.

(i) Pressures and reputations

Concentrating on the reports of first-ever heterosexual intercourse amongst young people, Ingham *et al.* (1991, 1992 and in preparation) report clear evidence of the effects of peer and media pressures of various kinds to become sexually experienced. Amongst males, peer pressure was given as the major reason for first experiences by roughly half of those sampled. The accounts provide many examples of how young men felt very strong pressure to 'become a man' through sexual initiation and, in many cases, it appeared that which particular woman served this function was almost immaterial! Even in cases where direct peer pressure did not seem to be such a powerful issue, respondents reported strong internal pressures to find out 'what it was like', having heard or read a lot about 'it' in the media. In such cases, the importance of reputations can be regarded as applying to 'self-as-audience' as much as to 'other-as-audience'.

These qualitative accounts provide data which conflict with those obtained in a large scale survey of Canadian young people (n = 38000), in which 'expected by friends' was given as the major reason for first intercourse by just 4% of the male respondents (King *et al.*, 1988). It is unlikely that cultural variations are sufficient to account for this difference.

On the other hand, the reported motivational factors amongst young females appear to place much less emphasis on reputational aspects, and considerably more emphasis on 'relationship' issues. Thus, well over half of the young women interviewed in the Southampton study cited this as the main motivation, and described their wish to 'give' something to a particular and valued partner (notwithstanding the fact that, in many cases, such partners *later* became rather less valued). Direct reputational issues featured much less amongst women than amongst men, (being reported as the major reason by 13% of the respondents) although many accounts were received of the difficulties of young women, within some social worlds, to withstand the strong pressures to avoid being labelled as a 'fridge', as 'tight', or through some other equally derogatory category. Lees (1986) has also discussed this issue in some detail, again based on qualitative material. Further, King *et al.*'s (1988) Canadian study reports 52% of women citing 'love' as their major motivation, with just 2% reporting that it was 'expected by friends'.

This area raises some interesting and challenging implications with regard to the encouragement of risk-reducing behaviours in some cultures. For example, in some African cultures (and some West Indian cultures in Europe) young men and women are expected to 'prove' their fertility prior to marriage so as to demonstrate that they are suitable partners. In such cases, attempts to encourage young people to adopt safer sexual practices will come into direct conflict with longstanding and important cultural phenomena.

(ii) Discourse and power
Some of the recent analyses of sexual activity (emanating primarily, but not exclusively from, feminist perspectives) have argued that considerably greater attention needs to be paid than has hitherto been the case to the 'discourses' which affect and 'control' human action. In particular, for example, Hollway (1984) identified a number of such discourses which affect heterosexual relationships and which are re-produced during each (or at least the vast majority of) heterosexual encounter. Thus, for example, a dominant discourse is the 'have-hold', in which the aim of young women is to 'acquire' and then 'hold on to' a suitable young man for the purposes of marriage and child-rearing. Such a discourse provides a ready scenario for young people to follow, being readily 'available' in magazines and other media outlets.

A further example is the 'male sexual drive' discourse, in which it is regarded as a 'given' that men need regular sexual outlets and that it is women's role in life to provide these. Examples of this discourse appeared in the accounts collected from young people regarding how they made assessments of the level of risk associated with potential partners. Some women, on justifying their partners' apparently quite high levels of previous sexual activity, referred to the fact that such behaviour is to be expected as normal for young men, and therefore not to be regarded as indicating potential risk (cf Woodcock *et al.*, 1992a).

A further illustration of the differential influence of discourses is provided by the analysis of the reports of how the young people felt after their first experience of intercourse. Whereas the young men, in over 90% of cases, reported that they had felt 'exhilarated', 'over the moon', and other similar positive emotions (despite some cases of physical disappointment), the vast majority of women reported feelings of regret. This was related to the contrast between what they had expected their first experience to be like (with someone they loved in the context of a longstanding and trusting relationship) and what they had actually experienced. What was particularly disturbing in these reports was the frequency with which these young women blamed themselves for these feelings of regret, despite it being clear from many of the accounts that they had, in fact, been relatively powerless in the situations involved (Ingham *et al.* 1991). Currie's work (1992) suggesting that women with low self-esteem are more likely to engage in higher risk behaviours is particularly relevant in this context.

Data from the Womens' Risk and AIDS Project (WRAP) in the UK lends strong support to the importance of taking into account the dominant discourses in this area, and especially those relating to male power. For example, the serious difficulties experienced by young women in successfully negotiating condom use is clearly illustrated (Holland *et al.*, 1991). Similar analyses have been reported from Australian work (Kippax *et al.*, 1990). Indeed, these authors argue that "...some common understandings underlying sexual encounters render negotiation not only impossible but largely unintelligible. The permissive discourse may possibly provide space for some negotiation, but...it is essential to develop a truly woman-centred discourse of sexuality out of which male sexuality can be problematised" (p. 533).

Although the bases of, and ideas surrounding, discourse analysis are relatively new in the discipline of psychology (cf Potter and Wetherall, 1987; Parker, 1991) they pose some important challenges. The integration of individual and societal levels of analysis is essential if real progress is to be achieved, especially in an area as replete with moral, ideological and emotional issues as the field of sexuality and sexual activity.

(iii) Negotiation
Little is known about the processes involved in the negotiation of sexual activities, despite it being clear that successful adoption of safer sexual practices will become increasingly important as the risk of HIV-infection increases. From the qualitative work published so far, there appears to be little evidence of actual negotiation taking place, with much of the work highlighting the implicit and explicit power relations within the couple. Women appear to be in a very weak position to 'negotiate' their preferred level and style of activity, even in cases where they are clearly well informed regarding what precautions they should be adopting.

RETHINKING PSYCHOLOGICAL APPROACHES

The recent work on sexual activity generated by the threats posed by HIV-infection has added some new dimensions to the earlier – primarily American based – work outlined at the start of this chapter. Of the three dominant approaches reviewed earlier, that involving the identification of sexual scripts is closest to the recent developments. The other two major approaches – those based on individual differences and 'rational' models of health behaviour – have been revealed to have some serious shortcomings if a full understanding of the area is to be obtained. Apart from the methodological issues already discussed, there are some major theoretical dimensions which need to be considered. Just two are briefly discussed here.

(i) The concept of rationality

In the light of the criticisms levelled at models based on conceptions of individual rationality, as well as considerations of the material obtained through personal accounts from young people, Ingham (1993) has speculated on some alternative ways of considering the concept of 'rationality' in the specific context of adopting safer sexual practices. These are:

(a) cases where the 'rational' response was well known by the respondent but regarded as personally unattainable (through not feeling able to exercise sufficient control over their behaviour);
(b) cases where the 'rational' response was regarded as unrealistic not as a result of personal weakness (as in (a) above) but by nature of the behaviour in question;
(c) cases where 'unsafe' behaviour was argued as being perfectly rational given the circumstances of the people involved;
(d) cases where taken-for-granted assumptions directly opposed the known rational response;
(e) cases where respondents acknowledged that behaving 'rationally' and 'safely' was, in effect, a choice to be made from amongst other options. Some of these respondents, however, whilst acknowledging this choice also reported that they 'were only young once', and intended to make the most of it (the very notion of choice itself is of course made problematic by the notion of discourse).

These reactions can be perfectly well integrated into analyses based on exploring the discourses available within which young people understand both the nature of sexual activity as well as the nature of being a young person. Thus, for example, defining oneself as relatively 'powerless', defining sexual activity as an overwhelming force, defining the nature of being young as characterised as 'irrational' and impulsive can all be regarded as social constructions, created and maintained through social discourses. This approach points to a fundamentally different way of thinking about the issues involved from those adopting assumptions that, given sufficient knowledge and incentives, people will behave in a rational and health preserving manner.

Other questioning of the 'rational' approach to health preservation has been undertaken. For example, Prieur (1990a, 1990b) has argued, based on her work with young gay men in Norway and New Mexico, that in the contexts of their lives – with no money, no home and no warmth – it is perfectly rational to seek comforts through sexual relationships. Brown *et al.* (1991) have suggested that the Health Belief Model "... does not lend itself to understanding maturational, developmental and perceptual constructs and the interaction between these constructs indigenous to this [adolescent] age group". These authors argue for an extension of the model to incorporate some "... innovative theoretical perspectives...", including greater recognition of interpersonal and interactional perspectives.

A more hopeful way of considering the area is to adopt some of the postulates of the so-called 'new social psychology' (Harré and Secord, 1978; Harré *et al.*, 1985) together with some of the even more recent developments in social psychology. By considering people as operating within social worlds, affected from within and without by powers and constraints (including discourses) alternative ways of approaching this whole area can be considered. Young people are clearly located within powerful and influential social worlds, which vary in nature according to locality, class, gender, race and other factors. By placing greater emphasis on these wider contexts, more attention is paid to the dynamic nature of the processes which create and maintain identities, and the role that sexual activity plays in these contexts. A major omission in the research so far has been the developmental implications of the transition from the social world of 'childhood' to that of 'adulthood' and the significance of sexual activity in this process. Such analyses would prove invaluable in helping to account for why some young people appear to adopt sexual lifestyles which place them at greater risk of pregnancy or infection than do others.

(ii) Relations with other disciplines

It follows from the above discussion that the traditional approaches by psychologists to many of the sorts of issues raised are severely ill-equipped to deal with them adequately. To consider just the individual level of behaviour, knowledge, attitudes, and so on (which by their nature questionnaires are bound to do) is to risk becoming blind to many other important and directly relevant issues. Rendering invisible some of the wider social processes involved is not only methodologically and theoretically mistaken, it also has important political implications (see, for example, Warwick and Aggleton's (1990) critique of (admittedly somewhat dated) psychological contributions to the understanding of 'adolescence'). Psychologists need to engage to a greater extent with colleagues from other disciplines, including sociologists and anthropologists, some of whom have much to offer.

POLICY IMPLICATIONS

Given the growing threats posed by HIV-infection (in addition to those posed by other STDs and unwanted pregnancies) it is imperative that suitable lessons are learned from the research in the area of young people and sexuality to inform and guide policy initiatives. There has been sustained and sharp criticism of the 'official' campaigns run up to now in many developed countries (see, for example, Rigby *et al.*, 1989; Aggleton, 1989; Moerkerk and Aggleton, 1990; Wilton and Aggleton, 1991). Many of these campaigns have been based on assumptions that accurate knowledge together with perceived threat are sufficient motivators to effect changes in behaviour. Whilst these may well be necessary (although even this is not certain, given the extent of rule-following behaviour which occurs without people being aware of why it is so), there is no doubt that they are not sufficient.

Although a full consideration of the policy implications of the sort of approach taken in this chapter is beyond its scope, some clear pointers can be highlighted. There must be a move away from mass campaigns in the media towards interventions which engage young people more directly in solving the issues which confront them. To do this effectively, talk and discussion would appear to be necessary, peer group 'education' could be extended, suitable facilitators need to be trained to work in different contexts, empowerment skills need to be encouraged amongst young women (and parallel 'depowerment' skills amongst men?) and efforts made to create closer links between parents/guardians and other agencies. Some of the interventions necessary require a rather longer time frame than others, but this should not be used as an excuse for inaction.

Of particular relevance in this endeavour are schools and colleges, since the vast majority of young people can be reached there. In the UK, for example, there is increasing concern amongst many agencies involved in the field that the current government policy is not helping by refusing to make sex education a compulsory component of the National Curriculum. The current (as at June 1993) position is that each state school must have a policy on sex education and that this should be revealed to parents, but the policy could simply state that the school concerned does not deal with these matters. In 1991, HIV was introduced as part of the National Curriculum, but in the science component. The fear is that placing the topic in this particular curriculum will encourage a purely biological treatment, and that the real and everyday implications of the virus will not be dealt with adequately. The inclusion of sex education through Personal and Social Development as compulsory subjects in schools would be of great benefit in ensuring that young people are better prepared than they appear to be at present for their subsequent sexual 'careers', and would also, by the way, provide encouragement and recognition to the many individuals and agencies who are attempting to face the difficult issues in a positive and creative manner. This is not just a problem in the UK; the political/moral climate in the US is similarly believed, by many in the field, to impose similar restraints on effective interventions, and recent government pronouncements in Uganda have restricted the activities of those agencies who have been encouraging the more widespread use of condoms amongst young people. It is also of interest to note that the (hardly radical) UK Royal College of Obstetricians and Gynaecologists has recently recommended not only compulsory sex education, but also compulsory coverage of related areas for all teachers during their initial training (RCOG, 1991).

Inclusion of sex education classes on their own would not of course solve all the problems. There are some major problems to be addressed, including the age at which issues should be raised, the format and style of the input, and so on. Input based around current age segregated classes raises particular problems, given that research has revealed the wide diversity of sexual awareness and experiences amongst young people of similar ages. Further, the diversity present in a multi-cultural society poses particular problems in achieving the balance between open and frank discussion of the issues, on the one hand, and not causing undue offence (and/or challenging cultural values), on the other.

The design and implementation of effective interventions are not easy tasks, but the alternative – a steady rise in the numbers of young people infected with HIV and the numbers of unwanted pregnancies – paints a very pessimistic scenario indeed.

Acknowledgements
The research reported from the Southampton study on young people was supported by a grant from the Economic and Social Research Council (grant number XA 44250012) to the author, for which grateful thanks are expressed.

REFERENCES

Abrams, D., Abraham, C., Spars, R. & Marks, D. (1990). AIDS invulnerability: relationships, sexual behaviour and attitudes among 16–19 year olds, in P. Aggleton, P. Davies and G. Hart (eds) *AIDS: Individual, Cultural and Policy dimensions*. Basingstoke, The Falmer Press.
Aggleton, P. (1989). Evaluating health education about AIDS, in P. Aggleton, G. Hart and P. Davies (eds) *AIDS: Social Representations, Social Practices*. Lewes, The Falmer Press.
Allen, I. (1987). *Education in Sex and Personal Relationships*. London: Policy Studies Institute.

Allgeier, E.R. (1984). The personal perils of sex researchers: Vern Bullough and William Masters, *SIECUS Reports*, **12**, 4, 16–19.

Anderson, R. & May, R.M. (1988). Epidemiological parameters of HIV infection, *Nature*, 9 June 1988, vol. 333 (6173).

Azjen, I. & Fishbein, M. (1980). *Understanding Attitudes and Predicting Social Behaviour.* Englewood Cliffs, NJ: Prentice Hall.

Brown, L.K., DiClemente, R.J. & Reynolds, S.A. (1991). HIV prevention for adolescents: utility of the Health Belief Model, *AIDS Education and Prevention*, **3**, 50–59.

Byrne, D. & Fisher, W.A. (eds) (1983). *Adolescents, Sex and Contraception.* Hillsdale, N.J.: Lawrence Erlbaum Associates.

Clift, S., Stears, D., Legg, S., Memon, A. & Ryan, L. (1989). *The HIV/AIDS Education and Young People Project*, Canterbury, Christ Church College (Report on Phase One).

Coxon, A. (1988). The numbers game – gay lifestyles, epidemiology of AIDS and social science, in P. Aggleton & H. Homans (eds) *Social Aspects of AIDS*. Lewes, The Falmer Press.

Currie, C. (1992). *Personal communication*, Research Unit in Health and Behavioral Change, University of Edinburgh.

Daugherty, L.R. & Burger, J.M. (1984). The influence of parents, church and peers on the sexual attitudes and behaviours of college students. *Archives of Sexual Behaviour*, **13**, 4, 351–359.

Day, S. (1988). Prostitute women and AIDS: anthropology, (editorial review). *AIDS*, **2**, 421–428.

Day, S. (1990). Prostitute women and the ideology of work in London, in D.A. Feldman (ed) *AIDS and Culture: the Global Pandemic.* New York: Praeger.

Farrell, C. (1978). *My Mother Said . . . the way young people learned about sex and birth control.* London: Routledge and Kegan Paul.

Fisher, W.A. (1990). Understanding and preventing adolescent pregnancy and sexually transmitted diseases/AIDS, in J. Edwards (ed) *Social Influence Processes and Prevention.* New York: Plenum Press.

Fisher, W.A., Byrne, D., White, L.A. & Kelley, K. (1988). Erotophobia-erotophilia as a dimension of personality. *J. of Sex Research*, **25**, 293–296.

Gagnon, J.H. (1977). *Human Sexualities.* Chicago: Scott Foresman.

Gagnon, J.H. (1986). Gender preference in erotic relations, the Kinsey scale and sexual scripts, unpublished manuscript based on a paper originally presented at the Conference on Homosexuality/Heterosexuality: the Kinsey Scale and Current Research, held at the Kinsey Institute, Bloomington, Indiana, May, 1986.

Gagnon, J.H. & Simon, W. (1973). *Sexual Conduct.* Chicago: Aldine.

Harré, R. & Secord, P. (1978). *The Explanation of Social Behavior.* Oxford: Basil Blackwell.

Harré, R., Clarke, D. & De Carlo, N. (1985). *Motives and Mechanisms.* London: Methuen.

Holland, J., Ramazanoglu, C., Scott, S., Sharpe, S. & Thomson, R. (1990). Sex, gender and power: young women's sexuality in the shadow of AIDS. *Sociology of Health and Illness*, **12**(3), 336–350.

Holland, J., Ramazanoglu, C., Scott, S., Sharpe, S. & Thomson, R. (1991). Between embarrassment and trust: young women and the diversity of condom use, in P. Aggleton, G. Hart & P. Davies (eds) *AIDS: Responses, Interventions and Care.* London: The Falmer Press.

Hollway, W. (1984). Gender difference and the production of subjectivity, in J. Henriques, W. Hollway, C. Urwin, C. Venn & V. Walkerdine *Changing the Subject: Psychology, Social Regulation and Subjectivity.* London: Methuen.

Ingham, R. (1990). WHO Schools KABP Pre-testing Report, unpublished report produced for the World Health Organisation, Geneva; Department of Psychology, The University of Southampton.

Ingham, R. (1993). Some speculations on the concept of 'rationality', in G. Albrecht (ed.) *Advances in Medical Sociology, vol IV A Reconsideration of Health Behavior Change Models.*

Greenwich, CT: JAI Press.

Ingham, R., Woodcock, A. & Stenner, K. (1991). Getting to know you...young people's knowledge of partners at first intercourse. *J. of Comm. and App Soc. Psych.*, 1, 2, 117–132.

Ingham, R., Woodcock, A. & Stenner, K. (1992). The limitations of rational decision making models as applied to young people's sexual behaviour, in P. Aggleton, G. Hart & P. Davies (eds) *AIDS: Rights Risk and Reason*. London: The Falmer Press, 163–173.

Ingham, R., Woodcock, A. & Stenner, K. (in prep.). Great expectations...planning for first ever intercourse, Department of Psychology, The University of Southampton.

Ingham, R., Woodcock, A. & Stenner, K. (in prep.). Sources of knowledge and attitudes about sex in families, Department of Psychology, University of Southampton.

King, A., Beazley, R., Warren, W., Hankins, C., Robertson, A. & Radford, J. *Canada, Youth and AIDS Study*, report produced by the Social Program Evaluation Group, Queen's University, Kingston, Ontario.

Kinsey, A.C., Pomeroy, W. & Martin, C. (1948). *Sexual Behaviour in the Human Male.* Philadelphia, Pa: Saunders.

Kippax, S., Crawford, J., Waldby, C. & Benton, P. (1990). Women negotiating heterosex: implications for AIDS prevention. *Women's Studies Int. Forum*, 13, 6, 533–542.

Lees, S. (1986). *Losing Out: Sexuality and Adolescent Girls.* London: Hutchinson.

Maticka-Tyndale, E. (1991). Variations in adherence to safer-sex guidelines by heterosexual adolescents. *J. of Sex Research*, 28, 1, 45–66.

Moerkerk, H. & Aggleton, P. (1990). AIDS prevention strategies in Europe: a comparison and critical analysis, in P. Aggleton, P. Davies & G. Hart (eds) *AIDS: Individual, Cultural and Policy Dimensions*. Basingstoke: The Falmer Press.

Mosher, D.L. & Cross, H.J. (1971). Sex guilt and premarital sexual experiences of college students. *J. Consult. Clin. Psych.*, 36, 1, 27–32.

Mosher, D.L. & Vonderheide, S.G. (1985). Contributions of sex guilt and masturbation guilt to women's contraceptive attitude and use. *The Journal of Sex Research*, 21, 1, 24–39.

Parker, I. (1991). *Discourse Dynamics: Critical Analysis for Social and Individual Psychology.* London: Routledge.

Potter, J. & Wetherall, M. (1987). *Discourse and Social Psychology: Beyond Attitudes and Behaviour.* London: Sage Publications.

Prieur, A. (1990a). Taking risks is rational behaviour; experiences from the use of qualitative research methods, paper presented at the International Conference 'Assessing AIDS Prevention' in Montreux, 29 October–1 November 1990.

Prieur, A. (1990b). Norwegian gay men: reasons for continued practice of unsafe sex. *AIDS Education and Prevention*, 2, 2, 109–115.

Rigby, K., Brown, M., Anagnostou, P., Ross, M.W. & Rosser, B.R.S. (1989). Shock tactics to counter AIDS: the Australian experience. *Psychology and Health*, 3, 3, 145–159.

Rosenstock, I.M. (1974). Historical origins of the Health Belief Model. *Health Education Monographs*, 2, 328–335.

Rosenstock, I.M., Strecher, V.J. & Becker, M.H. (1988). Social learning theory and the Health Belief Model. *Health Psychology Update*, 15, 175–183.

Royal College of Obstetricians and Gynaecologists (1991). *Report of the RCOG Working Party on Unplanned Pregnancy.* London: RCOG.

Schmidt, P. (1991). Perspectives from the Theory of Planned Behaviour for explaining sexual behaviour and evaluating prevention strategies, paper prepared for a Workshop of the EC Concerted Action on Sexual Behaviour and Risks of HIV Infection, Sesimbra, Portugal, (November 1991).

Sherr, L. (1987). An evaluation of the UK government health education campaign. *Psychology and Health*, 1, 1, 61–72.

Solomon, P.J., Doust, J.A. & Wilson, S.R. (1989). *Predicting the Course of AIDS in Australia and evaluating the effect of AZT: a first report*, Working Paper Number 3, National Centre for Epidemiology and Population Health, Australian National University, Canberra, Australia.

Thomson, R. & Scott, S. (1991). *Learning about Sex: Young women and the social construction of sexual identity.* London: Tufnell Press.

Warwick, I., Aggleton, P. & Homans, H. (1988). Young people's health beliefs and AIDS, in P. Aggleton & H. Homans (eds) *Social Aspects of AIDS.* Lewes: The Falmer Press.

Warwick, I. & Aggleton, P. (1990). 'Adolescents', young people and AIDS research in P. Aggleton, P. Davies, & G. Hart (eds) *AIDS: Individual, Cultural and Policy Dimensions.* Basingstoke: The Falmer Press.

Wilton, T. & Aggleton, P. (1991). Condoms, coercion and control: heterosexuality and the limits to HIV/AIDS education, in P. Agggleton, G. Hart & P. Davies (eds) *AIDS: Responses, Interventions and Care.* London: The Falmer Press.

Woodcock, A., Stenner, K. & Ingham, R. (1992a). Young people talking about HIV and AIDS: interpretations of personal risk of infection. *Health Education Research: Theory and Practice,* 7, 2, 229-247.

Woodcock, A., Stenner, K. & Ingham, R. (1992b). "All these contraceptives, videos and that": Young people talking about school sex education, *Health Education Research: Theory and Practice,* 7, 517-531

Zuckerman, M., Bone, R., Neary, R., Mangelsdorff, D. & Brustman, B. (1972). What is the sensation seeker? Personality trait and experience correlates of the Sensation Seeking Scales. *J. Consult. Clin. Psych.,* 39, 308-321.

Zuckerman, M., Tushup, R. & Finner, S. (1976). Sexual attitudes and experience: attitude and personality correlates and changes produced by a course on sexuality. *J. Consult. Clin. Psych.,* 44, 7-19.

SECTION III
Early Adulthood

REPRODUCTIVE FAILURE AND THE REPRODUCTIVE TECHNOLOGIES: A PSYCHOLOGICAL PERSPECTIVE

ROBERT J. EDELMANN AND KEVIN J. CONNOLLY

INTRODUCTION

Most people assume that the early adult phase of their lives will include childbearing and the raising of children (Regan and Roland, 1985). Indeed control is frequently exercised over the timing of such events, pregnancy being avoided until after certain life goals have been attained. Yet many couples find that they are unable to achieve pregnancy and that this important aspect of their lives is not within their control. It has been suggested that between one in seven and one in ten couples seek medical help in their efforts to conceive (Menning, 1980; Houghton, 1984) but precise figures are lacking. The most comprehensive estimates of the numbers of couples likely to experience a fertility problem at some time in their lives comes from data obtained for the National Center for Health Statistics in the U.S.A. (Hirsch and Mosher, 1987; Mosher, 1985, 1988). These suggest that the overall incidence of infertility (defined as the failure to achieve pregnancy after one year of regular intercourse without contraception) in women is approximately 13 per cent. There is no comparable data for the U.K. although Page (1989) recently suggested that betwen 20 and 35 per cent of couples take in excess of a year to conceive during their reproductive years. Infertility is thus a problem likely to be encountered by many young adults.

It has also been claimed that psychological difficulties accompany infertility in many couples attending infertility clinics (Seibel and Taymor, 1982; Bell, 1983). Whilst the relationship between such difficulties and infertility is not understood it is unlikely to be simple. Psychological factors may be a primary cause of infertility, although this view has not gone unchallenged (see reviews by Noyes and Chapnick, 1964; Edelmann and Connolly, 1986). Conversely infertility may have a marked impact upon psychological functioning. Thus Menning (1980) has described infertility as 'a complex life crisis, psychologically threatening and emotionally stressful' while Berger (1977, 1980a) goes as far as to suggest that 'a sense of despair must plague every couple who seek help for an infertility problem'. Other authors refer to health problems, loss of self-esteem, feelings of mourning, depression, guilt and frustration associated with failure to conceive (Pfeffer and Woollett, 1983; Bresnick, 1984). While not denying that infertility is an important and stressful experience, there is little evidence to suggest that infertility is commonly associated with major psychopathology and more recent research suggests that most couples cope effectively with the crisis of infertility.

Medical science has made great progress in the investigation and treatment of infertility over the past two decades. The number of births from Donor Insemination (DI) is increasing and *in vitro* fertilization (IVF) is more widely available. The number of babies born annually as a result of donor insemination in the USA is now likely to exceed the figure of 15,000 quoted by Snowden and Snowden (1984). The same authors estimate 2,000 to 2,500 such cases in the U.K., a figure which has almost certainly now been exceeded. While the DI technique is simple, the psychological issues encountered by the couple are likely to be complex. These include the male's adaptation to a child produced by donor insemination (or indeed the female's failure to conceive) and the secrecy associated with this means of producing a family (Edelmann, 1989).

Since the first intrauterine pregnancy was achieved (Steptoe, Edwards and Purdy, 1980) the use of *in vitro* fertilisation has developed rapidly throughout the world with 200 hundred IVF clinics (Salzer, 1986) in 15 countries (Mao and Wood, 1984) reported by the middle of the 1980s. The service has expanded even more rapidly since. Recently variations on the initial IVF procedure such as gamete intra-fallopian transfer (GIFT) have evolved and limited success with this procedure has been reported (Asch *et al.*, 1986). As with DI, the psychological implications of the medicalisation of re-production need to be considered (Edelmann, 1990).

This chapter will address three issues relating to reproductive failure: (1) the question of psychogenic infertility; (2) psychological difficulties consequent upon reproductive failure and (3) psychological issues raised by the developing reproductive technologies.

PSYCHOGENIC INFERTILITY

Over the past half century clinical observations and research reports have appeared in both the psychological and medical literature concerning possible psychological causes of infertility. This has generally been directed towards that group of patients whose infertility remains unexplained, no anatomical, physiological or pathological cause having been found after the completion of extensive diagnostic tests. The number of cases classed as unexplained has declined in recent years due to advances in investigative procedures and our developing understanding of reproductive biology. By the beginning of the 1980s, the highest estimate of unexplained infertility was quoted as rarely exceeding 18% (Harrison *et al.*, 1981) and most clinics would hope to obtain a lower rate. In our own studies, the figure for unexplained infertility after the first year of standard investigations is approximately 13% of clinic attenders (e.g. Edelmann *et al.*, 1991); a proportion of whom are subsequently diagnosed by more sophisticated investigative procedures.

Estimates of how many of these unexplained cases may be due to psychological factors has also been very variable ranging from 5% (Seibel and Taymor, 1882) to 50%

(Eisner, 1963). Indeed, the evidence suggesting psychological causes for infertility is not very convincing. In two reviews, published over twenty years apart similar negative conclusions were reached. Noyes and Chapnick (1964) commented that "...no firm evidence was found that a specific psychological factor can alter fertility in the normal infertile couple" (p. 555), while Edelmann and Connolly (1986) asserted that "On the basis of available evidence there appears little to support the suggestion that psychological factors play a part in the aetiology of childlessness" (p. 213).

The emphasis in the majority of the studies from which these conclusions are drawn was a search for psychological differences between individuals with unexplained infertility and those with explained or 'organic' infertility. Although some of these studies do indeed report such differences, methodological problems mean the results are open to question and doubt.

In many of the studies quoted in both reviews there is often no clear rationale for constructs that have been used to compare fertile and infertile couples. Thus while couples might differ in terms of attitudes or gender roles (Slade, 1981) it is difficult to gauge how such factors might be considered causal and any clear theoretical rationale for how the psychological variables measured might interfere with reproductive potential is usually lacking. It is clearly possible that psychological stressors may influence physiological and endocrinological function and so reduce the likelihood of conception for some couples. Indeed, it has been argued that a link or links may exist between psychological distress and related states and failure to conceive, in some cases via changes in physiological processes such as elevated prolactin levels (Edelmann and Golombok, 1989). Rarely, however, has psychological distress been assessed in studies comparing fertile and infertile groups.

A second difficulty relates to the fact that in studies finding differences between fertile and infertile couples the latter have often had a longstanding problem conceiving. For example, O'Moore *et al.* (1983) found differences between a group of infertile women whose mean duration of infertility was between 6 and 7 years and a fertile comparison group on a measure of anxiety. Given the reasonable assumption that infertility can be a distressing experience it is perhaps not surprising that some such couples are more anxious than their fertile counterparts.

Edelmann *et al.* (1991) report a study designed to avoid the methodological difficulties inherent in much of the earlier work addressing the question of psychogenic infertility. One hundred and thirty couples presenting with primary infertility were assessed on measures of personality and psychopathology at their first appointment at a specialist infertility clinic. In addition, comparable data were collected from three comparison groups of proven fertility and with intact families. Two of these groups had been referred for minor surgical procedures associated with sterilisation (tubal ligation and vasectomy), while the third group was composed of parents with children of nursery school age who were not seeking any medical treatment. The infertile group was subsequently divided into five subgroups on the basis of investigations made over the ensuing year (female cause, male cause, female and male cause diagnosed, unexplained and conceived). These data provide comparisons not only with fertile groups and test norms but also within the overall infertile group itself. The data were collected before the medical investigations began and a considerable time before diagnoses were made. If psychological factors are implicated in infertility then differences in the psychological profile of the unexplained subset compared to the subset diagnosed with organic causes would be expected.

In general, however, our findings gave no support to this hypothesis. The five subgroups did not differ on any of the measures taken; there were also few differences between the infertile set as a whole and the three comparison groups. There was also little indication of any differences between the scores obtained by the four groups and normative data available for the various tests. The one interesting exception to these findings related to elevated state anxiety scores obtained by women in the infertile group both in relation to the comparison groups and to the normative data available on the various tests. Given that this was relatively constant across the several infertility subgroups it seems reasonable to conclude that the elevated anxiety is a consequence rather than a cause of failure to conceive. Thus, even before medically related investigations begin, the difficulties these women experience in conceiving have already provoked considerable anxiety. This is further borne out by the fact that in a subsequent assessment of these women conducted some seven months later, anxiety had declined regardless of whether the couple had conceived or remained childless and regardless of whether or not a cause had been identified for their infertility (Connolly *et al.*, 1992).

Overall then, the evidence for psychogenic infertility is not convincing. It is of course possible that rather more subtle psychological parameters might be involved than those assessed by standardised psychological tests administered on a single occasion. It might also be argued that psychological parameters other than those assessed may be implicated. Any further research in this area clearly needs to investigate the possibility of combining endocrinological and psychological parameters with careful thought given to the optimal timing for such assessments. It is also possible that psychological variables may contribute to reproductive failure via their effects on physiological processes but that the rather simplistic notion of an 'infertile personality' has no support from this and similar studies.

PSYCHOLOGICAL EFFECTS OF REPRODUCTIVE FAILURE

Infertility is a deeply distressing experience for many couples. Mahlstedt, McDuff and Bernstein (1987) reported that 80% of their sample found infertility to be either stressful or extremely stressful, while Freeman *et al.* (1987) report that 49% of their infertile couples described infertility as the most upsetting experience of their lives. Other studies report evidence for elevated anxiety or depression scores for some infertile couples compared to controls. Thus Link and Darling (1986) found that 40% of wives and 16% of husbands had scores indicative of clinically significant depression while Harrison *et al.* (1984) report higher state anxiety scores for women but not for men in infertile partnerships in relation to controls.

Other studies have reported little if any difference between infertile individuals and fertile controls on measures of anxiety or depression (e.g. Paulson *et al.*, 1988). Different findings are no doubt due to some of the methodological difficulties discussed above. Indeed, the impact of infertility on cognitive functioning is likely to be a complex matter influenced by many variables.

Edelmann and Connolly (1986) identified four factors which they felt needed to be considered in any study of the impact of infertility on psychological functioning. Firstly, evidence suggested that the longer the known (diagnosed) period of infertility, the more likely it was that studies would reveal differences between fertile and infertile couples. Secondly, it was evident that the investigative procedures themselves were often distressing. Thirdly, although marked by an absence of research findings, comments in the literature suggested that whether the cause of infertility was attributed to the male or female might have a differential effect upon the couple concerned. Finally, the evidence reviewed suggested that a definite diagnosis was less distressing for the couple than continuing uncertainty. Since that review was published a number of reports have appeared which have helped to shed some light on the issues raised. Two areas in particular have been addressed; first, the impact of infertility upon the couple's relationship and second, the question of gender differences in the emotional impact of infertility and whether a diagnosis of male or female infertility has a differential impact upon the couple's emotional adjustment.

The Marital Relationship

A number of authors (e.g. Mahlstedt, 1985; Valentine, 1986; Woollett, 1985) have suggested that infertility and infertility testing can affect the couple's marital and sexual relationship. The need to take basal temperatures, time intercourse for the fertile period and carry out post-coital tests can be particularly disruptive (e.g. Bullock, 1974). Inevitably the couple will need to make a series of difficult decisions about whether or not to proceed with treatment; decisions made doubly difficult if one partner is more determined to have children (Pfeffer and Woollett, 1983). Marital happiness and satisfaction may also vary differentially at the various stages of infertility investigations. For example, Van Keep and Schmidt-Elmendorff (1975) note that women were least happy immediately prior to approaching the doctor, while men were least happy while waiting for a diagnosis.

Although it has been suggested that couples with normal sexual functioning prior to infertility may develop decreased coital frequency, orgasmic dysfunction or mid cycle male impotence (Pepperell and McBain, 1985), there is little evidence for marital or sexual difficulties in couples undergoing infertility investigations or treatment. Indeed a number of studies have noted the remarkably stable marital relationships of such couples (e.g. Johnston, Shaw and Bird, 1987; Takefman *et al.*, 1990). In our own research we have found evidence of stable marital relationships in couples approaching a specialist infertility clinic with little suggestion of any deterioration in these relationships over the course of a series of medical investigations, at least over a period of 7 to 9 months (Edelmann *et al.*, 1991; Connolly *et al.*, 1992). This observation should be interpreted cautiously since the finding may be due to an element of self-selection among the patients. It is possible that only those couples with stable relationships get as far as seeking medical help in their efforts to conceive. To investigate this possibility population rather than clinic based studies are needed. In this context Raval *et al.* (1987) suggest that because these couples are actively engaged in trying to resolve their difficulties, the process of investigation may in fact be beneficial for their relationship. Leiblum, Kemman and Lane (1987) have also argued that infertility may serve to improve a marital relationship by bringing a couple closer together through their shared problem. Infertility, however, is only likely to have supportive 'side effects' for stable marital relationships and where the problem is acknowledged by both partners as one that they share and which should be faced together. Thus, McEwan, Costello and Taylor (1987) note that infertile couples who shared a problem within their relationship showed less distress than those who sought support outside the relationship.

There is also little evidence of marital distress in couples undergoing treatment by donor insemination or *in vitro* fertilisation. Although there are a few cases of maladaptive responses to DI (e.g. Peyser, 1965) these are for the most part anecdotal and subjective. Once pregnancy is established or after delivery, problems are rare. It has also been reported that DI couples are happy, feel close to their children and express a desire to return for further inseminations (Snowden, Mitchell and Snowden, 1983). If those couples who present at infertility clinics are in general a self selected set tending to have more stable relationships it could well be argued that couples electing for DI or IVF could be subject to further selection and consequently in even more stable relationships. Indeed it is possible that couples in less than strong relationships effectively screen themselves out of a treatment programme during the counselling which precedes such interventions (see below). Thus, whilst infertility no doubt places a strain on some relationships, it seems that most couples attending specialist clinics or undergoing treatment show little evidence of marital disharmony.

Gender and Reactions to Infertility

Emotional reactions
Gender differences in emotional responsiveness to infertility have been reported in a number of studies. Reviewing this work Wright *et al.* (1989) concluded that women tended to report more distress than men. This seems to be a fairly consistent finding although methodological problems inherent in many studies (e.g. McGrade and Tolor, 1981; Raval *et al.*, 1987) may well mean that such gender differences are often incorrectly attributed to infertility. Examples of specific investigations include McGrade and Tolor's (1981) retrospective study in which they found that in a sample of 126 infertile couples women reported more emotional stress and tension, a greater deterioration of self image and more questioning of their sexuality than their husbands. It is interesting to note that this pattern of results was evident regardless of whether the couples had successfully conceived since initially seeking medical help and one might argue that the results merely reflect the well documented gender differences in symptom reporting. However, such an argument could not be used to explain findings from a study of 47 couples attending an infertility clinic (Raval *et al.*, 1987). In this study women reported significantly greater depression than men, and females' but not males' scores were elevated relative to normative data.

In a further study of 107 patients (45 men and 62 women) currently attending an infertility clinic, McEwan, Costello and Taylor (1987) reported that, using the recommended cut off score of 12 on the General Health Questionnaire (Goldberg, 1978), 40% of women and 13% of men experienced symptoms of clinical severity.

Although on balance the evidence suggests that women are more distressed by infertility than men the results must be interpreted with caution. It is recognised that negative life events elicit more distress in women than men (e.g. Al-Issa, 1982; Hammen, 1982). Thus, such findings may not be peculiar to infertility. Comparing males and females without having data on fertile controls or comparative normative data is likely to be misleading. Normative data for women always shows higher scores on variables such as anxiety and depression than are typical for men. Further, it can be argued that the greater reported incidence of distress in women is simply a result of reporting bias; many studies suggest that women are more prepared than men to admit to emotional distress (e.g. Spence, Deaux and Helmreich, 1985). The possibility that women are more adversely affected than their partners by a failure to conceive is clearly open to question and critical attention needs to be given to the methods used to address this issue. If we assume that the greater distress reported by women is more than a methodological artifact, what theoretical explanations might there be for such differences?

Explanations for gender differences
Differential reactions to infertility are frequently explained in terms of the social-isation process. Thus women who see their primary purpose in life as being motherhood and who cannot fulfill this by achieving one or more pregnancies are likely to feel stripped of their self-worth (Valentine, 1986). Despite alterations in gender roles precipitated by the womens movement gender differences in the impact of infertility may reflect women's greater psychosocial investment in reproduction resulting from social pressures concerning motherhood and marriage. As Mahlstedt (1985) comments: "for many women, having children is central to their identity. Society has been structured so that from the time they are very young, women think of themselves as – and others expect them to be – mothers" (p. 59).

One of the few attempts to place gender differences within a coherent theoretical framework is the sociobiological perspective proposed by Suarez and Gallup (1985). They note that women have greater genetic assurance than men because they have an absolute guarantee of sharing 50% of their genes with their offspring. Males, on the other hand, cannot be absolutely sure about paternity, consequently they should be less sensitive to reproductive failure. They further point out that women have a far more limited reproductive potential then men. Women are fertile for only a few days each month and release only a limited number of eggs during their reproductively active life. Men, potentially, are continuously fertile over a longer period and can produce hundreds of thousands of sperm on a daily basis. It is thus plausible to assume that because the woman has a relatively brief reproductive life and fertile period her distress at reproductive failure will be enhanced relative to that of her partner.

Women are also required to make a greater biological commitment when it comes to procreation (pregnancy, childbirth, breastfeeding and the lengthy process of child rearing). The socialisation pressures referred to previously no doubt serve to enhance these biological factors. Suarez and Gallup (1985) arguing from a sociobiological perspective make the case that the greater commitment of women to procreation will also make them more vulnerable to depression as a consequence of reproductive failure. Connolly and Edelmann (1988) failed to find evidence in support of this hypothesis from a retrospective survey of a clinic population over a 10 year period.

There are then feasible theoretical explanations for the possible gender differences in response to reproductive failure. It remains to be seen whether such apparent differences are indeed real and meaningful differences relating to infertility or merely a reflection of the inherent gender differences evident in normative data and sympto-matic of more general gender differences, or a reflection or gender differences in reporting symptoms. Clearly the issue is complicated; although there is some empirical evidence and feasible theoretical explanations for the notion that women are more affected by infertility than men, the latter are clearly not unaffected by reproductive failure. Indeed, there is evidence indicating that infertile males are likely to have lower self-esteem and greater anxiety in comparison with fertile controls (Kedem *et al.*, 1990). In this regard, a number of studies have noted that a diagnosis of male infertility may cause particular difficulties for both the male and female partner concerned.

Male infertility
Menning (1977) has suggested that in about 40 per cent of cases infertility is due to a problem with the female and around 40 per cent to a problem with the male, although information on male infertility is more sparse. In the remaining 20 per cent of cases both partners contribute to the problem. Clearly diagnosis has implications not only for the individual but also for that person's partner. Recent reports suggest that a diagnosis of male infertility may be more damaging for the couple concerned than a diagnosis of female infertility. In a retrospective study of over 800 couples Connolly, Edelmann and Cooke (1987) report greater emotional difficulties for both men and women when the cause of infertility was diagnosed to the man. Related to this, Berger (1980b) found a 63% incidence of transient impotence (lasting one to three months) following the discovery of azoospermia (absence of sperm in the semen) in a sample of 26 males. This may be due to the difficulties of treating azoospermia except by DI which is a means of addressing the problem of a couple's childlessness rather than a treatment for the male partner's infertility. In this context Owens and Read (1984) note that for their infertile sample an area of great concern was the lack of treatment for male infertility.

The possibility that male infertility is associated with particular psychological difficulties is also suggested by a recent longitudinal study (Connolly *et al.*, 1992). Over one hundred couples were assessed at their first appointment at a specialist infertility clinic and again some 7–9 months later when 65 per cent had been diagnosed (34 per cent male infertility; 8 per cent female infertility; 23 per cent both male and female problem) 19 per cent had conceived and 16 per cent remained unexplained. Over this period there was little evidence of psychopathology among the couples seeking treatment for infertility. Scores on the Dyadic Adjustment Scale (Spanier, 1976) suggested that the couples were from generally stable marriages; measures of depression, psychiatric morbidity and anxiety revealed generally low scores. Indeed, scores on tests of psychiatric morbidity and anxiety decreased between the initial and follow-up assessment for males and females as a whole regardless of diagnostic subgroup. The only exception was in those couples with a diagnosis of male infertility. Here, both psychiatric morbidity and anxiety increased for the males concerned between the initial and follow-up assessments. Social expectations and images of 'manhood' may well go some way to explain these results. Infertility and virility often become confused in relation to male infertility, so that as Mahlstedt (1985) comments, the man who is unable to father a child may feel that others doubt his masculinity.

The possibility that male infertility is associated with particular difficulties is an important issue in the context of the increasing use made of DI. Unlike treatments for several kinds of female infertility, DI is the only way of overcoming many cases of male infertility at present. This, in effect, bypasses rather than 'treats' the infertility. That is to say, it provides the couple with a means of having a child biologically related to the mother but not to her partner. Because in the case of DI the biological identity of one parent is known beyond doubt, there is a danger of some imbalance being built into the relationship between the natural mother, the social father and the child. Nevertheless, DI is now a very widely used method of alternative parenting. Some of the psychological issues, which are all too rarely addressed are considered in the following section.

DONOR INSEMINATION

The Warnock Committee's (1984) recent recommendation that in Britain DI should be confined to centres with trained psychological counsellors reccognises the complex emotional issues surrounding any decision that couples make when choosing DI. The aim of such counselling, as stated by the report, should be to enable patients "to understand their situation and to make their own decisions about what steps should be taken next" (p. 6 para 3.4). Ideally then the process of counselling may lead some couples to feel that DI is not the solution to their childlessness while facilitating acceptance for others. Menning (1981), for example, argues that couples will effectively screen themselves. Humphrey, Humphrey and Ainsworth-Smith (1991) also make an important distinction between screening (i.e. testing for the presence or absence of a certain quality) and vetting (a thorough appraisal of suitability). They argue in favour of the former, but not the latter, with respect to DI. The counsellor or psychologist's position is clearly not aimed at excluding couples who might become inadequate parents but to exclude those for whom DI might generate or exacerbate emotional problems. It is important to keep in mind that fertile couples are not required to undergo any assessment before attempting pregnancy. Similarly, exclusion from a DI programme should be the couple's decision albeit facilitated by skilled counselling.

Given these concerns relating to male infertility it is plainly important for the couples in question to be given guidance. Indeed, critics of DI have raised the possibility that the child may serve as a constant reminder of the man's sterility (Clamar, 1980) although the few available reports suggest that once a pregnancy is established, or after delivery, problems are rare. For example, it is frequently stated that divorce rates are low amongst couples electing for donor insemination (Clamar, 1980). There are, however, few well conducted empirical studies in this area, and most reports draw upon anecdotal and subjective 'findings'. As Humphrey and Humphrey (1987a) point out, there are few reliable figures available and carefully conducted follow-up studies are required to test these assertions. Conducting such studies is no easy matter however, given the assumption that secrecy is of paramount importance in relation to DI programmes. This involves donor confidentiality and the parents' frequently stated wish to keep their child's origins a secret, in order to protect the social father and the child. The issue of secrecy, in addition to the difficulty the social father might have adjusting to his inability to be the biological father of a child, raise issues concerning the psychological implications of donor insemination.

Secrecy and Donor Insemination

A number of reports document the widespread preference for secrecy voiced by DI couples themselves. Clayton and Kovacs (1982) in a survey of 50 Australian couples some 2 to 4 years after donor insemination report that 68 per cent had decided they would definitely not tell their child of its origins. Eighteen per cent were undecided and only 14 per cent had made up their mind to tell their child at some later date. These figures are not markedly dissimilar to those reported with similar samples in other cultures. Manuel, Chevret and Czyba (1980) report that 77 per cent of 72 DI couples in a French sample preferred absolute secrecy while Owens, Edelmann and Humphrey (1993) found that 74% of 76 couples with male infertility had no intention of telling a child conceived by DI about the mode of conception. Rowland (1985) in a further study in the U.K. found that 56 per cent of couples had already decided before undertaking DI that they would definitely not tell their child its origins. In this latter study 9 per cent of couples had decided they would tell their child and 36 per cent remained undecided suggesting that the figures would eventually come to resemble even more closely those reported by Clayton and Kovacs.

Whether the shift to greater openness which occurred in the case of adoption will also occur with donor insemination remains doubtful. The Warnock Committee (1984) which argued for a gradual move towards more openness prefaced this opinion by stating that the provision of information should not compromise the principle of anonymity. Information should only be given if specially requested and only if its provision was accompanied by appropriate counselling. Several decades ago secrecy was the watchword in the adoption field, whereas now, as Humphrey and Humphrey (1987b) note, parents with an adopted child aim to inform the child at an early age of its adoption and information regarding the genetic parents is now made available to adopted children. There is, however, an essential difference between DI and adoption. The former involves a fundamental difference which is built into the relationship between the genetic mother, the social father and the DI child, in the latter case both partners who raise the child are its social but not genetic parents. Whether secrecy or openness is more or less harmful to the child and its family is impossible to say at present. However, the very existence of secrecy makes it extremely difficult to answer the many questions which need to be addressed with regard to the DI child and his or her family.

Obviously tenuous links can be made with findings from the adoption literature, but the parallels are limited. In their review of the adoption literature Humphrey and Humphrey (1986) conclude that 'where the quality of surrogate family relationships is sufficient to meet the child's emotional needs, then there is no reason why ancestral knowledge should be a prerequisite of mental health' (p. 133). There is no reason to assume that, in the main, the quality of parenting in DI families will be any different from that in families sharing biological parentage. Nevertheless, in the absence of research, a doubt must remain given that male infertility seems to be associated with particular distress and, as Menning (1981) observes, family secrets are among the most pernicious and destructive forces in the family. If it was possible to gain a clearer idea of the difficulties which couples might encounter it would facilitate the provision of appropriate counselling. While counselling for couples contemplating donor insemination is considered to be essential, though not necessarily always available, counselling subsequent to DI is rare. The problems of secrecy make any careful and thorough assessment of the counselling needs of such couples difficult to ascertain. Although secrecy is not associated with IVF the situation regarding counselling needs in that area too is no clearer.

IN VITRO FERTILISATION

A number of studies have administered psychological tests to patients admitted to IVF programmes. Almost without exception these have found little if any difference between scores obtained by such couples and normative data or data from comparison groups (see Edelmann, 1990). Three recent studies will serve as examples. Chan *et al.* (1989) assessed 112 couples consecutively enrolled in the Hong Kong IVF/GIFT programme on measures of personality, anxiety, psychiatric morbidity and depression obtained during a pretreatment interview. The psychological profile of the women was similar to that of normal Chinese pregnant women. Newton, Hearn and Huzpe (1990) found that group means from a very large sample of IVF couples (947 women and 899 men) were well within the clinically normal range for data obtained by postal questionnaire administered some three months before their first IVF attempt. Finally, Edelmann, Connolly and Bartlett (1993) who assessed, on a range of psychological measures, one hundred and fifty two couples who were consecutive referrals for their first IVF cycle, found little variation from the normative range of these measures. Indeed, the only exception to these findings is the occasional report of elevated anxiety in women attending IVF clinics (e.g. Cook *et al.*, 1989; Johnston, Shaw and Bird, 1987). This is likely to be associated with clinic attendance rather than being a particular feature of IVF and is perhaps not surprising. As our own findings indicate, elevated anxiety is found before diagnosis and at first attendance at a specialist clinic; this declines subsequently in spite of the numerous potentially distressing investigative procedures and possible diagnostic outcomes which might be less than positive (Connolly *et al.*, 1992). Indeed, as Johnston, Shaw and Bird (1987) noted, the anxiety levels of their IVF couples were similar to data obtained by their colleagues from women attending an ante-natal clinic during the final two weeks of their pregnancy. Overall there seems to be little reason to assume that couples electing for IVF differ from the range of couples conceiving children by natural means. Indeed, it is possible that only those with stable characteristics and who enjoy stable relationships decide to proceed with IVF and hence submit themselves to the inevitable stressors associated with the procedure.

The Stressful Nature of IVF

Success rates of IVF are relatively low with figures between 12% and 20% representing the norm. A worldwide assessment of 50 IVF programmes revealed a 13% success rate per IVF cycle (Soules, 1985). Yet couples entering IVF treatment programmes tend to be overly optimistic about their chances of success (Johnston, Shaw and Bird, 1987; Reading, 1989). As Johnston, Shaw and Bird (1987) noted, all the men and women in their IVF sample overestimated the likelihood of success, although such optimism is unlikely to be peculiar to those attending IVF clinics. The authors relate their findings to evidence that denial or avoidance are used successfully as coping strategies by surgical patients generally. Overestimation may thus reduce the stress associated with the procedure.

A number of authors (e.g. Leiblum, Kemman and Lane, 1987; Mahlstedt, MacDuff and Bernstein, 1987) have commented on the tremendous emotional strains placed upon couples undergoing IVF. The IVF cycle lasts at least two weeks, involving about one week of outpatient monitoring and one week of clinic care, although aspects of the programme may vary considerably between clinics. Because there is a risk of failure at any of the various stages of the IVF procedure, each cycle of IVF has many potential points of anxiety and distress. These include concerns about the fertilisation process, fear of laparoscopy, pressure on the male to produce a semen sample on demand, anxiety at the time of embryo transfer and the results of pregnancy tests (Greenfeld and Haseltine, 1986). Such concerns and anxieties have been documented in a number of studies.

In the study by Callan and Hennessy (1986) the majority of the 77 women undergoing IVF who were interviewed associated some anxiety with each stage of the programme. The most anxiety provoking episodes were during the initial waiting at home, in hospital just prior to egg collection and during surgery for egg collection. This latter phase was also found to be associated with heightened anxiety in a further study by Johnston, Shaw and Bird (1987) who also found that the first visit to the IVF assessment clinic was a time of particular heightened anxiety. In addition, a general trend towards increasing stress and distress during the IVF treatment cycle was found by Reading, Chang and Kerin (1989), although overall scores remained low compared with normative data. Interestingly, these authors also note that greater distress (as measured by an index of grief) was apparent for women who discontinued at midcycle compared with those who completed the cycle even if they failed to achieve pregnancy. The emotional impact of unsuccessful IVF has been documented in a number of studies which refer to feelings of sadness, anger and depression (e.g. Baram *et al.*, 1988; Leiblum, Kemmann and Lane, 1987). Given the circumstances it would probably be unusual if such reactions were other than the norm for the couples concerned.

In addition to anxiety provoked during the procedure some authors have suggested that anxiety can vary over repeated treament cycles. Johnston *et al.* (1985) have argued that the first and final attempts at IVF are the most anxiety provoking; the first because of the unknown, the latter because it is seen as the 'last chance of pregnancy' for the couples concerned. However, the only empirical investigation to address this issue (Reading, Chang and Kerin, 1989) found no significant effects of repeated treatment upon psychological test results, although these findings were derived from a small sample (N = 37). *In vitro* fertilisation treatment is undeniably stressful for the couple concerned and sadness or depression would be neither unexpected nor unusual reactions to failed attempts. Most couples embarking on IVF are emotionally well adjusted and in stable relationships and thus probably have the coping resources to enable them to deal with the emotional demands involved. There is, however, a clear need to examine the counselling needs of such couples to decide how best to facilitate both their decision making (whether to embark upon IVF treatment and when to withdraw from treatment) and their ability to cope with the procedure and the likelihood of failed attempts.

COUNSELLING NEEDS

The recognition of counselling needs for infertile couples has been made explicit in Britain in two Government publications (Warnock Committee, 1984; Department of Health and Social Security, 1987). Certainly the importance attached to psychosocial support and counselling for involuntarily childless couples has increased over the last decade. Organisations offering support have been established in the U.S.A. (Resolve Inc, see Menning, 1980, 1984) and in Britain (National Association for the Childless – later renamed Issue). We have also discussed counselling needs in relation to in-voluntary childlessness in general (Edelmann and Connolly, 1986) and with regard to DI and IVF in particular (Edelmann, 1989, 1990). Although needs for counselling are widely acknowledged there is limited systematic research. Two studies have drawn upon the large body of research suggesting that adequate and appropriate psychological preparation can reduce distress for a wide range of surgical procedures. Thus Wallace (1984) found that providing patients about to undergo laparoscopic survery for infertility investigation with an informative preparatory booklet, reduced stress responses on measures of pre-operative fear and anxiety, heart rate and blood pressure, and post-operative anxiety. She also found reduced state anxiety on follow-up at both 1- and 6-weeks. In a further report Takefman *et al.* (1990) note that infertile couples given only descriptive information about investigative procedures reacted more positively to the investigation than those who received additional information relating to sexual and emotional reactions to the investigation. However, such studies can only be considered as preliminary and a range of questions remains to be answered. For example, we do not know what form psychological preparation or counselling should take, when it should be provided, or what the couples' needs are in terms of counselling provision.

Indeed, while counselling should be available, this does not necessarily imply that all couples should of necessity avail themselves of it. Many couples may have other resources available or may perceive counselling as a way of screening them from available treatment (IVF or DI) rather than as a means of helping their own decision making or providing them with support. This may be reflected in the findings by Bresnick and Taymor (1979) that of 212 couples offered infertility counselling, less than 30% accepted the referral and Shaw, Johnston and Shaw's report (1988) that when counselling was offered to couples undergoing IVF, only half took it up. The former result closely complements our own findings. When we asked 843 couples who had been seen at an infertility clinic over a 10 year period their retrospective responses to the question 'would you find (or would you have found) it useful to have help/guidance from someone other than the medical specialist?' Only 39.2% replied in the affirmative (Edelmann and Connolly, 1987). We have no way of knowing whether the proportion of infertile couples identified as requesting support would differ from the proportion of fertile couples who would welcome professional counselling to cope with other of life's difficulties (for a discussion of coping strategies employed by infertile couples see Callan and Hennessey, 1989).

In our own study (Edelmann and Connolly, 1987), we also found variations in the expressed preferences for when counselling would be most helpful. If the cause of infertility was attributed to the woman, the preference was for counselling within the first year, while if the cause was attributed to the male there was a preference for counselling after a year had elapsed. This may well relate to the issues discussed earlier concerning the particular difficulties which seem to be associated with male infertility. These men may feel the need to try to come to terms with the situation for themselves first before beginning to discuss it with others. This also emphasises the particular need for counselling provision in relation to DI even if this is only seen as a way of giving the couple, and particularly the male concerned, time to think through the implications of DI before embarking on such a course of action. A further interesting finding from our study was that if both the man and woman were diagnosed as contributing to the infertility then the preference was expressed for support through self-help groups. It appears that when both partners are 'responsible' for the difficulty this may in some way make discussion with others in a similar position more acceptable and more helpful.

Counselling for DI and IVF overlap in their focus. Counselling for such couples may not only serve a supportive function but may also facilitate their decision making, allowing some to, effectively, screen themselves from treatment. The issue of counselling needs after DI has rarely been addressed in the literature. One might assume that the needs of those who conceive will be very different from those who do not. Indeed, because of the issue of secrecy following successful conception with DI it is difficult to ascertain what the couples precise needs may be. Should the child eventually be told, and if so how, when and with what kind of message? As Humphrey and Humphrey (1986) observe, it is hard to know how to advise couples on the question of secrecy although as they acknowledge (Humphrey and Humphrey, 1987b) it is certainly an issue which should be discussed with all clients.

While counselling and support are also essential ingredients of an IVF programme there is limited research to date which addresses the many questions that arise. Thus we do not know the most appropriate stage of the IVF cycle at which support should be provided, what form of support is most useful or which couples might benefit most from this counselling. We have recently conducted a study (Connolly et al., 1993) addressing some of these issues. One hundred and fifty five couples who were consecutive referrals to an IVF clinic were allocated at random to one of two groups. One group received a standard form of counselling based on explaining the various procedures. Another group received, in addition, more extensive and structured counselling support. Counselling was provided at the first clinic visit, at the start of the treatment cycle and after either treatment failure or successful conception. Counselling provision was semi-structured, the same key dimensions being addressed with each client. The results showed the patients to be generally well adjusted with anxiety levels dropping over the course of treatment. Counselling compared to information alone did not lead to any enhanced reduction in levels of anxiety or depression. The nature and extent of counselling support needed by patients undergoing IVF may be quite modest. The challenge for future research is to identify when that support should be provided and which, probably small, proportion of patients might actually need such specialised support.

CONCLUDING COMMENTS

Since our review of the subject (Edelmann and Connolly, 1986) there has been a steady growth of interest in issues relating psychology to infertility. Although a clearer picture is slowly emerging, many of the methodological concerns we raised at that time are, unfortunately, still evident in a great deal of the research carried out to date. This probably accounts for many of the conflicting results obtained and although it clouds the picture certain conclusions now have a somewhat stronger basis. The case for the existence of psychogenic infertility remains unproven, though the balance of evidence is against it. The available studies show little evidence for psychological differences between fertile couples and those who have experienced difficulty in conceiving. It should be borne in mind however that the absence of gross differences on questionnaire measures does not rule out the possibility of subtle hormonal or endocrinological differences which might be mirrored by more sensitive psychological measures. Any future studies, therefore must measure both psychological and biological parameters, the choice of any such measures must be informed by sound theoretical propositions.

Evidence of widespread negative psychological sequalae to diagnosis of infertility also seems to be weaker than is implied by some of those who take up the more extreme positions in this field. It seems that, for the most part, couples presenting for medical investigations relating to their failure to conceive are emotionally stable and exist in a stable, secure relationship. These may well represent a self selected population in that only such couples present for investigation. Clearly infertility is a major life stressor for many but such couples nevertheless cope with their difficulties with little evidence of psychopathology or grave disturbance in interpersonal relationships (Connolly *et al.*, 1992). There are clearly exceptions to this rule and research could usefully be directed towards identifying 'at risk' couples. However, though the picture is generally positive the diagnosis of male infertility may carry a strong potential for psychological morbidity. This is of particular note given that DI, the 'treatment' in such cases, bypasses rather than treats the infertility problem. The secrecy surrounding DI may reflect the distress associated with male infertility but such secrecy also impedes research; we have no way of knowing how DI couples deal with secrecy nor, if they opt for openness, how they and their children might deal with the emotions involved.

The fact that certain couples might be 'at risk' emphasises the need for carefully formulated and organised counselling provision enabling such couples to effectively screen themselves from treatment. The issue of counselling has received scant attention from the research community and questions concerning the form of psychological preparation or support to provide, for whom and when remain to be answered. Research is slowly addressing the important issues but with rapid medical advances it is important not to lose sight of ethical, moral, legal and psychological concerns (Council for Science and Society, 1984).

REFERENCES

Al-Issa, I. (1982). Gender and adult psychopathology. In I. Al-Issa (ed) *Gender and psychopathology*. New York: Academic Press.

Asch, R.H., Balmaceda, J.P., Ellsworth, L.R. & Wong, P.C. (1986). Preliminary experiences with gamete intrafallopian transfer (GIFT). *Fertility and Sterility*, **45**, 366–371.

Baram, D., Tourtelot, E., Meuchler, E. & Huang, K.E. (1988). Psychological adjustment following unsuccessful **in vitro** fertilization. *Journal of Psychosomatic Obstetrics and Gynaecology*, **9**, 181–190.

Bell, J.S. (1983). Psychological aspects. In T.B. Hargreave (ed) *Male Infertility*. Berlin: Springer-Verlag.

Berger, D.M. (1977). The role of the psychiatrist in a reproductive biology clinic. *Fertility and Sterility*, **28**, 141–145.

Berger, D.M. (1980a). Infertility: A psychiatrist's perspective. *Canadian Journal of Psychiatry*, **25**, 553–559.

Berger, D.M. (1990b). Impotence following the discovery of azoospermia. *Fertility and Sterility*, **34**, 154–156.

Bresnick, E.K. (1984). A holistic approach to the treatment of infertility. In M.D. Mazor & H.F. Simons (eds) *Infertility: Medical, Emotional and Social Considerations*. New York: Human Sciences Press.

Bresnick, E. & Taymor, M.L. (1979). The role of counselling in infertility. *Fertility and Sterility*, **32**, 154–156.

Bullock, J.C. (1974). Introgenic impotence in an infertility clinic: An illustrative case. *American Journal of Obstetrics and Gynecology*, **124**, 476–478.

Callan, V.J. & Hennessey, J.F. (1986). IVF and adoption: The experiences of infertile couples. *Australian Journal of Early Childhood*, **11**, 32–36.

Callan, V.J. & Hennessey, J.F. (1989). Strategies for coping with infertility. *British Journal of Medical Psychology*, **62**, 343–354.

Chan, Y.F., Tsoi, M.M., O'Hoy, K.M., Wong, A., So, W.K. & Ho, P.C. (1989). Psychosocial evaluation in an IVF/GIFT program in Hong Kong. *Journal of Reproductive and Infant Psychology*, **7**, 67–77.

Clamar, A. (1980). Psychological implications of donor insemination. *American Journal of Psychoanalysis*, **40**, 853–856.

Clayton, C. & Kovacs, G. (1982). AID offspring. Initial follow-up study of 50 couples. *Medical Journal of Australia*, **?**, 338–339.

Connolly, K.J. & Edelmann, R.J. (1988). Depression and reproductive failure: A comment on Suarez & Gallup. *Journal of Social and Biological Structures*, **11**, 215–217.

Connolly, K.J., Edelmann, R.J. & Cooke, I.D. (1987). Distress and marital problems associated with infertility. *Journal of Reproductive and Infant Psychology*, **5**, 49–57.

Connolly, K.J., Edelmann, R.J., Cooke, I.D. & Robson, J. (1992). The impact of infertility investigations upon psychological functioning. *Journal of Psychosomatic Research*, **36**, 459–468.

Connolly, K.J., Edelmann, R.J., Bartlett, H., Cooke, I.D., Lenton, E. & Pike, S. (1993). An evaluation of counselling for couples undergoing treatment for in-vitro fertilization. *Human Reproduction*, **8** in press.

Cooke, R., Parsons, J., Mason, S. & Golombok, S. (1989). Emotional, marital and sexual functioning in patients embarking upon IVF and AID treatment for infertility. *Journal of Reproductive and Infant Psychology*, **7**, 87–94.

Council for Science and Society (1984). *Human Procreation: Ethical aspects of the new techniques.* Oxford: Oxford University Press.

Department of Health and Social Security (1987). *Human Fertilisation and Embryology: A Framework for legislation.* Cmd 259. London: Her Majesty's Stationary Office.

Edelmann, R.J. (1989). Psychological aspects of artificial insemination by donor. *Journal of Psychosomatic Obstetrics and Gynaecology*, **10**, 3–13.

Edelmann, R.J. (1990). Emotional aspects of *in vitro* fertilization procedures: A review. *Journal of Reproductive and Infant Psychology*, **8**, 161–173.

Edelmann, R.J. & Connolly, K.J. (1986). Psychological aspects of infertility. *British Journal of Medical Psychology*, **59**, 209–219.

Edelmann, R.J. & Connolly, K.J. (1987). The counselling needs of infertile couples. *Journal of Reproductive and Infant Psychology*, **5**, 63–70.

Edelmann, R.J., Connolly, K.J. & Bartlett, H. (1993). Factors influencing the psychological profile of couples presenting for IVF (manuscript submitted).

Edelmann, R.J., Connolly, K.J., Cooke, I.D. & Robson, J. (1991). Psychogenic infertility: Some findings. *Journal of Psychosomatic Obstetrics and Gynaecology*, **12**, 163–168.

Edelmann, R.J. & Golombok, S. (1989). Stress and reproductive failure. *Journal of Reproductive and Infant Psychology*, **7**, 79–86.

Eisner, B.G. (1963). Some psychological differences between fertile and infertile women. *Journal of Clinical Psychology*, **19**, 391–395.

Freeman, E.W., Rickels, K., Tausig, J., Boxer, A., Mastoianni, L. & Tureck, E.W. (1987). Emotional and psychological factors in follow-up of women after IVF-ET treatment: A pilot investigation. *Acta Obstetrica Gynecologica Scandinavica*, **66**, 517–521.

Goldberg, D. (1978). *Manual of the General Health Questionnaire.* Oxford: NFER-Nelson.

Greenfeld, D. & Haseltine, F. (1986). Candidate selection and psychosocial considerations of *in vitro* fertilisation procedures. *Clinical Obstetrics and Gynecology*, **29**, 119–126.

Hammen, C. (1982). Gender and depression. In I. Al-Issa (ed) *Gender and Psychopathology*. New York: Academic Press.

Harrison, R.F., O'Moore, A.M., O'Moore, R.R. & McSweeney, J.R. (1981). Stress profiles in normal infertile couples: Pharmacological and psychological approaches to therapy. In V. Insler & G. Betterndorf (eds) *Advances in Diagnosis and Treatment of Infertility*. Amsterdam: Elsevier-North Holland.

Harrison, R.F., O'Moore, A.M., O'Moore, R.R. & Robb, D. (1984). Stress in infertile couples. In R.F. Harrison, J. Bunnar & W. Thomson (eds) *Fertility and Sterility*. Lancaster: MTP Press.

Hirsch, M.B. & Mosher, W.D. (1987). Characteristics of infertile women in the United States and their use of infertility services. *Fertility and Sterility*, **47**, 618–625.

Houghton, P. (1984). Infertility: The consumer's outlook. *British Journal of Sexual Medicine*, **11**, 185–187.

Humphrey, M. & Humphrey, H. (1986). A fresh look at gyneacological bewilderment. *British Journal of Medical Psychology*, **59**, 133–140.

Humphrey, M. & Humphrey, H. (1987a). Marital relationships in couples seeking donor insemination. *Journal of Biosocial Science*, **19**, 209–219.

Humphrey, M. & Humphrey, H. (1987b). *Surrogate Families: The Handicap of Missing Parents*. London: Tavistock Press.

Humphrey, M., Humphrey H. & Aisworth-Smith, I. (1991). Screening couples for parenthood by donor insemination. *Social Science and Medicine*, **32**, 273–278.

Johnston, M., Shaw, R. & Bird, D. (1987). "Test-tube baby" procedures: Stress and judgements under uncertainty. *Psychology and Health*, **1**, 25–38.

Johnston, W.I.H., Oke, K., Spiers, A., Clarke, G.A., McBain, J., Bayley, C. *et al.* (1985). Patient selection for *in vitro* fertilization: Physical and psychological aspects. *Annals of the New York Academy of Sciences*, **442**, 490–503.

Kedem, P., Mikulincer, M., Mathanson, Y.E. & Bartoov, B. (1990). Psychological aspects of male infertility. *British Journal of Medical Psychology*, **63**, 73–80.

Keep van, P.A. & Schmidt-Elmendorff, H. (1975). Involuntary childlessness. *Journal of Biosocial Science*, **7**, 37–48.

Leiblum, S.R., Kemmann, E. & Lane, M.K. (1987). The psychological concomitants of *in vitro* fertilization. *Journal of Psychosomatic Obstetrics and Gynaecology*, **6**, 165–178.

Link, P.W. & Darling, C.A. (1986). Couples undergoing treatment for infertility: Dimensions of life satisfaction. *Journal of Sex and Marital Therapy*, **12**, 46–59.

Mahlstedt, P.P. (1985). The psychological components of infertility. *Fertility and Sterility*, **43**, 335–346.

Mahlstedt, P.P., MacDuff, S. & Bernstein, J. (1987). Emotional factors and the *in vitro* fertilisation and embryo transfer process. *Journal of In Vitro Fertilisation and Embryo Transfer*, **4**, 232–236.

Manuel, C., Chevret, M. & Czyba, J.C. (1980). Handling of secrecy by AID couples. In G. David & W.S. Price (eds) *Human Artificial Insemination and Semen Preservation*. New York: Plenum Press.

Mao, K. & Wood, C. (1984). Barriers to treatment of infertility by *in vitro* fertilization and embryo transfer. *The Medical Journal of Australia*, **140**, 532–533.

McEwan, K.L., Costello, C.G. & Taylor, P.J. (1987). Adjustment to infertility. *Journal of Abnormal Psychology*, **96**, 108–116.

McGrade, J.J. & Tolor, A. (1981). The reaction to infertility and the infertility investigation a comparison of the responses of men and women. *Infertility*, **4**, 7–27.

Menning, B.E. (1977). *Infertility: A Guide for the Childless Couple*. Englewood Cliffs, NJ: Prentice Hall.

Menning, B.E. (1980). The emotional needs of infertile couples. *Fertility and Sterility*, **34**, 313–319.

Menning, B.E. (1981). Donor insemination: The psychological issues. *Contemporary Obstetrics and Gynecology*, **18**, 155–172.

Menning, B.E. (1984). RESOLVE. Counselling and support for infertile couples. In M.D. Mazor & H.F. Simons (eds) *Infertility: Medical, Emotional and Social Considerations.* New York: Human Sciences Press.

Mosher, W.D. (1985). Reproductive impairments in the United States. 1965-1982. *Demography*, **22**, 415–429.

Mosher, W.D. (1988). Fecundity and infertility in the United States. *American Journal of Public Health*, **78**, 181–182.

Newton, C.R., Hearn, M.T. & B. Yuzpe, A.A. (1990). Psychological assessment and follow-up after *in vitro* fertilization: assessing the impact of failure. *Fertility and Sterility*, **54**, 879–886.

Noyes, R.W. & Chapnick, E.M. (1964). Literature on psychology and infertility. *Fertility and Sterility*, **15**, 543–558.

O'Moore, A.M., O'Moore, R.R., Harrison, R.F., Murphy, G. & Carruthers, M.E. (1983). Psychosomatic aspects of idiopathic infertility: Effects of treatment with autogenic training. *Journal of Psychosomatic Research*, **27**, 145–151.

Owens, D.J., Edelmann, R.J. & Humphrey, M. (1993). Male infertility and donor insemination: couples' decisions, reactions and counselling needs. *Human Reproduction* (in press).

Owens, D.J. & Read, M.W. (1984). Patients' experiences with and assessment of subfertility testing and treatment. *Journal of Reproductive and Infant Psychology*, **2**, 7–17.

Paulson, J.D., Harrman, B.S., Salerno, R.L. & Asmr, P. (1988). An investigation of the relationship between emotional maladjustment and infertility. *Fertility and Sterility*, **49**, 258–262.

Pepperell, R.J. & McBain, J.C. (1985). Unexplained infertility: A review. *British Journal of Obstetrics and Gynaecology*, **92**, 569–580.

Peyser, M.R. (1965). Untoward effects of artificial insemination. *New York State Journal of Medicine*, **6**, 1876–1879.

Pfeffer, N. & Woollett, A. (1983). *The Experience of Infertility.* London: Virago Press.

Raval, H., Slade, P., Buck, P. & Lieberman, B.E. (1987). The impact of infertility on emotions and the marital and sexual relationship. *Journal of Reproductive and Infant Psychology*, **5**, 221–234.

Reading, A.E. (1989). Decision making and *in vitro* fertilization: the influence of emotional state. *Journal of Psychosomatic Obstetrics and Gynaecology*, **10**, 107–112.

Reading, A.E., Chang, L.C. & Kerin, J.F. (1989). Psychological state and coping styles across an IVF treatment cycle. *Journal of Reproductive and Infant Psychology*, **7**, 95–103.

Regan, M.C. & Rowland, H.E. (1985). Rearranging family and career priorities: Professional women and men of the eighties. *Journal of Marriage and the Family*, **47**, 985–992.

Rowland, R. (1985). The social and psychological consequences of secrecy in artificial insemination by donor (AID) programmes. *Social Science and Medicine*, **21**, 391–396.

Saltzer, L.P. (1986). *Infertility: How couples can cope.* Boston, Massachusetts: G.K. Hall & Co.

Seibel, M.M. & Taymor, M.L. (1982). Emotional aspects of infertility. *Fertility and Sterility*, **37**, 137–145.

Shaw, P., Johnston, M. & Shaw, R. (1988). Counselling needs, emotional and relationship problems in couples awaiting IVF. *Journal of Psychosomatic Obstetrics and Gynaecology*, **9**, 171–180.

Slade, P. (1981). Sexual attitudes and social role orientations in infertile women. *Journal of Psychosomatic Research*, **25**, 183–186.

Snowden, R., Mitchell, G.D. & Snowden, E. (1983). *Artificial Reproduction: A social investigation.* London: Allen & Unwin.

Snowden, R. & Snowden, E. (1984). *The Gift of a Child.* London: Allen & Unwin.

Soules, M.R. (1985). The *in vitro* fertilization rate: let's be honest with one another. *Fertility and Sterility*, **43**, 511–513.

Spanier, G.B. (1976). Measuring dydadic adjustment: New scales for assessing the quality of marriage and similar dyads. *Journal of Marriage and the Family*, **38**, 15–28.

Spence, J.T., Deaux, K. & Helmreich, R.L. (1985). Sex roles in contemporary American society. In G. Lindzey & E. Aranson (eds) *Handbook of Social Psychology*. Vol 2 (3rd ed.). New York: Random House.

Steptoe, P.C., Edwards, R.C. & Purdy, J.M. (1980). Clinical aspects of pregnancy established with cleaving embryos grown *in vitro*. *British Journal of Obstetrics and Gynaecology*, **87**, 757–781.

Suarez, S.D. & Gallup, G.G. (1985). Depression as a response to reproductive failure. *Journal of Social and Biological Structures*, **8**, 279–287.

Takefman, J.E., Brender, W., Boivin, J. & Tulandi, T. (1990). Sexual and emotional adjustment of couples undergoing infertility investigation and the effectiveness of preparatory information. *Journal of Psychosomatic Obstetrics and Gynaecology*, **11**, 175–290.

Valentine, D.P. (1986). Psychological impact of infertility: Identifying issues and needs. *Social Work in Health Care*, **11**, 61–69.

Wallace, L.M. (1984). Psychological preparation as a method of reducing the stress of surgery. *Journal of Human Stress*, **10**, 62–69.

Warnock Committee (1984). *Report of the Committee of Inquiry into Human Fertilisation and Embryology*. London: HMSO.

Woollett, A. (1985). Childlessness: Strategies for coping with infertility. *International Journal of Behavioral Development*, **8**, 473–482.

Wright, J., Allard, M., Lecours, A. & Sabourin, S. (1989). Psychosocial distress and infertility: A review of controlled research. *International Journal of Fertility*, **34**, 126–142.

PSYCHOLOGICAL PERSPECTIVES ON YOUNG ADULTS' HEALTH BEHAVIOUR: SOME IMPLICATIONS FOR HEALTH PROMOTION

SIMON MURPHY AND PAUL BENNETT

INTRODUCTION

Many writers have called for a lifecycle approach to the study of behaviour, including that related to health (e.g. Bryman *et al.*, 1987; Allat *et al.*, 1987). The Black Report (Townsend and Davidson, 1988), for example, argues 'that any satisfactory explanation (of health) must build essentially on the ideas of the cumulative dispositions and experience of the lifetime and multiple causation" (p. 104). Nevertheless, there is little coherent theoretical development based on empirical research, relating changes in health and health behaviour to life stage issues. Most research has been confined to childhood and adolescence. This rather exclusive focus may result from theory which sees a strong biological influence upon behaviour at these ages (Flavell, 1970). This biological basis can give directionality, inevitability and a certain uniformity to the cognitive and behavioural changes that are studied. Adult development on the other hand is rooted more firmly in social experience. Here, normative experiences vary greatly between individuals and social groups. Although there may be universal sequences of life events, there are a variety of ways of experiencing and responding to them (Erikson, 1959). This neglect of the adult phase of the lifecycle continues despite a theoretical acceptance that psychological development does not end at adolescence (Rodeheaver and Datan, 1981) and a lack of evidence to suggest strong stability between many childhood and adult health behaviours (Mechanic, 1979).

A lack of a developmental focus is compounded by more general theoretical and research problems. The majority of the relevant empirical research focuses on single health risk behaviours, the so called 'holy four' of diet, drinking, smoking and exercise (McQueen, 1987). Taken together, these are often used as a measure of lifestyle but with little examination of their relationship with other health behaviours. This concentration on single risk factors associated with morbidity and mortality remains despite the fact that health risk behaviours are not found in isolation (Badura, 1984; Kaplan, 1984; Belloc and Breslow, 1972; Harris and Gutren, 1979; Langlie, 1979) and clear evidence that they interact to predict health and disease (e.g. Breslow and Enstrom, 1980). In addition, there is a frequent failure to examine the social context of health behaviour (Bunton, Murphy and Bennett, 1991; Dean, 1989). This is surprising given theories which see health not as a static element but a response to social (Herzlich, 1973) and environmental influences (Anderson, 1984).

These issues make a review of a life cycle perspective on young adults' health behaviours particularly problematic, and emphasise the need to formulate a conceptual framework to guide related theory and research. Firstly, there is a need to define 'young adults' in terms of developmental tasks. Psychologists have identified such developmental tasks as entering into an intimate relationship, marriage, beginning family responsibilities and developing the groundwork for an occupation or career (Erikson, 1959; Havinghurst, 1973; Pikunas, 1976). Women's experiences of these tasks have been shown to differ considerably from those of men, with far less separation between the spheres of work and family (Rubin, 1980). These tasks represent the development of the adult role (Levinson, 1986). However, it should be noted that such a definition is largely based on research conducted with white middle class Americans.

The basis for a conceptual framework can be identified in a number of areas. Mendoza (1990) defines lifestyles as an outcome of the interaction between reactions learned via socialisation and the prevailing social conditions. Similar definitions are provided by Milo (1981) and Abel (1991). Milo sees lifestyles as patterns of behaviour, whose availability is determined by socio-economic circumstances and the ability to choose one behaviour over another. Abel (1991) has asserted that this approach has a basis in the work of Max Weber who defined lifestyle as the 'stylisation of life' used for particular social groups to evolve and maintain status within society. This stylisation, Abel argues, allows us to differentiate groups of individuals that hold similar and meaningful patterns of behaviours, attitudes, norms and values. It arises from the determinants of life chances and life conduct; in other words the structural conditions one lives within and the personal choices one makes.

This separation between life chances and conduct is present implicitly or explicitly in much of the literature examining health inequalities in terms of cultural/behavioural or materialist/structuralist analysis (Whitehead, 1988; Townsend and Davidson, 1988). The former attempts to explain patterns of health in terms of the different behaviours that social groups adopt and the latter by the social conditions people live under. Much of the theoretical development and research conducted in this area tends to concentrate on one of these aspects to the exclusion of the other. However, the distinction between these approaches has been questioned by a number of writers who argue that behaviour can not be examined outside its social context (Blane, 1985; Blaxter, 1983). The interaction between these variables remains complex and a number of explanatory theories which have attempted to link them have been criticised as inadequate (e.g. Blaxter and Paterson, 1982; Pill and Stott, 1985).

The present chapter represents an attempt to identify some of the social and individual determinants of health behaviours of young adults. In doing so we realise that many of the factors we have attempted to isolate for the purpose of clarity are in fact strongly inter-related. Equally, concepts of health and appropriate behaviour have strong generational biases. Differences between young adults and older people may represent as much inter-generational differences (for example, in terms of education) as time or stage related changes. We also acknowledge that to review adequately all the relevant literature is not possible within the confines of such a brief and wide-ranging chapter. We therefore focus on particular issues as exemplars and, where possible, we have identified related reviews for the interested reader.

AN INTERACTIVE MODEL OF HEALTH BEHAVIOUR

The explanatory model adopted by the World Health Organisation cited by Mendoza (1990) identifies four interacting factors which combine to determine health behaviours; genetic or acquired individual features; the micro-social environment such as family friends and work, the macro-social environment such as economics and the media, and the physical environment. The final dimension, the physical environment, has more limited psychological relevance, particularly in relation to young adults, and due to space limitations will not be discussed here. Taking this as a broad structure, the influence of each factor on young adults' health behaviours will be reviewed. In doing so, we hope to indicate areas for potential further exploration within health psychology.

Individual Features

Three broad categories of literature appear to be relevant to this area; formal predictive models of health behaviour (e.g. Ajzen and Fishbein, 1980) the implications of age-related cognitive developments on health behaviour (e.g. Rodeheaver and Datan, 1981), and adult constructions of health and health maintaining factors (e.g. Blaxter, 1990).

The first strand of research stems from an endeavour to develop formal psychological models in an attempt to explain why people engage in a variety of health behaviours. With few exceptions, these have not been age specific and are thought to effect behaviour throughout the adult lifespan. Models include the theory of reasoned (Ajzen and Fishbein, 1980) or planned (Ajzen, 1985) behaviour, the Health Belief Model (HBM; Becker, 1974) and social learning theory, in particular that relating to the multi-dimensional health locus of control (MHLC) and value for health (Lau and Ware, 1982; Wallston et al., 1978).

The theory of reasoned action has been found to explain significant percentages of variance in a variety of health and other behaviours. For example, in a recent meta-analytic review of 85 studies, Sheppard et al. (1988) calculated a mean R of 0.67. Despite this success the model is not without its critics. Sarver (1983), for example, suggested that the model does not include the necessity for the *opportunity* for behaviour consonant with beliefs and attitudes. He also identifies the limitations of the model in explaining routine behaviours, such as tooth brushing. As a partial response to such criticism, Ajzen (1985) has further developed the theory of planned behaviour, which includes a dimension of behavioural control, similar to Bandura's notion of self-efficacy. Adding variables similar to perceived control contributes to better prediction of behavioural intentions concerning dental hygiene (McCaul et al., 1988) and both intentions and behaviours concerning alcohol use (Schlegel, Crawford and Sanborn, 1977) and breast self examination (Ronis and Kaiser, 1989).

The HBM is also relatively weak in predicting long term health behaviours such as exercise and tooth brushing or discontinuing undesirable behaviours (Kirscht, 1983). However, it is more successful in predicting behaviours which are not repetitive and where health considerations are closely linked to the action, such as attendance at screening (e.g. Calnan, 1984). The HBM may be more pertinent to the middle years, when there are more cues to action than in the younger years. In addition, health consequences of behaviours such as smoking are accorded little consideration by young people when initiating smoking but may become more salient in later years.

Finally, the MHLC has been used to predict a wide range of health behaviours in young adults including tobacco and alcohol consumption (Winefield *et al.*, 1989; Calnan, 1989) and engaging in physical activity (Carlson and Petti, 1989; Calnan, 1989). Whilst the model seems to hold for a variety of behaviours, in that high internal scores are associated with higher engagement in 'healthy' behaviours and higher chance scores are associated with lower involvement in such behaviours, the percentage of variance in any outcome measure explained by the MHLC has generally been low. Whilst such results may be partly explained by a failure to take into account individual's value for health (see Wallston, chapter 4) the results do suggest that the MHLC may be a better predictor of discrete behaviours such as attendance at screening (e.g. Norman, 1990), than more generalised 'lifestyle' behaviours. In addition, although younger people typically report higher Internal MHLC scores than middle-aged and older persons they also rate their value for health as lower (Bennett *et al.*, in press; Calnan, 1989) and therefore may be less motivated to engage in health protective behaviours.

These formal psychological models may be developed further by taking account of age-related cognitions and lay beliefs rooted in the life cycle. Cognitive developments central to adulthood are characterised by the dialectic between remembrance and anticipation (Rodeheaver and Datan, 1981). The former lead to increasing perceptions of competence and control over one's life; the latter to feelings of vulnerability as experiences are judged in terms of 'time left'. This suggests that young adults experience a period of both behavioural entrenchment, as autonomy and control are exerted, but also potential behavioural change as they come to confront perceptions of morbidity and mortality. Cognitive developments at this stage are also closely tied to changes in important others (Erikson, 1959). This involves responses to the influence of same age peers, partners, and parents as they move from middle to old age. These influences grow in importance as the individual changes from active assimilator to passive accommodator of the social changes around them.

A third group of studies has attempted to construct models of lay perceptions of health and a minority have examined how these differ according to life stage. For example, Blaxter (1990) found that young adults were most likely to pinpoint health as being associated with an absence of 'bad habits' such as smoking and drinking, reflecting conventionally defined causes of illness rather than concepts of health. Although younger women identified fitness as a component of health, they also placed emphasis on concepts of energy and vitality or a combination of the two. These included concepts such as liveliness and alertness exemplified by not staying in bed and having good relationships with family and friends. For men and women approaching middle age concepts of health became much more complex and diffuse, emphasising a more rounded state encompassing both physical and mental well being. This included such things as being happy and relaxed and living life to the full. The idea of vitality remained, but for older men this was expressed in terms of enthusiasm for paid work and for older women, the ability to tackle house work. Women in particular, defined health in terms of social fulfilment including their attitude towards, and their ability to get on with, others.

The Micro-Social Environment

The importance of the micro-social environment's influence on behaviour is illustrated by Cullen (1979), who in a study of working class households found that respondents felt that ninety percent of their waking day involved no real choices but involved an adaption to a relatively stable long term environment. Various attempts have been made to assess the impact of the social environment and life events on health behaviours and health. Some (e.g. Holmes and Rahe, 1967) have argued that life changes *per se* are stressful, whilst others have questioned this assumption and focused on negative life experiences as predictors of ill health (Vinokur and Selzer, 1975; Sarason, Johnson and Siegel, 1978). Both approaches fail to take into account modifying factors which interact with events to determine outcome. For example, supportive social networks may serve both to reduce stress and facilitate health enhancing behaviours (Cohen and Syme, 1985; Turner, 1983). Gottlieb and Green (1984) found that married men and women (and those with a good social network) used less tobacco and alcohol at times of stress. Conversely, Harrell (1986) reported that increasing dissatisfaction with marital life or perceived conflict between one's partner's work and marriage was linearly associated with alcohol consumption.

Peer and Family Influence

Family socialisation forms the basis of many of our health beliefs and behaviours (Fleck, 1975). Mechanic (1980) and Lau (1988), amongst others have also identified peers as important socialising agents, although the relative influence of the family and peers remains unclear. A longitudinal study by Lau *et al.* (1990) concluded that the parental influence is strongest and will persist unless the child is exposed to important social models whose beliefs and behaviour differ to those of their parents during what they term 'windows of vulnerability'. Two of these 'windows' occur when a person sets up a home environment for themselves or with a significant other away from parental control. The influence of a 'significant other' on young adults is supported by Backett (1990) who found interactional and situational constraints on men's and women's opportunities to talk to each other about their health and in the acceptability of health concepts that can be raised in the home environment. For example, whilst women found many contexts to raise issues of health such as diet, exercise and preventive health behaviour, men felt they could only discuss issues directly related to illness or to physical fitness or sports.

Because of the complex nature of the roles in family life, a number of theorists have called for an examination of the contextual and situational aspects of health behaviours in families (Alonzo, 1979; Graham, 1985). If this is done over time, changes in the social context of each member can also be examined. For example, Backett (1990) found very different patterns of health behaviours between the sexes. Young men were much more likely than young women to exercise regularly. For many women, routine exercise came below other family commitments, despite them expressing a desire to exercise. Women with young children report having the least time for leisure activities (Deem, 1982; Green *et al.*, 1986; OPCS, 1982).

Literature examining the role of women within the family and the implications for their own health represents a rich source of theory and data (see for example Graham, 1984; Oakley, 1974). However, as Oakley (1987) suggests, "both the official statistics and the social scientists have inflated gender-specific links between men and work and women and the home – so the key processes of the jigsaw to do with women and work and men and the home are missing" (p. 25). Nevertheless, the evidence suggests that many women have day-to-day control over a number of health related factors within the household although related 'policies' may result from negotiation by family members. For example, although many women still control the content of individual meals (as they do the cooking), families' overall diet is often a negotiated compromise between the needs of differing factions (Kerr and Charles, 1983). Food choice is not a didactic top-down decision. Mintel (1991) found that children between the ages of five and twelve have a significant influence on their parents shopping choice. Parents food choice may also be influenced by children's health needs and eating habits, such as vegetarianism. In addition, many parents attempt to provide a 'healthy' role model. This may lead to health enhancing behavioural change by parents, but more often than not leads to furtive behaviour (Backett, 1990) to avoid children observing smoking and poor dietary habits.

Maintenance of health damaging behaviour may also result from the pressures of parenthood, particularly where material circumstances are poor and resources are low. A number of studies (e.g. Graham, 1976) have identified smoking as a convenient way to relieve tension while supervising a child and to cope with excessive workloads. Jacobson (1981) found that working class women were well aware of the danger to their health from smoking. However, they placed the health needs of their family above their own and gave time and effort into running the family under difficult circumstances rather than attempting to stop smoking. In addition, parents in difficult circumstances may ensure an adequate diet for their child by sometimes doing without food themselves (Burghes, 1980). Of course, family related life events may also contribute more positively to lifestyle change. For example, Waterson and Murray-Lyon (1989) found that about a fifth of women, predominantly aged below 35 years, who smoked before pregnancy stopped during the pregnancy, and an even greater percentage stopped drinking more than the recommended 10 units per week. A smaller percentage of fathers reduced their consumption of tobacco and alcohol (Waterson *et al.*, 1990).

Surprisingly perhaps, parental death, even when premature, has been found to have little impact on the next generation's health behaviour (Backett, 1990). This may reflect a belief that successive generation's lives are very different in terms of social attitudes and material circumstance. Consequently, children view their parents' behaviour and any consequent morbidity to disease as a response to harsher social conditions and a result of erroneous cultural beliefs and a lack of education. In other words, individual's view health risk against socio-economic and cultural circumstances (see also Blaxter and Paterson, 1982). In addition, adult respondents viewed their lives as more structured, moderate and sensible than in their youth. One further inter-generational factor cannot be ignored. Older parents can influence their children's health in more direct ways if they become physically dependent on them. This can result in re-negotiation of support networks, exercise and leisure time, and family diet.

It can also result in increased pressure over family commitments. Care for declining parents often falls to women and changes existing interaction patterns (Yeandle, 1984) as well as restricting the time and material resources necessary for healthy behaviours (Graham, 1984).

Paid Employment
Material working conditions and work-related stress have been shown to have an important influence on health. The Black Report (Townsend and Davidson, 1988) stated that "the variable of occupational class is in itself multifaceted and its influence probably varies according to age or stage in the life-cycle" (p. 104). The steepest gradient in mortality between age and occupation was in the under 45s. Few studies, however, have examined how these factors combine to produce this increase in relative risk. Indeed it is possible that there are no factors specific to those under 45 years which make them particularly vulnerable to work stress. These data may represent a survival effect; that is, those who survive to 45 years are less vulnerable to adverse life circumstances including those related to the work environment. Alternatively, young adults may encounter more stresses, and be affected to a greater degree, due to higher levels of job mobility, advancement, and perhaps disillusionment, at this time.

There is strong evidence that work stress is linked to a number of unhealthy methods of stress reduction. For example, Ames and Janes (1987) found heavy drinking in North American blue collar workers to be related to job alienation, job stress, inconsistent social controls and the evolution of a drinking culture. Men are more likely to engage in alcohol consumption than women (Staats and Staats, 1982). Bromet *et al.* (1988) found lack of job control combined with high job demands (i.e. conditions of high strain) to be associated with high levels of alcohol consumption. Relocation stress can result in a number of negative emotional states with accompanying increased alcohol or drug use (Gaylord and Symons, 1986). A similar picture is found for smoking. Westman, Eden and Shirom (1985) reported high numbers of work hours, lack of control and support were each positively associated with smoking intensity. More recently, Karasek (1990) found increased smoking to be associated with job change in women but not men. A more positive coping behaviour, exercise, was found to be applicable to men but not women by Gottlieb and Green (1984).

Also important in this context is how work is used to adapt to 'life-cycle squeezes' (Moen *et al.*, 1983) when a family's financial demands become greater than its resources. Oppenheimer (1974, 1982) has identified three such squeezes, the first when young couples attempt to set up homes together, the second in middle age when supporting older children and the third in retirement. This often means that one person has to work longer or a partner has to go out to part- or full-time work. This can result in deleterious consequences for, more often than not, women's health. For example, Arber *et al.* (1985) found full time working mothers under 40 showed many more symptoms of ill health than part-time workers. They also found that the beneficial effects of work outside the home were dependent on social circumstances and family responsibilities, with the most detrimental effects experienced by women with insufficient financial resources to help support their multiple roles.

The Macro-Social Environment

Numerous studies of differences in the health status of social classes have pointed to the role of socio-economic factors in preventing or increasing rates of ill health (e.g. Marmot *et al.*, 1991; Townsend and Davidson, 1988; Whitehead, 1988). Reviewing the influence of micro-social environments highlights the often confusing relationship between socio-economic status and health. As a multifaceted variable it includes not only income, property, savings, and housing but other factors such as education and work experiences. What is clear is that even when incomes increase in society as a whole those at the lower end of the socio-economic scale experience relatively smaller health gains in relation to overall developments. The Black Report calls this 'the maintenance of big differences in life chances against the dynamic background of a growing economy' (p. 122).

The influence of socio-economic status on many health related behaviours such as smoking, alcohol consumption, diet and exercise has been well documented (Townsend and Davidson, 1988; Whitehead, 1988). Lack of money for example has been found to be the major factor in restricting healthy food choices (Lang, 1984; Graham, 1984) and working class men (in particular young men) drink and smoke more in relation to those in higher socio-economic groups (e.g. Bennett, Smith and Nugent, 1991; Marmot, Shipley and Rose, 1984). Quality of life, in part mediated by material circumstances, may also moderate motivation to engage in health protective behaviours. As one young adult respondent in a recent interview study suggested, "a wish to sustain life has to be coupled with a will towards life. If you don't like what you've got you won't try to keep it very long" (Bremble, Bennett and Morgan, 1992).

Despite these acknowledged differences in risk behaviour varying with socio-economic satatus, differences in mortality and morbidity cannot be explained simply by behavioural factors. In a second major study of British civil servants Marmot *et al.* (1991) found that differences in death rates from CHD between different grades could not be accounted for by variations in smoking obesity, serum cholesterol, blood pressure or physical activity. Similarly, Blaxter (1990) concluded that income and the quality of housing were the primary determinants of the health of much of the population. It was amongst those who were not environmentally vulnerable that harmful behavioural habits such as smoking appeared to have a greater effect. In short, behavioural factors have a considerably stronger influence on the health of those in good material circumstances than those in poorer circumstances.

Perceived health status may also be more linked to social class and occupation than lifestyle. Abel *et al.* (1989) found that high perceived health status in higher socio-economic status groups was not substantially mediated by participation in healthy lifestyles. Concepts of health have also been shown to vary depending on the individuals socio-economic position. A French study by d'Houtaud and Field (1984), for example, found that manual workers had basic concepts of health, such as absence of illness. Only further up the socio-economic scale did concepts such as personal enjoyment become more frequently reported.

SOME IMPLICATIONS FOR HEALTH PROMOTION

Over the last two decades a number of major health promotion initiatives have focused on the prevention of coronary heart disease. These are of particular interest in that they have directly attempted to change the behaviours of young adults, as behaviour established at this time may have a profound effect on the later health (through family health practices) of them and their children. In addition, they still provide the best documented studies of the effectiveness of health promotion programmes directly informed by psychological theories including social learning theory (Bandura, 1977), McGuire's (1984) model of persuasive communication as well as the theory of reasoned action and HBM. Although the details of programmes differed, a number of core manipulations were common to the two most widely known programmes in North Karelia (Puska *et al.*, 1985) and Stanford (Farquhar *et al.*, 1977). The Stanford Project involved a high profile publicity campaign and individual counselling for a group of people found to be at particularly high risk for coronary heart disease (CHD). The North Karelia Project also involved media campaigns in addition to a number of environmental changes, education programmes and risk factor screening programmes. In both interventions, media output was phased in an attempt to be maximally effective. The first phase comprised information about the health costs of risk behaviours such as smoking, a diet high in saturated fat and so on. This was not intended to result in change; more to alert the population of the benefits of such change. The next phase involved vicarious modelling and skills teaching. Thus, for example, television programmes were transmitted showing how 'ordinary' people were able to stop smoking. This phase of the media campaign was followed by triggers or cues to action to either promote or maintain any appropriate behavioural change.

Attention was also given to changing social norms. For example, in North Karelia much was made of the fact that the recommended diet was in fact more traditional to North Karelia than the, then, present high fat diet and a vegetarian athlete was used as an example that eating meat was not the only way to be strong. Environmental contingencies were also set up to enhance or maintain behaviour change. For example, in North Karelia, shops were encouraged to display 'No smoking' signs, low fat sausages were produced at a local sausage factory and the county dairy actively promoted low fat products. The manipulation of control and marketing has been further developed in the United Kingdom in the Heartbeat Wales project (Nutbeam and Catford, 1987), which negotiated with producers and retailers to develop healthy eating restaurants (low fat choices, no smoking area and so on), food labelling, the sale of low fat dairy and meat products and so on. In addition, project members negotiated with brewers to encourage the sale of low alcohol drinks in their public houses and to promote the concept of a 'healthy pub' with non-smoking bars, increased provision of soft drinks, coffee etc. These manipulations perhaps represent the increasing importance placed on changing both individual behaviour and the context of the behaviour.

All the interventions made extensive use of 'lay' opinion leaders to promote change. In North Karelia and Wales, these comprised individuals, particularly doctors and nurses, identified as opinion leaders who were asked to promote appropriate behavioural change. In the Stanford project, a number of people found to be within the tenth percentile for risk for CHD were identified, received individual counselling in behaviour change techniques, and were then asked to educate friends and colleagues about how to minimise their risk for CHD. Each person reported discussing health related issues with, on average six other people.

Evaluation of the effectiveness of these programmes, and by extension, the utility of the theories underpinning their development has proven difficult. In North Karelia, following a five year intervention phase there was evidence of significant reductions in smoking amongst North Karelian men in comparison to smoking levels in a contiguous comparison area, although the levels of women's smoking had *risen* at the same rate as this area. Levels of serum cholesterol reduced significantly in men (but not women) but no more than in the control area. A relative lowering of systolic (but not diastolic) blood pressure was found for both men and women. However, it is difficult to attribute these to behavioural changes as nearly 10% of the North Karelian population had been screened (and presumably treated if necessary) for raised blood pressure. In addition, Salonen (1987) one of the principal investigators questioned whether even these changes could be attributed to the programme. He suggested that the results may be attributable, at least in part, to naturally occurring differential changes in CHD morbidity rates in the intervention and control areas, changes in the North Karelian population (with an influx of urbanities), and a general increase in the standard of living. The assessment of effectiveness of the Stanford project ran into similar problems of interpretation, in particular due to differentially greater drop out amongst high risk subjects and the possible differential priming and reactive effects of repeated measurements and feedback on risk status in intervention and control subjects (Leventhal *et al.*, 1980). Many of these research issues have been resolved in the later Stanford Five Communities Project (Farquhar *et al.*, 1985 and 1990). However, it is likely that the use of traditional quasi-experimental designs will never provide an unambiguous result indicating success or failure of these programmes (Nutbeam *et al.*, 1993).

The majority of health promotion programmes which are rooted in theory, have attempted to directly change components of individual behaviour, such as attitudes, values, motives and intentions. More recently, theories of behavioural change that have been discussed within health promotion (see for example, *Health Education Research, Theory and Practice*, 1991, part 2, special edition on theory) have shifted from pure psychological models of change to more socio-psychological models. This is represented by an increasing emphasis on the socio-cultural influences on behaviour change. We have previously argued (Bunton, Murphy and Bennett, 1991) that whilst it is crucial to be able to identify (and indeed to modify) individual, inner elements, there is a danger of treating such features as static entities. Individual elements of belief, value, attitude and intention exist and are constructed, maintained or changed through social interaction (Douglas, 1971). In health promotion, as perhaps in health psychology, there is a need to develop further lines of research and interest, towards a further understanding of collective behaviour in organisational and community settings. From this approach health behaviour would be examined as an aspect of the collective production of community – as a dynamic product, and organisational, community and other sub-cultures would become important foci for interventions. Reviewing young adults' health behaviour has questioned the assumption of relatively stable features of social life in which health beliefs, attitudes and value are maintained. Instead, we must look at how routine aspects of health behaviour are accomplished, maintained and the part they play in the organisation of everyday activities.

Active, self-regenerating belief systems and their social and economic underpinnings form part of the social processes which are central to any analysis of behaviour change. Such an approach requires alternative methods of planning and evaluating health promotion programmes which supplement, rather than replace, more psychologically orientated features of the other models. Understanding health behaviour as an interaction between individual features, the micro and the macro-social environment, and different stages in the life cycle raises a number of implications for health promotion. To begin with, designing effective health promotion initiatives may require an understanding of the beliefs and cognitions of differential groups in society, in terms of both life cycle stages and social and material circumstances. As we have suggested, the interaction between age and material conditions result in a variety of beliefs about what constitutes health, as well as offering different opportunities for health enhancing and health damaging behaviours. These differences are particularly pronounced between men and women and additionally across socio-economic groups. Health promotion may therefore need to adopt highly targeted initiatives. For example, the need to address structural elements is much more pronounced amongst working class groups. Additionally, the needs of working class women are very different to working class men and are tied to particular stages of the life cycle. There is also a need to fully address the context of behaviour.

One particular concern of health promotion has been understanding the process of transmission of information stemming from health promotion programmes. This is brought into sharp focus by the potential effects of the social processes of dissemination. At present a dominant paradigm within health promotion has been to measure the effects of the *agent* of intervention – the education programme, community project, mass media campaign or multi-level demonstration project – on some outcome measure. This approach tends to assume that change in behaviour is either mostly or solely the result of outside intervention. It places emphasis on the success or failure of the communication and intervention strategy at the expense of an understanding of the manner in which messages and programmes are received and responded to.

A more dynamic view of social reproduction, depicts social structures as the outcome, not of individual actions, but of recurrent collective social practices (Giddens, 1979). From this point of view social structures are maintained largely by the outcome of collective and negotiated forms of interaction. Families, workplace institutions and communities continually reproduce more or less stable features of the social world. Socialisation, particularly in adult life, is the process of the acquisition of a new set of interpretive procedures (Cicourel, 1971; Speier, 1971). Such acquisition is achieved continuously by taking part in the reproduction of social life in many different settings. Richards (1976) has identified some recurrent problems when these processes are ignored. These problems arise as a result of failure to account for social structure and subcultural process. A number of health promotion initiatives suggest ways forward using more interactive methods. Work conducted by Dorn (1983) and Warwick *et al.* (1988) has pointed to ways of incorporating social processes and context into health initiatives. Health initiatives themselves have been shown to be capable of using cultural processes instead of working against them. Recent examples of the health promotion initiatives within the workplace have begun to move beyond the individual to encompass the psycho-social context (Terris, 1977; Godin and Shepard, 1984; Mullen, 1992) by taking a symbolic interactionism perspective to examining how meanings emerge in the work environment.

In conclusion, both health psychology and health promotion needs to more fully address the concept of life cycle. In doing so, one is forced to examine the elements of age, socially constructed perceptions and the large influence of the social environment on behaviour. Educational strategies should be closely tied to research on belief systems and the social context of behaviour. The use of action research, phased or episodic research and evaluation work would be particularly important here. Strategies should be designed within the cultural context using people's own beliefs and practices to inform and implement them. Perhaps most importantly future developments in theory and 'research' may well require an interactionism perspective to understand the social processes that influence health behaviour and to determine the outcome of health promotion initiatives. The World Health Organisation has pointed to a multi-level approach to health promotion. This covers enabling factors such as skills for adopting healthy behaviours (WHO, 1986), developing appropriate public health policies, (WHO, 1988) and an explicit concern with the development of political economic, social, and physical environments which are supportive of health (WHO, 1991). Many of these ideas, although theoretically developed require practical application. Health psychologists may have a powerful influence on bringing these ideas to reality.

Acknowledgements
Many thanks to Christopher Smith for his comments on this chapter and to Ruth Miller and Sue Avery for typing it.

REFERENCES

Abel, T., Cockerham, W.C., Lueschen, G. & Kunz, G. (1988). Health lifestyles and self-direction in employment among American men: A test of the spill over effect. *Social Science and Medicine*, **28**, 1269–1274.

Abel, T. (1991). Measuring Health Lifestyles in a Comparative Analysis: Theoretical Issues and Empirical Findings. *Social Science and Medicine*, **32**, 889–908.

Ajzen, I. (1985). From intentions to action: a theory of planned behavior. In J. Kuhl & J. Beckman (eds) *Action control: from cognition to behaviour*. Heidelberg: Springer.

Ajzen, I. & Fishbein, M. (1980). *Understanding attitudes and predicting social behaviour*. Englewood Cliffs, NJ: Prentice Hall.

Allat, P., Keil, T., Bryman, A. & Bytheway, B. (eds) (1987). *Women and the Lifecycle*. London: Macmillan Press.

Alonzo, A. (1979). Everyday illness behaviour: a situational approach to health status alleviations. *Social Science and Medicine*, **13A**, 397–404.

Ames, G.M. & Janes, C.R. (1987). Heavy and problem drinking in an American blue-collar population: Implications for prevention. *Social Science and Medicine*, **25**, 949–960.

Anderson, R. (1984).Health Promotion an overview. European Monographs on *Health and Education Research*, **6**, 1–76.

Arber, S., Gilbert, G. & Dale, A. (1985). Paid employment and women's health a benefit or a source of role strain? *Sociology of Health and Illness*, **7**, 375–400.

Backett, K. (1990). Studying Health in Families: A Qualitative Approach. In Cunningham, S. Burly & N. McKeganey (eds) *Readings in Medical Sociology*. London: Routledge.

Badura, B. (1984). Social epidemiology in theory and practice. *European Monographs on Health Education Research*, **5**.

Bandura, A. (1977). *Social Learning Theory*. Englewood Cliffs, NJ: Prentice Hall.

Baronowski, T. & Nader, P. (1986). Family Health Behaviour. In D. Turk & R. Kerns (eds) *Health Illness and Families: A Life Span Perspective*. Wiley: New York.

Belloc, N. & Breslow, L. (1972). Relationship of physical health status and health practices. *Preventive Medicine*, **1**, 409–421.

Becker, M.H. (1974). *The health belief model and personal health behavior*. Thorofare, NJ: Charles B. Slack.

Bennett, P., Smith, C. & Nugent, Z. (1991). Patterns of drinking in Wales. *Alcohol and Alcoholism*, **26**, 367–374.

Bennett, P., Moore, L., Smith, A., Murphy, S. & Smith, C. (in press). Health locus of control and value for health as predictors of dietary behaviour. *Psychology and Health*.

Blane, D. (1985). An Assessment of the Black Report's Explanations of Health Inequalities. *Sociology of Health and Illness*, **7**, 423–445.

Blaxter, M. (1983). The causes of disease: women talking. *Social Science and Medicine*, **17**, 59–64.

Blaxter, M. & Paterson, E. (1982). *Mothers and daughters: a three generational study of health attitudes and behaviours*. London: Heinemann.

Blaxter, M. (1990). *Health and Lifestyles*. London: Tavistock.

Bremble, A., Bennett, P. & Morgan, M. (1991). Explaining health behaviours: a pilot study. *Unpublished manuscript*.

Breslow, L. & Enstrom, J.E. (1980). Persistence of health habits and their relationship to mortality. *Preventive Medicine*, **9**, 469–483.

Bromett, E.J., Dew, M.A., Parkinson, D.K. & Schulberg, H.C. (1988). Predictive effects of occupational and marital stress on the mental health of a male workforce. *Journal of Organisational Behaviour*, **9**, 1–13.

Bryman, A., Bytheway, B., Allat P. & Keil, T. (eds) (1987). *Rethinking the Life Cycle*. London: Macmillan Press.

Bunton, R., Murphy, S. & Bennett, P. (1991). Theories of behavioural change and their use in health promotion: Some neglected areas. *Health Education Research, Theory and Practice*, **6**, 153–162.

Burghes, L. (1980). '*Living from hand to mouth: a study of 65 families living on supplementary Benefit*' Child Poverty Action Group/Family Services Unit.

Calnan, M. (1984). The health belief model and participation in programmes for the early detection of breast cancer. *Social Science and Medicine*, **19**, 823–830.

Calnan, M. (1989). Control over health and patterns of health related behaviour. *Social Science and Medicine*, **29**, 131–136.

Carlson, B.R. & Petti, K. (1989). Health locus of control and engagement in physical activity. *American Journal of Health Promotion*, **3**, 32–37.

Cicourel, A.V. (1971). The Acquisition of social structure: toward a developmental sociology of language and meaning. In J. Douglas (ed) *Understanding Everyday Life*. London: Routledge and Kegan Paul.

Cohen, S. & Syme, L. (1985). *Social Support and Health*. New York: Academic Press.

Cullen, I. (1979). Urban social policy and problems of family life: the use of an extended diary method to inform decision analysis. In C. Harris (ed) The sociology of the family: new directions in Britain. *Sociological Review Monograph 28*. University of Keele.

d'Houtard, A. & Field, M. (1984). The image of health: variations in perception by social class in a French population. *Sociology of Health and Illness*, **6**, 30–60.

Dean, K. (1989). Self care Components of Lifestyles: The Importance of Gender, Attitudes and the Social Situation. *Social Science and Medicine*, **29**, 137–157.

Deem, R. (1982). Women, leisure and inequality. *Leisure Studies*, **1**, 29–46.

Dorn, N. (1983). *Alcohol, Youth and the State*. London: Croom Helm.

Douglas, M. (ed) (1971). *Understanding Everyday Life: Toward the Reconstruction of Sociological Knowledge*. London: Routledge and Kegan Paul.

Erikson, E.H. (1959). Identity and the life cycle: Selected papers. *Psychological Issues*, **1**, 50–100. New York: International Universities Press.

Farquhar, J.W., Fortman, S.P., Maccoby, N., Haskell, W.L., Williams, P.T., Flora, J.A.,

Taylor, C.B., Brown, B.W., Solomon, D.S. & Hulley, S.B. (1985). The Stanford five city project: design and methods. *American Journal of Epidemiology*, **122**, 323–334.

Farquhar, J.W., Maccoby, N., Wood, P.D., Alexander, J.K., Breitrose, H., Brown, Jr. B.W., Haskell, W.L., McAlister, A., Meyer, A.J., Nash, J.D. & Stern, M.P. (1977). Community education for cardiovascular health. *Lancet* June 4, 1192–1195.

Farquhar, J.W., Fortmann, S.P., June, F.A., Barr Taylor, C., Haskell, W.L., Williams, P.T., Maccoby, N. & Wood, P.D. (1990). Effects of Communitywide Education on Cardiovascular Disease Risk factors. The Stanford Five-City Project. *Journal of the American Medical Association*, **264**(3), 359–365.

Flavell, J.H. (1970). Cognitive Changes in Adulthood in L.R. Goulet & P.B. Baltes (eds) *Lifespan Developmental Psychology – Research and Theory*. London: Academic Press.

Fleck, S. (1975). Unified Health Services and Family-focused Primary Care. *International Journal of Psychiatry in Medicine*, **6**, 501, 515.

Gaylord, M. & Symons, E. (1896). Relocation stress: a definition and a need for services. *Employee Assistance Quarterly*, **2**, 21–36.

Giddens, A. (1979). *Central Problems in Sociological Theory: Action Press, Structure and Contradiction in Social Analysis*. London: MacMillan.

Godin, G. & Shepard, R. (1984). Physical Fitness – Individual or Societal Responsibility? *Canadian Journal of Public Health*, **75**, 200–203.

Gottlieb, N.H. & Green, L.W. (1984). Life events, social network, life-style, and health: An analysis of the 1979 National Survey of personal health practices and consequences. *Health Education Quarterly*, **11**, 91–105.

Graham, H. (1976). Smoking in pregnancy: the attitudes of expectant mothers. *Social Science and Medicine*, **10**, 399–405.

Graham, H. (1984). *Women Health and the Family*. Brighton: Harvester Press.

Graham, H. (1985). Providers, Negotiators and Mediators: Women as the hidden carers. In T. Lewin & V. Olesen (eds) *Women Health and Healing*. London: Tavistock.

Green, E., Hebron, S. & Woodward, D. (1986). *Leisure and Gender. A Study of Sheffield Women's Experiences*. Report to the ESRC/Sports Council Joint Panel on Leisure Research London.

Harrell, W.A. (1986). Do liberated women drive their husbands to drink? The impact of masculine orientation, status inconsistency, and family life satisfaction on male liquor consumption. *International Journal of the Addictions*, **21**, 385–391.

Harris. D. & Gutren, S. (1979). Health Protective Behaviour: An exploratory study. *Journal of Health and Social Behaviour*, **2**, 17–29.

Havinghurst, R.J. (1973). Social Roles, Work, Leisure and Education in C. Eisdorfer & M.P. Lawton (eds) *The Psychology of Adult Development and Ageing*. Washington: American Psychology Association.

Herzlich, C. (1973). *Health and Illness: a social psychological analysis*. London: Academic Press.

Holmes, T.H. & Rahe, R.H. (1967). The Social Readjustment rating Scale. *Journal of Psychosomatic Research*, **11**, 213–218.

Jacobson, B. (1981). *The Lady Killers: Why Smoking is a Feminist Issue*. London: Pluto Press.

Kaplan, R. (1984). The connection between clinical health promotion and health status: a critical overview. *American Psychologist*, **39**.

Karasek, R. (1990). Lower health risk with increased job control among white collar workers. *Journal of Organisational Behaviour*, **11**, 171–185.

Kerr, M. & Charles, N. (1983). *Attitudes to the Feeding and Nutrition of Young Children: Preliminary Report*. University of York.

Kirscht, J.P. (1983). Preventive health behavior: a review of research and issues. *Health Psychology*, **2**, 277–301.

Lang, T. (1984). *Jam Tomorrow?* Food Policy Unit: Manchester Polytechnic.

Langlie, J. (1979). Interrelationships among Preventative Health Behaviours: A test of

Competing Hypotheses. *Public Health Reports*, **94**, 216–225.

Lau, R. (1988). Beliefs about Control and Health Behaviour. In D. Gochman (ed) *Health Behaviour: Emerging Research Perspectives*. New York: Plenum.

Lau, R., Jacobs Quandrel, M. & Hartman, K. (1990). Development and change of young Adults Preventive Health Beliefs and Behaviour: Influence from Parents and Peers. *Journal of Health and Social Behaviour*, **31**, 240–259.

Lau, R.R. & Ware, J.E. Jr (1981). Refinements in the measurement of health-specific locus-of-control beliefs. *Medical Care*, **19**, 1147–1158.

Leventhal, H., Safer, M.A., Cleary, P.D. & Gutmann, M. (1980). Cardiovascular risk modification by community-based programs for lifestyle change: comments on the Stanford study. *Journal of Consulting and Clinical Psychology*, **48**, 150–158.

Levinson, D.J. (1986). A conception of adult development. *American Psychologist*, **41**, 3–13.

Marmot, M.G., Davey Smith, G., Stansfeld, D., Patel, C., North, F., Head, J., White, I., Brunner, E. & Feeney, A. (1991). Health inequalities among British civil servants: The Whitehall II study, *Lancet*, **337**, 1387–1392.

Marmot, M.G., Shipley, M.J. & Rose, G. (1984). Inequalities in health – specific explanations of a general pattern? *Lancet*, **1**, 1003–1006.

McCaul, K.D., O'Neil, H.K. & Glasgow, R.E. (1988). Predicting the performance of dental hygiene behaviours: an examination of the Fishbein and Ajzen model and self-efficacy expectations. *Journal of Applied Social Psychology*, **18**, 114–128.

McGuire, W.J. (1984). Public communication as a strategy for inducing health-promoting behaviour change. *Preventive Medicine*, **13**, 299–319.

McQueen, D. (1987). Research in health behaviour, health promotion and public health. Research unit in Health and Behavioural change Working Paper: Edinburgh.

Mechanic, D. (1980). Education, Parental Interest and Health Perception and Behaviour. *Inquiry*, **17**, 331–338.

Mechanic, D. (1979). The Stability of health and illness behaviour: results from a 16 year follow up. *American Journal of Public Health*, **69**.

Mechanic, D. (1975). Some problems in the measurement of stress and social readjustment. *Journal of Human Stress*, **1**, 43–48.

Mendoza, R. (1990). Concept of healthy lifestyles and their determinants. *2nd European Conference on Health Education*, Warsaw 7–9 June.

Milo, N. (1981). *Promoting health through public policy*. Philadelphia: Davis.

Mintel, (1991). *Children The Influencing Factor*. London: Mintel International Group Ltd.

Moen, P., Kain, E. & Elder, G.H. (1983). Economic Conditions and Family Life. In R. Nelson & F. Skidmore (eds) *American Families and the Economy*. Washington DC: National Academic Press.

Mullen, K. (1992). A question of balance: health behaviour and work context among male Glaswegians. *Sociology of Health and Illness*, **14**(1), 73–97.

Nutbeam, D. & Catford, J. (1987). The Welsh Heart programme evaluation strategy: progress, plans and possibilities. *Health Promotion*, **2**, 5–18.

Nutbeam, D., Smith, C., Murphy, S. & Catford, J. (1993). Maintaining evaluation designs for long-term community-based health promotion programmes: Heartbeat Wales Case study. *Journal of Epidemiology and Community Health*, **47**, 127–133.

Norman, P. (1990). Social learning theory and the prediction of attendance at screening. *Psychology and Health*, **5**, 231–239.

Oakley, A. (1987). Gender and generation: the life and times of Adam and Eve. In P. Allat, T. Keil, A Bryman & B. Bytheway (eds) *Women and the Lifecycle*. London: Macmillan Press.

Oakley, A. (1974). *The Sociology of Housework*. London: Martin Robertson.

Office of Population Census and Surveys (1982). *General Household survey 1980*. London: OPCS.

Oppenheimer, V. (1974). The life-cycle squeeze. *Demography*, **11**, 227–245.

Oppenheimer, V. (1982). *Work and the Family.* New York: Academic Press.

Pikunas, J. (1976). *Human Development: An Emergent Science.* New York: McGraw-Hill.

Pill, R. & Stott, N. (1985). Preventative procedures and practices among British working class women. *Health Education Research, Theory and Practice,* 1, 111–119.

Puska, P., Nissinen, A., Tuomilehto, J., Salonen, J.T., Koskela, K., McAlister, A., Kottke, T.E., Maccoby, N. & Farquhar, J.W. (1985). The community-based strategy to prevent coronary heart disease: conclusions from the ten years of the North Karelia Project. *Annual Review of Public Health,* 6, 147–193.

Richards, N.D. (1976). Towards redefinition of health education and the role of social sciences. *Community Health,* 7, 135–143.

Rodeheaver, D. & Datan, N. (1981). Making It: The dialectics of middle age. In R.M. Lerner & Busch-Rossnagel (eds) *Individuals as producers of their development: A life span perspective.* London: Academic Press.

Ronis, D.L. & Kaiser, M.K. (1989). Correlates of breast self-examination in a sample of college women: analysis of linear structural relations. *Journal of Applied Social Psychology,* 19, 1068–1084.

Rubin, L.B. (1980). Women of a certain age. *Society,* 17, 68–76.

Salonen, J.T. (1987). Did the North Karelia project reduce coronary mortality? *Lancet,* August 1, 269.

Sarver, V.T. (1983). 'Ajzen and Fishbein's Theory of Reasoned Action': a critical assessment. *Journal for the Theory of Social Behaviour,* 13, 155–163.

Sarason, I.G., Johnson, J.H. & Siegel, J.M. (1978). Assessing the impact of life changes: development of the life experiences survey. *Journal of Consulting and Clinical Psychology,* 46, 932–946.

Schlegel, R.P., Crawford, C.A. & Sanborn, M.D. (1977). Correspondence and medicational properties of the Fishbein model: An application to adolescent alcohol use. *Journal of Experimental and Social Psychology,* 13, 421–430.

Sheppard, B.H., Hartwick, J. & Warshaw, P.R. (1988). A theory of reasoned action: a meta-analysis of past research, with recommendations for modifications and future research. *Journal of Consumer Research,* 15, 325–343.

Speier, M. (1971). The everyday world of the child. In J. Douglas (ed) *Understanding Everyday Life.* Routledge and Kegan Paul.

Staats, T.E. & Staats, M.B. (1982). Sex differences in stress: measurement of differential stress levels in managerial and professional males and females. *Southern Psychologist,* 1, 9–19.

Terris, M. (1977). Strategy for Prevention. *American Journal of Public Health,* 67, 1026–1027.

Townsend, P. & Davidson, N. (eds) (1988). *Inequalities In Health: the Black Report.* Penguin Books, also comprising The Health Divide, edition V.

Turner, R. (1983). Social Support and psychological distress in H. Kaplan (ed) *Psychological Stress.* New York: Academic Press.

Vinokur, A. & Seltzer, M.L. (1975). Desirable versus undesirable life events. Their relationship to stress and mental distress. *Journal of Personality and Social Psychology,* 32, 329–337.

Wallston, K.A., Wallston, B.S. & De Vellis, R. (1978). Development of the multi-dimensional health locus of control. *Health Education Monographs,* 6, 160–170.

Warwick, I., Aggleton, P. & Hommans, H. (1988). Constructing common sense – young people's beliefs about AIDS. *Sociology of Health and Illness,* 10(3), 213–233.

Waterson, E.J., Evans, C. & Murray-Lyon, I.M. (1990). Is pregnancy a time of changing drinking and smoking patterns for fathers as well as mothers? An initial investigation. *British Journal of Addiction,* 85, 389–396.

Waterson, E.J. & Murray-Lyon, I.M. (1989). Drinking and smoking patterns amongst women attending an antenatal clinic – II During pregnancy. *Alcohol and Alcoholism,* 24, 163–173.

Westman, M. Eden, D. & Shirom, A. (1985). Job stress, cigarette smoking and cessation: conditioning effects of peer support. *Social Science and Medicine,* 20, 637–644.

Whitehead, M. (1988). *The Health Divide* 1988 edition also comprising The Black Report, Penguin Harmondsworth.

Winefield, H.R., Winefield, A.H., Tiggeman, M. & Goldney, R.D. (1989). Psychological concomitant of tobacco and alcohol use in young Australian adults. *British Journal of Addiction*, **84**, 1067–1073.

World Health Organisation (1986). *Ottawa Charter for Health Promotion: Report on the International Conference on Health Promotion*. WHO/Health and Welfare/Canadian Public Health Association.

World Health Organisation (1988). *Adelaide Recommendations: Report of the Second International Conference on Health Promotion*. WHO/Australian Department of Community Services and Health.

World Health Organisation (1991). *Sundsvall Statement on Supportive Environments for Health*. WHO/United Nationals Environment Programme/and the Nordic countries.

Yeandle, S. (1984). *Women's Working Lives: Patterns and Strategies*. London: Tavistock.

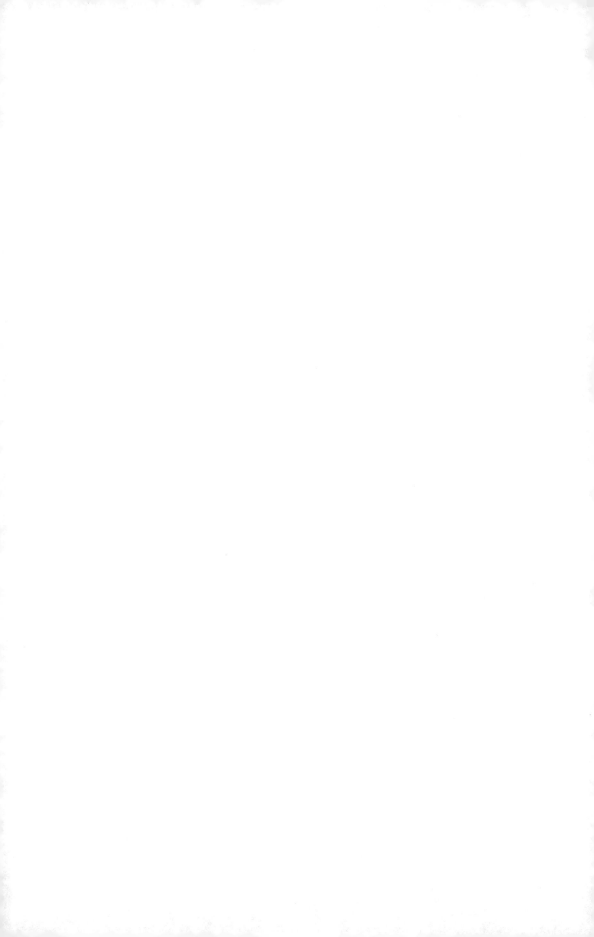

SECTION IV
Mid Life

MENSTRUATION AND MENOPAUSE: THE MAKING OR BREAKING OF WOMAN?

INTRODUCTION

Women's health, and women's illness, have for centuries been tied to the body. The womb has been regarded as a source of madness, melancholia and mercurial desire. The vagaries of reproduction have been said to rule women's lives, with the menarche and menopause defining the extent of a life cycle that marks women as different, and in many eyes, deficient. In both popular and academic discourse, factors associated with reproduction have been seen to be deleterious; reproduction considered only as a dysfunction, as a source of lability or as the root of a debilitating syndrome.

In the late twentieth century the confident pronouncements on the adverse influence of female reproduction which previously littered the annals of medical history are invariably viewed with disbelief or amusement. We in the West no longer confine or condemn women because of their reproductive cycle. We no longer locate health (or ill health) in the wandering womb. We no longer fear the fecundity of woman. Our new psychology of health is a liberal enlightened discipline, where reductionist theories are decried, and notions of equality are part of the current zeitgeist. Liberal theorists and feminist critics have debunked many of the myths which have shrouded the female body for centuries, claiming that menstruation and the menopause are not inevitability negative events, and that the theories which continue to assert so are misogynistic and misguided (see Sayers, 1982).

In such a climate it is easy to understand why problems associated with female reproduction are often ignored. Psychologists who concern themselves with the myriad influences on human behaviour rarely refer to it (Ussher, 1989). In an attempt to distance ourselves from the misogynistic pronouncements of the nineteenth century medics who reduced all female madness to the womb, we have appear to have adopted a strategy of denial. Men and women are treated similarly in research and theory (if women are not ignored altogether – see Squire, 1989), and the notion of femininity as being biologically influenced is generally impugned.

Yet an understanding of female reproduction, and specifically an understanding of the potential influence of the menstrual cycle and menopause, is an essential component of any analysis of women's health. Both because of its biological reality and the cultural discourse which mediates its effects, reproduction has a significant influence on women's identity. This chapter will examine the current state of knowledge associated with female reproduction, focussing on menstruation and the menopause, in order to demonstrate their salience for health psychology. The social and academic discourse which is associated with reproduction will be examined, drawing on both historical and cross cultural examples. It will be argued that the position of reproduction as negative and debilitating has widespread influence on the beliefs and behaviour of women and men, health professionals and lay people alike. The various theories posited to explain both 'normal' and 'abnormal' experiences of reproduction will be critically examined, with particular reference to PMS and the "menopausal syndrome." It will be argued that whilst reproduction cannot be ignored, neither can it be privileged above all other factors as a potential influence on women's lives. In this light, a positive and empowering framework within which experiences of menstruation and menopause can be conceptualised will be discussed.

THE GENEALOGY OF REPRODUCTIVE MYTHS

Current discourses concerning female reproduction which have passed unquestioned into the rhetoric of health psychologists are not historically invariant. From the time of Hippocrates, through to the evolution of the modern science of medicine in the nineteenth century, reproduction has been a source of concern for learned men, considered in the light of its supposed deleterious effects and insidious influence on women. The following examples are illustrative.

> "The monthly activity of the ovaries...has a notable effect upon the mind and body; wherefore it may become an important cause of mental and physical derangement...It is a matter of common experience in asylums, that exacerbations of insanity often take place at menstrual periods."
> Maudsley, 1873: 88

> "Every body of the least experience must be sensible of the influence of menstruation on the operations of the mind. In truth, it is the moral and physical barometer of the female constitution."
> Burrows, 1828

> "the reproductive organs...are closely interwoven with erratic and disordered intellectual, as well as moral, manifestations."
> Maddock, 1854: 177

Such views are not atypical or unusual and are perhaps most notable for the *lack* of controversy they have traditionally given rise to. The consequences of this negative discourse have included the exclusion of women from education or work, for fear that it would damage their reproductive ability, or because reproduction was believed to weaken the mind (Sayers, 1982). It has lead to a concentration of medical interventions on sexuality or control of the womb, through clitoredectomy, leeching of the vagina, or the 'bed-rest cure' (Ussher, 1989); and the continued attribution of female distress and discontent to internal bodily pathological processes.

This view of reproduction, and particularly menstruation as negative, was not confined to Western society. Anthropological texts are littered with comments concerning the necessity of controlling or confining the menstruating woman, who was said to spoil crops, foul food, sour wine, and if inadvertently found to be in proximity to the sexual member of man, wreak potentially dire consequences. The taboo on sex during menstruation (Weidegar, 1976; Laws, 1990) testifies to the fear of impotence or symbolic castration which the bleeding woman implied. To protect further against the influence of the dangerous blood, and mark their entry into the hazardous state of womanhood, menarcheal girls have reportedly been subjected to a gamut of ritualistic confinements at the advent of their first menstrual period.

> Among many Brazilian tribes a girl at her first menstrual period is suspended in a hammock under the roof of the hut and subject to the most severe fumigation as well as being starved. Thus among the Guarinis the girls were sewn up in their hammock in the same manner as those tribes sew up corpses, only the smallest opening being left to allow them to breathe; they were suspended over the fire in that condition for several days . . . It not infrequently happens that the unfortunate girls die under the severity of the process of disinfection to which they are subject. (Briffault, 1927; cited by Laws, 1990)

Such confinement is not peculiar to adolescence: throughout the life cycle women have experienced the direct consequences of the menstrual taboo. In many societies women are literally confined to menstrual huts (Frazer, 1938), in others debarred from cooking or crossing the path of men. Underlying the menstrual taboos is the notion of uncleanliness, of contamination, and the danger of the menstruating woman, leading to purification rituals on an individual level, as is the case with many Indian or orthodox Jewish women (Weidegar, 1976), or on a societal level should a woman break the restrictions imposed:

> Among the Dogsan of East Africa the menstrual taboo is so strong that a woman in this condition brings misfortune to everything she touches. Not only is she segregated in an isolated hut and provided with special eating utensils, but if she is seen passing through the village a general purification must take place (Hays, 1972).

Repercussions of ignoring the taboo can be dire:

> A young woman was solemnly tried on the charge of having eaten a fish while she was unclean (menstruating); she was condemned and executed in the presence of the people, by being thrown from a rock into the river (Briffault, 1927).

The menopausal woman does not escape the constructions and taboos, despite the fact of her womb having ceased to bleed. She has been described as irrational, frustrated, asexual, liable to madness, dried up and spent. Her womb is seen as being as liable to inflict misery when 'arid' and 'barren', as when it was in the first flush of reproductive youth. If historically menarche was believed to mark the onset of uterine madness, menopause did not herald the end, a release for the reproductive chains, but a new set of difficulties:

> women become insane during pregnancy, after parturition, during lactation; at the age when the catemenia (menses) first appear and when they disappear (the menopause). The sympathetic connection between the brain and uterus is plainly seen by the most casual observer.
>
> G. Fielding Blandford, 1871 (cited by Hunter, 1990c)

The death of the reproductive faculty is accompanied...by struggles which implicate every organ and every function of the body
Smith, 1848 (cited by Showalter, 1979).

TWENTIETH CENTURY FICTIONS

In the late twentieth century the focus and content of concerns associated with reproduction has shifted: fear of menstrual blood is not so loudly proclaimed, and the womb is no longer thought to wander. However, the underlying belief remains that the menstruating or menopausal woman is vulnerable. Reproduction is still often seen as negative in popular and professional discourse.

This representation is perhaps most clearly seen in modern medical texts, which have been subjected to scrutiny by a member of feminist scholars (Kitzinger, 1983; Martin, 1987; Laws, 1990), wherein the very language used to describe menstruation is seen as pejorative.

In rapid succession the reader is confronted with "degenerate", "decline", "withdrawn", "spasms", "lack"..."weakened", "leak", "deteriorate", "discharge", and after all that, "repair"...these are not neutral terms; rather they convey failure and dissolution... unacknowledged cultural attitudes can seep into scientific writing through evaluative words (Martin, 1987)

The derogatory description of female reproductive function, where menstruation is described in terms of 'catastrophic disintegration', has been compared by Martin with a text on male reproductive physiology, clearly not viewed as degenerative, described below to illustrate the different bias in the language:

The mechanisms which guide the *remarkable* cellular transformation from spermatoid to mature sperm remain uncertain...perhaps the most *amazing* characteristic of spermato-genesis is its *sheer magnitude*: the normal male may manufacture several millions of sperm per day (*original emphasis*) (Martin, 1987: 48)

The message is clear: women's reproduction is a curse – men's is a miracle. The 'vaginal atrophy', the 'senile pelvic involution', the degeneration of the body is not described in men. As Reitz (1981) has argued "we do not have 'testicular insufficiency' to match 'ovarian sufficiency' or 'senile scrotum' to match 'senile ovaries'". The language used betrays the beliefs.

Further, this negative view of menstruation and menopause is not confined to medical texts. It penetrates popular discourse, and is internalised by women who experience reproduction as negative. Menarche is associated with silence and secrecy, and often with shame; menstruation is regarded as a cause of distress, whilst the menopause is often seen as a deficiency disease, described by a leading proponent as a 'living decay' (Wilson, 1966). Consider for example these recent comments on menstruation and menopause in popular media:

PMS stands for premenstrual syndrome, but it could stand for Periods, Murder, and Shop-lifting. '*More*' *magazine*, Summer 1988
(cited by Nicolson, 1992: 192).

At least 40 percent of women who menstruate have some degree of PMS: about 10 per cent have severe problems with it. PMS is also, probably, an unhelpful hidden factor in many women's lives: accidents, poor performance and anti-social behaviour are markedly more common in women just before menstruation *Nursing Standard*, 27.11.87.

The fact is that many (menopausal) women are suffering from a definite deficiency disorder, just like diabetes or those with underactive thyroids. *Daily Telegraph* 31.1.89.

Rather than wait for the menopause to attack, it is now possible, with a simple test, to determine the degree of estrogen deficiency and to take HRT to forestall any unpleasantness. *Observer* 18.3.84
(cited by Hunter, 1990c)

Self help books can reinforce the message, declaring for example that 'if you suffer from the premenstrual syndrome, you are likely to work less efficiency for a few days each month' (Shreeve, 1984). A view analogous to that in a medical text that 'women's ability to work reduces to a quarter of normal by menopause' (Achte, 1970; cited by Hunter, 1990c). Women's own view of their reproductive cycles and their bodies are dismissed by many medical texts, implicitly asserting the medical 'expert' view as the only one which is valid. As one recent gynaecology textbook argues, 'previous gynaecological history is best learned about from clinical records if obtainable. Gynaecological pathology and terminology are mysterious to most women' (Garrey *et al*., 1978). The doctor clearly knows best, and as outlined below what he (sic) advises is invariably pharmacological intervention to right the imbalanced body. The opposing view, that reproduction has little deleterious effect on the majority of women, does appear in certain medical texts, and is a view held by many individual practitioners. But it is clearly the doom laden negative perspective which has penetrated popular discourse. Perhaps this is because the popular press are less likely to publish a story declaring 'Menstruation has no effect on women's lives' than they are to print the 'Raging hormones makes women mad' tale.

Silence and Secrecy

In view of the above, it is perhaps not surprising to find that women in general do not view menstruation positively, and that one of the most salient features associated with menstruation in popular discourse is the insistence on silence and secrecy. Adolescent girls rate secrecy as their most pressing concern (Williams, 1983). Advertisements focus on the concealing properties of sanitary products, the fact that 'nobody will know you're having a period', and tampons are sold in coloured boxes or wrapped in individual bright wrappers, masqueraded and disguised, so that their identity as a sanitary product remains unseen. Equally, euphemisms disguise the word 'menstruation' itself. Girls talk of 'reading a book', 'grandma is here' 'red letter day' (Ernster, 1975), rather than of menstruation. Boys use euphemisms too, but adopt those which are more obviously derogatory 'on the rag', 'blood and sand', 'in season'. The impact is the same: menstruation itself is unspeakable. This silence and subterfuge also extends to menarche and adolescent menstruation, as evidenced in the following extracts:

When my mother was thirteen she came home from school convinced that, like her sister, she has a severe haemorrhage. She told her mother she was bleeding and was bundled into the kitchen. 'How could you have mentioned that in front of your father?' Her mother found her a sanitary towel. 'It's your periods. Put that on. It'll go on until you're forty' (Lee, 1984; quoted by Laws, 1990)

It was her mother who made the fuss. Her mother who taught her to creep down from her bedroom when everyone else was asleep, to burn evidence on the fire in the dark, tiptoeing so she should not wake her father, would not have to invent a sudden thirst or hunger to explain her midnight wanderings about his house. It was imperative that he should not know. She had started wearing Tampax not for her own comfort but for the sake of more perfect secrecy. So her father should not know that the blood curse was on his house and on his possessions.
(Maitland, 1981)

What is central to these extracts is the shame, fear, misinformation and mythology associated with menstruation. That negative attitudes towards menstruation are common in both young women and men (Brookes, Ruble and Clarke, 1977) is perhaps therefore not surprising. The pervasiveness of these negative attitudes across the gender divide clearly indicates the peculiar position adopted by menstruation as a negative signifier. In a study of men's attitudes to menstruation Laws (1990) concluded that two specific messages are '(a) that women's genitals are disgusting/ produce disgusting substances (this is expressed in the attention to sanitary towels), and (b) that women are ruled by their hormones'.

Negative stereotyping, and associated negative attitudes towards reproduction, may reflect the attention given by both medical and psychological researchers to the premenstrual syndrome and the menopausal syndrome, wherein the notion of reproductive fallibility is reified within psychiatric nosology. They also reinforce the legitimacy of experts to advise and intervene in the arena of reproductive health.

REPRODUCTIVE SYNDROMES

Premenstrual Syndrome

The Premenstrual syndrome (PMS), said by some to affect as many as 95% of women (see Ussher, 1989), has reinforced the notion to menstruation as a source of madness, badness or weakness. First described as premenstrual tension by Frank in 1931, renamed PMS in the 1970s because of the wide array of symptoms, and more recently 'late luteal phase disorder' (LLPD) as part of the campaign for inclusion in the Diagnostic and Statistical Manual of the American Psychiatric Association (DSM-III-R) (Spitzer *et al.*, 1989), the connection between reproduction and debilitating symptoms has now become enshrined in psychiatric nosology. PMS is said to include a range of up to 150 different symptoms, including moodiness, anxiety, elation, irritability, depression, tiredness, lack of concentration, hostility, aches and pains, swelling, diarrhoea and constipation (Moos, 1969). Yet despite confident claims, there is no agreement over core symptoms necessary or sufficient for diagnosis, and there are widely differing symptom profiles across individual women (Ussher, 1989). Comparison across studies is made difficult by the fact that the premenstrual phase of the cycle is variously defined as between 1–15 days before menstruation (Asso, 1983). As there is no evidence for the existence of an identifiable hormonal substrate underlying PMS, which would allow for a categorical physical diagnosis, its presence is inevitably determined by the existence of behavioural disturbance and negative symptomatology. But this is also a problematic issue.

Menstrual cycle mood change

Fluctuations in mood have been one of the most commonly reported effects of PMS, but the results of empirical research are contradictory. One problem arises from the fact that negative mood has been shown to increase in either the *premenstrual* (Golub, 1976; Moos *et al.*, 1969; Taylor, 1979; Warner and Bancroft, 1990) or *menstrual* (Englander-Golden, Whitmore and Dienstbier, 1978; Golub and Harrington, 1981; Wilcoxen Schrader and Sherif, 1976) phase of the cycle, whilst others have claimed that there is in fact no evidence for consistent cyclical variations in mood in most women (Abplanalp, 1979; May, 1976; O'Neil, Lancee and Freeman, 1984; Ussher, 1987).

One of the explanations for this disagreement is the demonstrated discrepancy between retrospective and daily mood evaluations (Rubinow *et al.*, 1984; Ainscough, 1990). Peri-menstrual distress recorded on retrospective questionnaires is often not found on daily ratings, resulting in many false positives in diagnosis (Hamilton and Gallant, 1990) i.e. women who are categorised as 'PMS sufferers' when there is no identifiable reason for doing so. Standardised questionnaires, such as the Moos Menstrual Distress Questionnaire (MDQ), have also been criticised for their concentration on negative symptoms, which don't allow women to report any positive feelings or experiences (Parlee, 1973), thereby producing biased results. It has also been argued that explicitly labelling mood questionnaires as being related to the menstrual cycle will actually induce evidence of cyclical changes in affect, possibly as a result of women fulfilling experimenter expectations, whilst non-specific mood questionnaires will show no such pattern (Golub and Harrington, 1981; Slade, 1984; Olasov and Jackson, 1987). Individual differences between women, or differences between cycles, provide further explanation for the conflicting evidence over the existence of PMS.

Behavioural disturbance

The association between menstruation and behaviour is presented as further evidence for the validity of PMS as a concept, as women's apparent inability to achieve as much as men, or their propensity to experience psychological problems, is attributed to menstruation (Ussher, 1991). Yet recent research has argued that the claims for any variation in performance during the menstrual cycle, either in the laboratory or in the work-place, are largely unfounded (see Sommer, 1992, for a review). Variations in performance are only found on subtests, and may be attributable to chance. Equally, the contention that a wide range of female 'madness or badness' can be attributed to menstruation has been contested. The assertion of researchers that accidents (e.g. Lees, 1965), violent or criminal behaviour (e.g. Greene and Dalton, 1953; Coppen and Kessel, 1963; Lewis, 1990), psychiatric admissions (e.g. Luggin *et al.*, 1984), or suicides (e.g. Glass *et al.*, 1971) increase during the para-menstrual phase has been refuted, on the basis that the studies above are methodologically unsound or present spurious unreplicated findings (Parlee, 1973; Ussher, 1989). Methodological difficulties in the research, such as retrospective designation of phase definition, or absence of statistical analysis of results, has also been highlighted.

For example, Katrina Dalton's (1960a) assertion that school girls' academic and examination performance is so severely affected by menstruation that examiners should be informed of menstrual cycle phase, has not been supported by empirical research (Bernstein, 1977; Sommer, 1972; Richardson, 1992, Walsh *et al.*, 1981). The study (Dalton, 1960a) repeatedly cited as evidence that 'students become mentally duller' during the premenstrual phase has been criticised for containing no statistical analysis of what may be chance results (Gannon, 1981; Sommer, 1982). Yet despite this, many adolescent girls still attribute performance difficulties to menstruation (Richardson, 1992; Wilson and Key, 1989).

Much of the research which attests to a deleterious relationship between menstruation and aspects of behaviour has been found to be difficult to replicate, and often questionable in terms of its underlying assumptions. It has been argued that any connection between menstruation and an event such as an examination failure (cf. Dalton, 1960a) or an accident may be due to a third factor, such as stress (Gannon, 1981; Sommer, 1982). The publication of these results, which is facilitated by the likelihood that only research with statistically significant results will be published (only 2% of published papers contain statistically non-significant results), leads to the 'file-drawer problem' (where non-significant results languish unpublished), and the consequent perpetuation of potentially misleading conclusions about menstrual cycle effects (Sommer, 1982). Equally, research which attests to the absence of a significant relationship between menstruation and behaviour is marginalised or ignored, and successive generations of researchers seek to discover an association which may be fictitious (Ussher, 1992a).

Deconstructing PMS

One of the consequences of the conflicting evidence, and the failure of empirical research studies to confirm the existence of physical, psychological or behavioural disturbance during the para-menstruum, has been the development of critiques which challenge the very existence of a premenstrual syndrome. It has been argued that PMS is merely a means of pathologising women's anger, discontent or deviant behaviour (Laws, 1990), particularly that which does not conform with the stereotypical feminine role, in the same way that hysteria and neurasthenia were used to pathologise women in the late nineteenth century. It has been argued that the very notion of reproductive syndromes continues the tradition of blaming the body (Ussher, 1992b), and confirms underlying misogynistic beliefs about the infirmity or danger of woman. Violence and anger are incongrous with notions of femininity, and so are conveniently attributed to hormones. Female underachievement does not need to be explained by recourse to social or political factors if hormones are seen to be the root cause.

It has also been argued (Ussher, 1989) that the concept of a premenstrual syndrome is invalid, as neither criterion for a syndrome – that there be a fixed group of symptoms, or a common but not invariant set of symptoms, (Walsh, 1985) – can be satisfied. Alternatively, criteria for a syndrome could be satisfied if the various symptoms shared a greater concordance amongst themselves than each has with other symptoms, with statistical analysis confirming the strength of the interrelationships (Walsh, 1985). Ussher (1989) has argued that 'this could not be said to be the case with the possible symptoms found in the premenstrual syndrome, as many are part of other diagnosed syndromes, such as anxiety or depression, in similar groupings'. It is also impossible to identify categorically the most important 'ingredients' of a supposed premenstrual syndrome, which has been suggested as a means of overcoming the other difficulties (Kinsbourne, 1971), as there is, as yet, little agreement concerning the essential features of PMS – with over 150 possible symptoms, which can occur in any combination for individual women. Even LLPD, the new DSM III-R diagnostic category, does not contain an exclusive list of symptoms which all women who may receive the diagnosis would experience.

It could thus be argued that the very existence of PMS cannot be justified on any grounds, its function being to categorise many different symptoms and behaviours under one all encompassing, yet vague and questionable umbrella term. The danger inherent in the notion of PMS as a psychiatric syndrome is that it can be seen to *cause* the symptoms and behaviours, rather than merely being a descriptive term.

Despite these critiques, women's reports of premenstrual symptomatology, and professional investment in the notion of a syndrome, has led to the firm adherence to the disease model as a means of conceptualising menstruation, and the adoption of a wide range of both physical and psychological aetiological theories, which clearly have serious implications in the assessment and treatment of individual women.

Aetiological explanations for PMS

Hormonal theories and therapies for PMS
The most influential theories, in terms of their penetration of popular and academic discourse, are those which assert an hormonal substrate underlying menstrual complaints. Supposed menstrual cycle debilitation or mood variation has been attributed to:

* deficiencies in beta endorphins (Giannini *et al.*, 1990)
* elevations in the biogenic amine plasma epinephrine (Odink *et al.*, 1990)
* elevated estrogen (Backstrom and Carstensen, 1974)
* plasma monoamine oxidase activity (Klaiber *et al.*, 1974)
* renin aldosterone (Janowski *et al.*, 1973)
* Interaction between steroids and gamma-amniobutyric acid (Majewska, 1987)
* prolactine-progesterone interaction (Benedek-Jazman and Hearn-Sturtevart, 1976)
* pyrodoxine deficiency (Herzberg *et al.*, 1970; Brush, 1977)
* peptide hormones (Butt, Watts and Holder, 1983; Halbreich and Endicott, 1981)
* prostaglandins (Craig, 1980; Jakubowicz, 1983)
* sodium-potassium abnormalities (Varma, 1983)
* melatonin secretion (Parry *et al.*, 1990)
* genetically transmitted vulnerability (Taghavi, 1990)
* dopamine deficiency (Haspels, 1983)

Equally, a wide range of physical interventions have been said to be effective in treating PMS. These can be differentiated on the basis of those which operate on an hormonal level, those which are based on psycho-tropic intervention (e.g. anti-depressants), and those which aim at altering fluid or electrolyte imbalance. They include:

* oestrogen (Shaw, 1983)
* progesterone (Dalton, 1969; Kerr, 1977; Halbreich, 1990)
* implants of estrodiol (Magos *et al.*, 1984)
* oral contraceptives (Herzberg *et al.*, 1970)
* fluoxetine (Rickels *et al.*, 1990; Metz, 1990)

* prostaglandin inhibitors and precursors (Puolakka and Makarainen, 1985; Wood and Jakubowicz, 1980)
* dygesterone (Varma, 1983)
* bromocriptine (Benedek-Jazman and Hearn-Sturevart, 1976)
* amytriptyline (Tavhavi, 1990)
* clomipramine (Eriksson *et al.*, 1990)
* alprazolam (Robinson and Garfinkel, 1990)
* lithium (Mattson and von Schoultz, 1974; Singer, Chen and Shou, 1974; Horrobin *et al.*, 1973)
* nortriptyline (Feder, 1989; Harrison *et al.*, 1989)
* diuretics (O'Brien *et al.*, 1979)
* pyridoxine (Abraham and Hargrove, 1980)

However, as the few double blind controlled studies which have been carried out (e.g. Sampson, 1979; Andersch and Hahn, 1983; Maddocks *et al.*, 1986) have failed to show any of these biochemical interventions to be consistently more effective than a placebo, the argument for their efficacy must be questioned.

Despite the equivocal data, menstrual myths continue. Many women still report that they suffer from PMS, or that menstruation affects them in a detrimental way, despite the evidence to the contrary from 'objective' measures, such as mood questionnaires or performance tests. Even women who *do* report menstrual cycle mood or behavioural change don't do so in every cycle, suggesting that it is not a stable phenomena (Asso, 1983). Psychological explanations may go some way towards explaining these contradictions.

Psycho-social theories of PMS

One possible explanation for any apparent association between menstruation and mood or behavioural change is the influence of life stress. It has been demonstrated that menstrual and premenstrual distress are related to undesirable events (Siegal, Johnson and Sarason, 1979; Wilcoxon, Schrader & Sherif, 1976) and that increases in life stress results in increases in menstrual cycle complaints (Koeske, 1977; Ussher, 1987; Clare, 1983; Warner and Bancroft, 1990). Thus life stressors may be a more important indicator of mood than menstrual cycle phase (Mansfield, Hood and Henderson, 1989). These theories also allow for the fact that women who do report premenstrual symptomatology do not report symptoms in every cycle, as there are likely to be monthly changes in social circumstances (Clare, 1983).

A further argument is that menstruation may be acting as a stressor for some women (Jensen, 1982; Ussher and Wilding, 1992), increasing the risk of negative affect when external stressors are increased, or making the woman more vulnerable. The mechanism underlying this may be the perception of increases in physiological activation (e.g. Asso and Braier, 1982; Little and Zahn, 1974; Ussher and Wilding, 1991) which are interpreted as negative because of the negative attitudes associated with menstruation (Koeske, 1980). There is some evidence that attribution of negative symptomatology varies during the cycle, with symptoms being attributed to the menstrual cycle premenstrually yet attributed to environmental factors inter-menstrually (Koeske, 1977; Bains and Slade, 1988; McFarland, Ross and DeCourville, 1987) and that life events may be perceived or experienced as more stressful when they occur in the Peri-menstrual period (Schmidt *et al.*, 1990). These studies suggest that women may inappropriately attribute negative moods caused by a third factor such as stress to menstruation, and hereby reinforce their own belief in the existence of a premenstrual syndrome.

This notion of attributional bias and socially mediated expectations may also explain the absence of significant associations between behavioural change and menstrual cycle phase. Sommer (1972) considered that "Studies using response measures based on self report and social behaviours indicate a behavioural decrement associated with the premenstrual and menstrual phases. Studies utilizing objective performance measures generally fail to demonstrate menstrual cycle related changes". Women may *believe* that their performance suffers in the paramenstruum, when in reality there is no evidence that it does (Sommer, 1992). In this vein, researchers who have examined the role of cognitive or personality factors have reported that women who report PMS score more highly on measures of neurotic personality than non-sufferers (Backstrom and Hammarback, 1986; Ussher, 1987), although Gannon (1981) has claimed that this is due to the similarities between the diagnostic scales used to assess PMS and neuroticism. It has also been suggested that women who engage more in 'A' type behaviour and are therefore more likely to be reactive to stressors are more likely to report symptoms of PMS (Martini and Fee, 1983; Ussher, 1987). This has lead to the claim that stress and personality factors may combine to 'sensitize premenstrual symptoms in women', resulting in a diagnosis of PMS (Heilbrun and Frank, 1989).

Psychologists have put forward other cognitive or personality factors as explanations for individual differences between women in menstrual cycle symptomatology. These include trait anxiety (Picone and Kirkby, 1990), locus of control (Scott-Palmer and Skevington, 1981), negative attitudes or expectations (Rodin, 19786; Woods, Dery and Most, 1982), presence of persistent mental disorder (Harrison *et al.*, 1989), borderline personality disorder (Hamilton and Gallant, 1990), rejection of femininity (Levitt and Lubin, 1967), and emotional instability (Sheldrake and Cormack, 1976). What these different explanations suggest is that many underlying state or trait factors may contribute to the likelihood of an individual woman being diagnosed (by self or others) as suffering from PMS. Whether this means that PMS itself is a valid or reliable construct, rather than an pathologising umbrella term applied to a multifarious range of almost random symptoms and states, is unclear.

THE MENOPAUSE

The myth of the menopausal syndrome

The notion of reproduction as source of distress and debilitation is not confined to menstruation. The menopause is treated similarly in modern medical discourse. Negative symptoms experienced during the climacteric, the mid-life period during which cessation of menstruation occurs, have been attributed to what has been termed the 'menopausal syndrome' (Utian and Seer, 1976). The physical symptoms said to be associated with the menopause include vasomotor symptoms (hot flushes), vaginal dryness, somatic symptoms (i.e. dizziness), osteoporosis, headaches, and rheumatism, whilst psychological symptoms include depression, irritability, lack of confidence, decreased libido, and poor concentration (see Greene, 1984; Hunter, 1990a). Estimates of prevalence vary from between 10 and 95% of women (Holte, 1989).

Factors such as methodological inadequacies in sampling, failure to distinguish between symptoms due to the hormonal changes of the menopause and symptoms due to other factors, or errors in measurement, have been put forward as explanations for these widely varying estimates (McKinlay and McKinlay, 1973; Kaufert and Syrotuik, 1981; Greene, 1984; Holte, 1989).

As with PMS, the notion of a menopausal syndrome has come under criticism, partly because it has been contended that the high rates of psychological symptoms reported by researchers are only found in studies of women attending clinics (Holte, 1989). Those who examine general population samples in menopausal research, have reported that vasomotor and somatic difficulties are not uncommon, but that there is no evidence for increased psychological symptoms associated with the menopause (e.g. Neurgarten and Kraines, 1965; McKinlay and Jeffreys, 1974; Greene, 1984; Hunter, Battersby and Whitehead, 1986). In a review of prospective studies carried out in Europe and North America, where pre and post-menopausal women were compared, Hunter (1990a) concluded that only hot flushes and vaginal dryness could be related to the menopause, and that there was no evidence for an association between the menopause and emotional problems.

Not only has the notion of negative psychological symptoms as a normal part of the menopause been challenged (Matthews *et al.*, 1990), the author of a recent review of the literature concluded 'if anything, women in the post-menopausal years show *less* evidence of psychiatric disturbance than younger women' (Ballinger, 1990). However the proliferation and dominance of the biomedical view of the menopause, and belief in the notion of the menopausal syndrome has continued.

Hormonal theories and therapies for menopausal complaints

The notion of the menopausal syndrome as a 'deficiency disease' related to falling levels of estrogen has been the dominant model for many years (e.g. Wilson, 1966). In addition to declining estrogen levels, other biological factors have also been implicated, including:

* cortisol secretion, prolactin and thyroid stimulating hormone (Ballinger, Smith and Hobbs, 1985)
* androgen (Sherwin and Gelfand, 1987)
* changes in feedback mechanisms in the hypothalmic pituitary axis (Eagles and Whalley, 1985)
* anomalous brain substrates (Herzog, 1989)
* brain catecholamine turnover (Molnar, Takacks and Bazsane, 1988).

It is therefore not surprising that the most common form of intervention for menopausal symptoms is hormone replacement therapy (HRT) (Walling, Anderson and Johnson, 1990; Stuenkel, 1989). Hailed as a panacea for all ills during the 1970s and 1980s, HRT became the treatment of choice for a whole gamut of physical and psychological problems experienced by women. Stadel and Weiss (1975) claimed that it was being taken by 51% of menopausal women in North America for a minimum of three months and a median time of 10 years. A more recent estimate suggested that 7% of menopausal women in Britain currently take HRT (Hunter, 1990b). Yet despite this apparently low figure, there is still a great faith in the almost magical efficacy of

HRT in prolonging youth, as is illustrated by this recent newspaper quote from the British Conservative MP Theresa Gorman,

> Everyone comments on how rosy my skin is. I can nearly always tell if someone is taking HRT by the quality of their skin.
> *Daily Telegraph* 31.1.89

The use of HRT for menopausal symptoms is, however, controversial. A World Health Organisation report (1981) concluded that vasomotor symptoms and vaginal dryness were the only menopausal symptoms which could be related to hormonal changes, and that prescribing HRT for psychological symptoms was inappropriate. In support of that position, Greene (1984) reviewed ten clinical trials and concluded that hot flushes and vaginal dryness were the only symptoms to be relieved by HRT, observing that in three of the trials a placebo was as effective as HRT in reducing *all* symptoms. There is also controversy concerning the possible links between HRT and cancer (Stuenkel, 1989; Rothert *et al.*, 1990), suggesting that manipulating hormones should be done with caution.

The other common medical intervention for menopausal complaints is hysterectomy. Yet this kind of surgery often has little impact upon the physical or psychological symptoms experienced by women, and is carried out on the basis of women's subjective reports of symptoms such as heavy bleeding (Kincey and McFarland, 1984) – reports which have been demonstrated to be often erroneous as women have knowledge of only their own 'normal' bleeding. For example, a study by Hodges (1984) where blood was measured during menstruation, found that women's reports of heavy or light bleeding did not correspond with the actual amount of blood lost. Some women who lost a lot of blood defined themselves as moderate or light, and others with a small amount of blood loss described their periods as heavy.

Psycho-social theories of the menopause

The biomedical model of menopausal symptomatology is not the only one. Both social and psychological theories have been put forward offered to explain distress and discontent experienced by women during the mid-life period. These models do not deny the reality of the physical concomitants of the menopause, but advocate a less reductionist analysis of associated psychological symptoms.

Whilst the menopause *per se* may not inevitably result in symptomatology for women, there are certainly incidences of depression and anxiety in many women during the climacteric (Ussher, 1991). Yet this does not lead inevitably to a 'raging hormones' explanation, for psychological symptoms may not be any different from that experienced at any other stage of the life cycle. Supporting this argument, depression in menopausal women has been demonstrated as being related to factors including 'family and socio-economic experiences of mid-life' (Notman, 1984), life stress (Hunter, Battersby and Whitehead, 1986; Greene, 1984), associated with multiple roles of women (McKinlay, McKinlay and Brambilla, 1987), or with past depression, or cognitive and social factors (Hunter, 1990b). It has also been argued that negative cultural views of female ageing produce negative attitudes towards the menopause (Beyene, 1986), which may underlie any symptomatology.

The other side of this argument is that a number of factors have been shown to be correlated with *positive* mental health in the menopause, including employment

(Wilbur *et al.*, 1990), children leaving home (Glen, 1975; Neurgarten, 1979; Lowenthal, 1975), and positive attitudes towards female aging (Patterson and Lynch, 1988; Lennon, 1987; Berkun, 1986). It could be argued that psychological symptoms during the climacteric could be conceptualised as reactions to many of the life stressors which affect women at any time of the life cycle.

PSYCHOLOGICAL RESPONSES TO REPRODUCTIVE SYNDROMES

In contrast to the bio-medical explanations of symptomatology which lead almost directly to a physical treatment, the psychological theories offered to explain distress associated with menstruation or menopause suggest a diverse range of approaches: including specific psychological therapies, information provision or education, and multifactorial approaches. Specific psychological interventions advocated for PMS have included stress management (Picone and Kirkby, 1990; Asso, 1988b), cognitive-behavioural therapy (Kuczmierczyk, 1989; Slade, 1989), relaxation and rational emotive therapy (Morse *et al.*, 1989), or exercise (Gannon, 1988).

For menopausal symptoms,

* psychotherapy (Cundo, 1984; Channon and Ballinger, 1982)
* counselling (Patterson and Lynch, 1988)
* self help on an individual or group basis (Hunter, 1990b)

have been advocated. However, firm conclusions cannot be reached regarding the relative efficacy of these different approaches, as research in this area is still in its infancy. As Slade (1989) has noted in relation to PMS, 'in comparison with the extensive trials of medication, specific psychological interventions have been scarce'. Individual interventions, such as those discussed above, have not been assessed in controlled studies where comparisons can be made between treatments, or where psychological therapy can be compared with either medication or with a waiting list control group. One controlled study reported by Slade (1989) as an intervention for PMS, involving a combination of problem solving, autogenic training, anxiety and anger control stragegies, combined with modification of cognitions and attributions associated with menstruation, did suggest significant positive improvements. Further research is clearly needed to ascertain exactly how these psychological interventions are proving effective.

Based on the premise that symptoms associated with menstruation or menopause are related to misattribution of bodily sensations, or negative attitudes and beliefs, it has been suggested that education, information provision and self help groups may be an effective and empowering means of alleviating distress (Hunter, 1990c; Ussher, 1992d). The provision of educational material which would facilitate coping strategies that women could develop on a self help basis would also obviate the need for professional intervention for those women who experience mild symptomatology, and avoid the tendency of framing women's experiences within a medicalized framework (Ussher, 1992b). Research is needed to assess the merits of this approach in relation to other forms of intervention before firm conclusions can be made regarding efficacy.

One of the problems facing health psychologists dealing with reproductive symptomatology is the recognition that there is a biological component to the woman's experience, even if that biology is not *cause* of the distress. This has lead to the suggestion that psychological approaches to assessment and treatment, if used in isolation, are not enough. In an attempt to reconcile the different aetiological theories and to acknowledge individual differences between women, multifactorial models have been suggested, which recognise that symptomatology associated with reproduction is multiply determined, and allow biological and psycho-social factors to be addressed in a context that does not privilege one or the other. These more individualised, multi-disciplinary models have now been suggested in relation to PMS (Ussher, 1992a; Parlee, 1991; Asso, 1988a; Alberts and Alberts, 1990; Rubinow and Schmidt, 1989), and the menopause (Atchison and El-Guebaly, 1987; McKinlay and McKinlay, 1986).

From a practical point of view, a multi-factorial model involves assessing an individual woman's needs, and applying an intervention, or development of be-havioural coping strategies accordingly. It would involve both physical and psycho-logical assessment, in a framework where no singular approach was adopted for all women. Implicitly, this model accommodates the critiques of the very existence of the reproductive syndromes (Palee, 1991; Ussher, 1989; Laws, 1990; Nicolson, 1992), since it recognises no single entity of PMS or menopausal syndrome, and acknowledges that a multitude of different factors may be the root cause of difficulties.

In the light of this approach, one woman presenting to a psychologist or physician with 'PMS' may be experiencing stress at work, or difficulties in an unsupportive relationship, exacerbated by her perception of menstruation as a time of tension, causing her to attribute the most salient source of negative affect to her cycle. Another woman may be particularly perceptive to bodily sensations or to changes in state, and interpret negatively perceived premenstrual increases in arousal because of her expectation that they be so construed. Secrecy and silence confirm her belief that menstruation is difficult, and prevent her from engaging with discourses which challenge her negative cognitions.

Neither woman *has* 'PMS' – an illness which is the *cause* of her difficulties. But each could benefit from an empowering reanalysis of her current situation, which would include an assessment of the role of reproduction. This may result in a realisation of the misattribution of symptoms, following education or supportive counselling; a direction of attention to underlying difficulties; therapy focussing on specific symptoms and experiences associated with reproduction; or the adoption of self help coping strategies to deal with distress. Within this framework, reproduction is no longer viewed as the sole source of misery, but is considered in relation to the many factors which impinge upon and determine a woman's experience.

CONCLUSION

Reproduction is clearly a central aspect of women's experience. Viewing menstruation and the menopause as sources of insanity and infirmity within both popular and academic discourse inevitably has an influence on a woman's interpretation of reproduction as being negative. It encourages the attribution of negative affect, of apparent failure, to the body. That this continues in the late twentieth century through the widespread acceptance of PMS and the menopausal syndrome is testimony to the deeply engrained belief that the female body is a source of madness or badness.

Yet whilst it is necessary to refute the myths associated with female reproduction, we must also acknowledge that many individuals do experience symptoms which appear to be associated with menstruation or the menopause. For these women a critical analysis and deconstruction of the existence of reproductive syndromes cannot be enough. For many women such an approach may be analogous to the age-old and frequently criticised response to female complaints 'it's all in your mind, dear'. So whilst it can be acknowledged that the needs of women as a group may not be served as by the faith in the existence of the reproductive syndrome, individual women's needs cannot be ignored.

Education, information provision, and self-help groups may provide relief for many women, but more focussed intervention in the form of therapy or counselling, with or without a medical component, may be necessary for some. A multi-factorial, multi-disciplinary approach may offer the most positive means of facilitating this intervention, since the whole range of biological, social and psychological variables affecting a woman's experience can be considered. In taking a critical perspective of the inevitably biologically driven woman, it is important to acknowledge that women expressing difficulty associated with menstruation or menopause are no more imagining their problems than women in distress at any other stage of the life cycle. Advice and intervention should therefore be tailored accordingly, with reproduction being just one part of the equation, not magnified or ignored.

REFERENCES

Abplanalp, J.M. (1979). Psychoendocrinology of the Menstrual cycle: 11. The relationship between enjoyment of activities, moods and reproductive hormones. *Psychosomatic Medicine*, **41**, 605–615.

Abraham, S. & Hargrove, C. (1980). Effects of vitamin B6 on premenstrual symptomatology on women with premenstrual syndromes: A double blind cross over study. *Infertility*, **3**, 150–64.

Ainscough, C.E. (1990). Premenstrual emotional changes: A prospective study of symptomatology in normal women. *Journal of Psychosomatic Research*, **34**, 35–45.

Alberts, P.S. & Alberts, M.S. (1990). Unvalidated treatment of premenstrual syndrome. Special Issue: Unvalidated, fringe, and fraudulent treatment of mental disorders. *International Journal of Mental Health*, **19**, 69–80.

Andersch, B. & Hahn, L. (1983). Progesterone treatment of premenstrual tension: a double blind study. *Journal of Psychosomatic Research*, **29**, 489–493.

Asso, D. (1983). *The Real Menstrual Cycle*. London; John Wiley & Sons.

Asso, D. (1988a). Physiology and psychology of the normal menstrual cycle. In: M. Brush & E. Goudsmit (Eds) *Functional Disorders of the Menstrual Cycle*. Chichester; John Wiley.

Asso, D. (1988b). Psychological and physiological changes with the menstrual cycle: implications for counselling. *Counselling Psychology Quarterly*, **1**, 2&3, 263–273.

Asso, C. & Braier, J. (1982). Changes with the menstrual cycle in psycho-physiological and self-report measures of activation. *Biological Psychology*, **15**, 95–107.

Atchison, B. & El-Guebaly, N. (1983). The joint mature women's clinic or menopause revisited. *Canadian Journal of Psychiatry*, **28**, 640–645.

Backstrom, T. & Carstensen, H. (1974). Estrogen and progesterone in plasma in relation to premenstrual tension. *Journal of Steroid Biochemistry*, **5**, 257.

Backstrom, T. & Hammarback, S. (1986). Definition and determinants of the premenstrual syndrome. Paper presented at the 8th international congress of the International Society of Psychosomatic Obstetrics and Gynaecology. March.

Bains, G.K. & Slade, P. (1988). Attributional patterns; mood and the menstrual cycle. *Psychosomatic Medicine*, 50, 469–476.

Ballinger, C.B. (1990). Psychiatric aspects of the menopause. *British Journal of Psychiatry*, 156, 773–787.

Ballinger, C.B., Smith, A.H. & Hobbs, P.R. (1985). Factors associated with psychiatric morbidity in women – a general practice survey. *Acta Psychiatrica Scandinavica*, 71, 272–280.

Benedek-Jazmann, L. & Hearn-Sturtevart, M. (1976). Premenstrual tension and functional infertility: Aetiology and treatment. *Lancet*, i, 1095–1098.

Berkun, C.S. (1986). On behalf of women over 40: Understanding the importance of the menopause. *Social Work*, 31, 378–384.

Bernstein, B.E. (1977). Effect of menstruation on academic performance among college women. *Archives of Sexual Behaviour*, 6, 289–296.

Beyene, Y. (1986). Cultural significance and physiological manifestations of menopause a biocultural analysis. Special Issue: Anthropological approaches to menopause: Questioning received wisdom. *Culture, Medicine and Psychiatry*, 10, 47–71.

Briffault, R. (1972). *The mothers: a study of the origins of sentiments and institutions*. Vol II. London; George Allen & Unwin.

Brookes, G., Ruble, D. & Clarke, C. (1977). College women's attitudes and expectations concerning menstrual related change. *Psychosomatic Medicine*, 39, 288–98.

Brush, M.G. (1977). The possible mechanisms causing the premenstrual tension syndrome. *Current Medical Research and Opinion*, 4, Suppl 4, 9–15.

Burrows, G. (1828). Commentaries on Insanity. London; Underwood.

Butt, W., Watts, J. & Holder, G. (1983). The biochemical background to the premenstrual syndrome. In R. Taylor (ed.) *Premenstrual Syndrome*. London; Medical News Tribune.

Channon, L.D. & Ballinger, S.E. (1982). Some aspects of sexuality and vaginal symptoms during menopause and their relations to anxiety and depression. *British Journal of Medical Psychology*, 59, 173–180.

Clare, A. (1983). Psychiatric and social aspects of premenstrual complaints. *Psychological Medicine Monographs*, Suppl 4, 58.

Coppen, A. & Kessel, N. (1963). Menstruation and personality. *British Journal of Psychiatry*, 11, 155–167.

Craig, G.M. (1980). The premenstrual syndrome and prostaglandin metabolism. *British Journal of Family Planning*, 6, 74–7.

Cundo, P. (1984). Menopause as an evolutive crisis: From a public health service experience. *Eta-evolutiva*, 17, 42–51.

Dalton, K. (1960a). Effect of menstruation on schoolgirls weekly work. *British Medical Journal*, 1(5169), 326–328.

Dalton, K. (1960b). Menstruation and accidents. *British Medical Journal*, 2, 1425–6.

Dalton, K. (1969). *The Menstrual Cycle*. Harmondsworth; Penguin.

Eagles, J.M. & Whalley, L.J. (1985). Ageing and affective disorders: the age at first onset of psychiatric disorders in Scotland 1969–1978. *British Journal of Psychiatry*, 147, 180–187.

Englander-Golden, P., Whitmore, M. & Dienstbier, R. (1978). Menstrual cycle as a focus of study and self-report of moods and behaviours. *Motivation and Emotion*, 2, 75–86.

Eriksson, E., Lisjo, P., Sundblad, C., Andersson, K. *et al.* (1990). Effect of clomipramine on premenstrual syndrome. *Acta Psychiatrica Scandinavica*, 81, 87–88.

Ernster, V. (1975). *American Menstrual experiences*. Sex Roles, 1, 3–13.

Feder, R. (1989). "Treatment of premenstrual depression with nortriptyline: A pilot study": Comment. *Journal of Clinical Psychiatry*, 50, 393.

Frank, R.T. (1931). The normal causes of premenstrual syndrome. *Archives of Neurology and Psychiatry*, 26, 1053–7.

Frazer, J.G. (1938). *The Golden Bough: A study in magic and religion*. London; Macmillan.

Gannon, L. (1981). Psychological and physiological factors in the development, maintenance, and treatment of menstrual disorders. In: S.N. Hayes & L. Gannon (eds) *Psychosomatic disorders: A psychophysiological approach to etiology and treatment.* New York: Praeger.

Gannon, L. (1988). The potential role of exercise in the alleviation of menstrual disorders and menopausal symptoms: A theoretical synthesis of recent research. *Women and Health,* **14,** 105–127.

Garrey, M., Govan, A.D.T., Hodge, C. & Callander, R. (1978). *Gynaecology Illustrated.* Edinburgh; Churchill Livingstone.

Giannini, A.J., Martin, D.M. & Turner, C.E. (1990). Beta-endorphin decline in late luteal phase dysphoric disorder. *International Journal of Psychiatry in Medicine,* 20, 279–284.

Glass, G., Heninger, G., Lansky, M. & Talan, K. (1971). Psychiatric emergency related to the menstrual cycle. *American Journal of Psychiatry,* **128,** 705–11.

Glen, N. (1975). Psychological well-being in the post-parent stage, some evidence from national surveys. *Journal of Marriage and the Family,* 37, 105–10.

Golub, S. & Harrington, D. (1981). Premenstrual and menstrual mood changes in adolescent women. *Journal of Personality and Social Psychology,* **41,** 961–965.

Golub, S. (1976). The magnitude of premenstrual anxiety and depression. *Psychosomatic Medicine,* **38,** 4–11.

Greene, J.G. (1984). *The social and psychological origins of the climacteric syndrome.* Aldershot; Gower.

Greene, R. & Dalton, K. (1953). The premenstrual syndrome. *British Medical Journal,* 1, 1007–14.

Halbreich, U. (1990). Treatment of premenstrual syndromes with progesterone antagonists (e.g. RU-486): Political and methodological issues. *Psychiatry,* **53,** 407–409.

Halbreich, U. & Endicott, J. (1981). Possible involvement of endorphin withdrawal or imbalance in specific premenstrual syndromes and post-partum depression. *Medical Hypotheses,* 7, 1045–58.

Hamilton, J.A. & Gallant, S. (1990). Problematic aspects of diagnosing premenstrual phase dysphoria: recommendations for psychological research and practice. *Professional Psychology: Research and Practice,* **21,** 60–68.

Harrison, W.M., Endicott, J., Nee, J., Glick, H. *et al.* (1989). Characteristics of women seeking treatment for premenstrual syndrome. *Psychosomatics,* 30, 405–411.

Haspels, A. (1983). Premenstrual syndrome – a view from the continent. In R. Taylor (ed.) *Premenstrual Syndrome.* London; Medical News Tribune.

Hays, H.R. (1972). *The dangerous sex: The myth of feminine evil.* Pocket Books; New York.

Heilbrun, A.B. & Frank, M.E. (1989). Self-preoccupation and general stress level as sensitizing factors in premenstrual and menstrual distress. *Journal of Psychosomatic Research,* **33,** 571–577.

Herzberg, B., Johnson, A., Brown, F. & Beck, A. (1970). Self-rating scale for depression, oral contraceptives and premenstrual depression. *Lancet,* i, 775.

Herzog, A.G. (1989). Perimenopausal depression: Possible role of anomalous brain substrates. *Brain Dysfunction,* **2,** 146–154.

Hodges, S. (1987). The psychology of menstruation: how heavy is heavy? Paper presented at the Women and Psychology conference, July; Brunel University, London.

Holte, A. (1989). *The Norwegian Menopause project: A six year prospective follow-up of psychosocial and biological indicators of health, symptoms and quality of life in normal women.* Unpublished research paper. Department of Behavioural Sciences in Medicine, Oslo, Norway.

Horrobin, D., Manku, M., Nassur, B. & Evered, D. (1973). Prolactin and fluid and electrolyte balance. In J.L. Pasteels & C. Robyn (eds.) *Human Prolactin.* Exerpta Medica; Amsterdam.

Hunter, M. (1990a). Emotional well-being, sexual behaviour and hormone replacement therapy. *Maturitas,* 7, 299–314.

Hunter, M. (1990b). Psychological and somatic experience of the menopause: A prospective study. *Psychosomatic Medicine*, 52, 357-367.

Hunter, M. (1990c). *The Menopause*. London; Pandora Press.

Hunter, M., Battersby, R. & Whitehead, M. (1986). Relationship between psychological symptoms, somatic complaints and menopausal status. *Maturitas*, 3, 217-228.

Jakubowicz, D. (1983). the significance of prostoglandins in the premenstrual syndrome. In R. Taylor (ed.) *Premenstrual Syndrome*, London; Medical News Tribune.

Janowski, D., Berens, S., Davis, J. & Vanderbilt, U. (1973). Correlations between mood, weight and electrolytes during the menstrual cycle: a renin-aldosterone hypothesis of premenstrual tension. *Psychosomatic Medicine*, 35, 143-54.

Jensen, B. (1982). Menstrual cycle effects on task performance examined in the context of stress research. *Acta Psychologica*, 50, 159-178.

Kaufert, P.A. & Syrotuik, J. (1981). Symptom reporting at the menopause. *Social Science and Medicine*, 15, 173-184.

Kerr, G. (1977). The management of the premenstrual syndrome, *Current Medical Research and Opinion*, 4, Suppl 4, 29-34.

Kincey, J. & McFarland, T. (1984). Psychological aspects of hysterectomy. In A. Brooke & L. Wallace (eds) *Psychology and Gynaecological Problems*. London; Tavistock.

Kinsbourne, M. (1971). Cognitive deficit: experimental analysis. In J. McGaugh (ed) *Psychobiology*. New York; Academic Press.

Kitzinger, S. (1983). *Women's experience of sex*. London; Dorling Kindersley.

Klaiber, E., Broverman, D., Vogel, W. & Kobayashi, Y. (1974). Rhythms in plasma MAO activity, EEG, and behaviour during the menstrual cycle. In M. Ferin, F. Halberg, R. Richard & R. Vande Wiele (eds.) *Biorhythms and Human Reproduction*. New York; John Wiley & Sons.

Koeske, R. (1977). *The interaction of social-cognitive and physiological factors in premenstrual emotionality*. (unpublished doctoral dissertation, Caregie, Mellon University).

Koeske, R. (1980). Theoretical perspectives on menstrual cycle research: the relevance of attributional approaches for the perception and explanation of premenstrual emotionality. In A.J. Dan, E. Graham & C. Beecher (eds) *The Menstrual Cycle vol I*. New York; Springer.

Kuczmierczyk, A.R. (1989). Multi-component behavioural treatment of premenstrual syndrome: A case report. *Journal of Behaviour Therapy and Experimental Psychiatry*, 20, 235-240.

Laws, S. (1990). *Issues of blood*. London; MacMillian.

Lees, P. 61965). The vulnerability to trauma of women in relation to periodic stress. Abstract. *The Medical Commission on Accident Prevention*; second annual report.

Lennon, M.C. (1987). Is menopause depressing? An investigation of three perspectives. *Sex Roles*, 17, 1-16.

Levitt, E. & Lubin, B. (1967). Some personality factors associated with menstrual complaints and menstrual attitudes. *Journal of Psychosomatic Research*, 11, 267-70.

Lewis, J.W. (1990). Premenstrual syndrome as a criminal defense. *Archives of Sexual Behavior*, 19, 425-441.

Little, B.C. & Zahn, T.P. (1974). Changes in mood and autonomic functioning during the menstrual cycle. *Psychophysiology*, 11, 579-80.

Lowenthal, M. (1975). Psychosocial variations along the adult life course: frontiers for research and policy. *The Gerentologist*, 15, 6-12.

Luggin, R., Bensted, L., Petersson, B. & Jacobsen, A. (1984). Acute psychiatric admission related to the menstrual cycle. *Acta psychiatrica Scandinavica*, 69, 461-5.

Maddock, A. (1854). *The Education of Women*. From: On Mental and Nervous Disorders. London; Simpkin, Marshall & Co.

Maddocks, S., Hahn, P., Moller, F. & Reid, R.L. (1986). A double blind placebo controlled trial of progesterone vaginal suppositories in the treatment of premenstrual syndrome. *American Journal of Obstetrics and Gynaecology*, **154**, 573–581.

Magos, A.L., Collins, W.P. & Studd, J.W. (1984). Management of the premenstrual syndrome by subcutaneous implants of oestradiol. *Journal of Psychosomatic Obstetrics and Gynaecology*, 3, 93–99.

Maitland, S. (1981). *Daughters of Jerusalem*. London; Pavanne.

Majewska, M.D. (1987). Actions of steroids on neuron: Role in personality, mood, stress, and disease. *Integrative Psychiatry*, 5, 258–273.

Mansfield, P., Hood, K. & Henderson, J. (1989). Women and their husbands; Mood and arousal fluctuations across the menstrual cycle and days of the week. *Psychosomatic Medicine*, 51, 66–80.

Marini, D. & Fee, R. (1983). Relative personality differences in high versus low menstrual symptom reporters. Paper given to the Society for the Scientific Study of Sex, University of Pennsylvania.

Martin, E. (1987). *The Woman in the Body*. Milton Keynes; Open University Press.

Matthews, K.A., Wing, R.R., Kuller, Lewis-H. & Meilahn, E.N. (1990). Influences of natural menopause on psychological characteristics and symptoms of middle-aged healthy women. *Journal of Consulting and Clinical Psychology*, 58, 345–31.

Mattson, B. & von Schoultz, B. (1974). A comparison between lithium, placebo and a diuretic in premenstrual tension. *Acta Psychiatrica Scandinavica*, Suppl 255, 75–83.

Maudsley, H. (1873). *Body and Mind*. Macmillan; London.

May, R. (1976). Mood shifts and the menstrual cycle. *Journal of Psychosomatic Research*, 20, 125–130.

McFarland, C., Ross, M. & deCourville, N. (1987). Women's theories of menstruation and biases in recall of menstrual symptoms. *Journal of Personality and Social Psychology*, 57, 522–531.

McKinlay, J.B. & Jeffreys, M. (1974). The menopausal syndrome. *British Journal of Preventative and Social Medicine*, 28, 108–115.

McKinlay, J.B., McKinlay, S.M. & Brambilla, D. (1987). The relative contributions of endocrine changes and social circumstances to depression in mid-aged women. *Journal of Health and Social Behaviour*, 28, 345–363.

McKinlay, S. & McKinlay, J. (1973). Selected studies of the menopause. *Journal of Biosocial Science*, 5, 533–555.

McKinlay, S.M. & McKinlay, J.B. (1986). Aging in a "healthy" population. *Social Science and Medicine*, 23, 531–535.

Metz, A. (1990). Fluoxetine treatment of premenstrual syndrome. *Journal of Clinical Psychiatry*, 51, 260.

Molnar, G., Takacs, I. & Bazsane, Z. (1988). Endocrine changes in endogenous psychoses of climacteric and involution. *European Journal of Psychiatry*, 2, 147–158.

Moos, R. (1969). Typology of menstrual cycle symptoms. *American Journal of Obstetrics and Gynaecology*, 103, 390–402.

Moos, R.H., Kopell, B.S., Meleges, F.T., Yalom, I.D., Lunde, D.T., Clayton, R.B. & Hamburg, D.A. (1969). Fluctuations in symptoms and moods during the menstrual cycle. *Journal of Psychosomatic Research*, 13, 37–44.

Morse, C., Bernard, M.E. & Dennerstein, L. (1989). The effects of rational-emotive therapy and relaxation training on premenstrual syndrome: A preliminary study. *Journal of Rational Emotive and Cognitive Behavior Therapy*, 1, 798–110.

Morse, C.A., Dennerstein, L., Varnavides, K. & Burrows, G.D. (1988). Menstrual cycle symptoms: Comparison of a non-clinic sample with a patient group. *Journal of Affective Disorders*, 14, 41–50.

Neurgarten, B. (1979). Time, age and the life cycle. *American Journal of Psychiatry*, **136**, 1887–94.

Neurgarten, B. & Kraines, R.J. (1965). Menopausal symptoms in women of various ages. *Psychosomatic Medicine*, **27**, 266–273.

Nicolson, P. (1992). Menstrual cycle research and the constructing of female psychology. In J.T.E. Richardson (ed) *Cognition and the Menstrual Cycle*. Springer Verlag; New York.

Notman, M.T. (1984). Psychiatric disorders of menopause. *Psychiatric Annals*, **14**, 448–453.

O'Brien, P., Craven, D. & Selby, S. (1979). Treatment of premenstrual syndrome by spirolactone. *British Journal of Obstetrics and Gynaecology*, **86**, 142–7.

O'Neil, M., Lancee, W. & Freeman, J. (1984). Fluctuations in psychological distress during the menstrual cycle. *Canadian Journal of Psychiatry*, **29**, 373–378.

Odink, J., Van der Ploeg, H.M., Van den Berg, H., Van Kempen, G.M. *et al.* (1990). Circadian and circatrigintan rhythms of biogenic amines in premenstrual syndrome (PMS). *Psychosomatic Medicine*, **52**, 346–356.

Olasov, B. & Jackson, J. (1987). Effects of expectancies on women's reports of moods during the menstrual cycle. *Psychosomatic Medicine*, **49**, 65–78.

Parlee, M. (1973). The premenstrual syndrome. *Psychological Bulletin*, **80**, 454–65.

Parlee, M. (1991). The social construction of premenstrual syndrome: a case study of scientific discourse as cultural contestation. Paper presented at conference on 'The good body: Asceticism in contemporary culture', Institue for the Medical Humanities, The University of Texas Medical Branch at Galveston, Galveston, Texas.

Parry, B.L., Berga, S.L., Kripke, D.F., Klauber, M.R. *et al.* (1990). Altered waveform of plasma nocturnal melatonin secretion in premenstrual depression. *Archives of General Psychiatry*, **47**, 1139–1146.

Patterson, M.M. & Lynch, A.Q. (1988). Menopause: Salient issues for counselors. *Journal of Counseling and Development*, **67**, 185–188.

Picone, L. & Kirkby, R.J. (1990). Relationship between anxiety and premenstrual syndrome. *Psychological Reports*, **67**, 43–48.

Puolakka, J. & Makarainen, L. (1985). 6: keto-prostaglandin f loc and thornboxane in premenstrual syndrome: the effect of treatment with prostaglandin synthesis premenstrually (unpublished manuscript). Cited in W. Harrison, L. Sharpe & J. Endicott; Treatment of premenstrual symptoms. *General Hospital Psychiatry*, **7**, 54–65.

Reitz, R. (1981). *Menopause: A Positive Approach*. London; Unwin.

Richardson, J.T.E. (1992). The menstrual cycle, cognition and paramenstrual symptomatology. In J.T.E. Richardson (ed) *Cognition and the Menstrual Cycle*. London; Springer Verlag.

Rickels, K., Freeman, E.W., Sondheimer, S. & Albert, J. (1990). Fluoxetine in the treatment of premenstrual syndrome. *Current Therapeutic Research*, **48**, 161–166.

Robinson, G.E. & Garfinkel, P.E. (1990). Problems in the treatment of premenstrual syndrome. *Canadian Journal of Psychiatry*, **35**, 199–206.

Rodin, J. (1976). Menstruation, reattribution and competence. *Journal of Personality and Social Psychology*, **33**, 345–53.

Rothert, M., Rovner, D., Holmes, M., Schmitt, N. *et al.* (1990). Women's use of information regarding hormone replacement therapy. *Research in Nursing and Health*, **13**, 355–366.

Rubinow, D.R., Roy-Byrne, P., Hoban, C., Gold, P.W. & Post, R.M. (1984). Prospective assessment of menstrually related mood disorders. *Journal of Psychiatry*, **141**, 684–686.

Rubinow, D.R. & Schmidt, P.J. (1989). Models for the development of symptoms in premenstrual syndrome. *Psychiatric Clinics of North America*, **12**, 53–68.

Sampson, G. (1979). Premenstrual tension: a double blind controlled trial of progesterone and placebo. *British Journal of Psychiatry*, **135**, 209–15.

Sayers, J. (1982). *Biological Politics: Feminist and Anti-Feminist Perspectives*. London; Tavistock.

Schmidt, P.J., Rosenfeld, D., Muller, K.L., Grover, G.N. *et al.* (1990) A case of autoimmune thyroiditis presenting as menstrual related mood disorder. *Journal of Clinical Psychiatry*, **51**, 434–436.

Scott-Palmer, J. & Skevington, S. (1981). Pain during childbirth and menstruation: a study of locus of control. *Journal of Psychosomatic Research*, **25**, 151-5.

Shaw, D. (1983). Hormones, amines and mood. In R. Taylor (ed.) *Premenstrual Syndrome*. London; Medical News Tribune.

Sheldrake, P. & Cormack, M. (1976). Variations in menstrual cycle symptom reporting. *Journal of Psychosomatic Research*, **20**, 169-177.

Sherwin, B.B. & Gelfand, M.M. (1987). The role of androgen in the maintenance of sexual functioning in oophorectomized women. *Psychosomatic Medicine*, **49**, 397-409.

Showalter, E. (1987). *The Female Malady*. London; Virago.

Shreeve, C. (1984). *the Premenstrual Syndrome*. Wellingborough; Thorsons.

Siegal, J., Johnson, J. & Sarason, I. (1979). Life changes and menstrual discomfort. *Journal of kPsychosomatic Medicine*, **5**, 41-46.

Singer, K., Cheng, R. & Schou, M. (1974). A controlled evaluation of lithium in the premenstrual tension syndrome. *British Journal of Psychiatry*, **124**, 50-51.

Slade, P. (1984). Premenstrual emotional changes in normal women: fact or fiction? *Journal of Psychosomatic Research*, **28**, 1-7.

Slade, P. (1989). Psychological therapy for premenstrual emotional symptoms. *Behavioural Psychotherapy*, **17**, 135-150.

Smith, W. Tyler (1848). The climacteric disease in women.

Sommer, B. (1972). Menstrual cycle changes and intellectual performance. *Psychosomtic Medicine*, **34**, 263-269.

Sommer, B. (1982). Cognitive behaviour and the menstrual cycle. In R.C. Friedman (ed) *Behaviour and the Menstrual Cycle*. New York; Marcel Dekker.

Sommer, B. (1992). Cognitive performance and the menstrual cycle. In: J.T.E. Richardson (ed) *Cognition and the Menstrual Cycle*. London; Springer Verlag.

Spitzer, R.L., Severino, S.K., Williams, J.B. & Parry, B.L. (1989). Late luteal phase dysphoric disorder and DSM-III-R. *American Journal of Psychiatry*, **146**, 892-897.

Squire, C. (1989). *Significant Differences: Feminism in Psychology*. London; Routledge.

Stadel, B. & Weiss, N. (1975). Characteristics of menopausal women: A survey of King and Pierce counties in Washington, 1973-1974. *American Journal of Epidemiology*, **102**, 206-16.

Stuenkel, C.A. (1989). Menopause and estrogen replacement therapy. *Psychiatric Clinics of North America*, **12**, 133-152.

Taghavi, E. (1990). Premenstrual syndrome in three generations responds to antidepressants. *Australian and New Zealand Journal of Psychiatry*, **24**, 276-279.

Taylor, J. (1979). The timing of menstruation related symptoms assessed by a daily symptom rating. *Acta Psychiatrica Scandinavica*, **60**, 87-105.

Ussher, J. (1987). Variations in performance, mood and state during the menstrual cycle. Unpublished PhD thesis, University of London.

Ussher, J.M. (1989). *The Psychology of the Female Body*. London; Routledge.

Ussher, J.M. & Wilding, J. (1991). Performance and state changes during the menstrual cycle, conceptualised within a broad band testing framework. *Social Science and Medicine*, **32**, 525-534.

Ussher, J.M. (1991). *Women's Madness: Misogny or Mental Illness?* Hemel Hempstead; Harvester Wheatsheaf.

Ussher, J.M. & Wilding, J. (1992). Interactions between stress and performance during the menstrual cycle in relation to the premenstrual syndrome. *Journal of Reproductive and Infant Psychology*, **10**, 83-101.

Ussher, J.M. (1992a). The demise of dissent and the rise of cognition in menstrual cycle research. In J.T.E. Richardson (ed) *Cognition and the Menstrual Cycle*. New York; Springer Verlag.

Ussher, J.M. (1992b). Reproductive rhetoric and the blaming of the body. In P. Nicholson & J.M. Ussher (eds) *The Psychology of Women's Health and Health Care*. London; Macmillan.

Ussher, J.M. (1992c). Sex differences in performances: fact, fiction or fantasy? In D. Jones & A. Smith (eds) *Studies in Human Performance. Vol III.* New York; Erlbaum.

Ussher, J.M. (1992d). Research and theory related to female reproduction: implications for clinical psychology. *British Journal of Clinical Psychology*, **31**, 129–152.

Utian, W.H. & Serr, D. (1976). The climacteric syndrome. In P.A. Van Keep, R.B. Greenblatt & M. Albeaux-Fernet *Consensus on Menopause Research.* Lancaster; MTP Press.

Varma, T. (1983). Hormones and electrolytes in the premenstrual syndrome. In R. Taylor (ed.) *Premenstrual Syndrome.* London; Medical News Tribune.

Walling, M., Andersen, B.L. & Johnson, S.R. (1990). Hormonal replacement therapy for post-menopausal women: A review of sexual outcomes and related gynecologic effects. *Archives of Sexual Behaviour*, **19**, 119–137.

Walsh, K. (1985). *Understanding Brain Damage.* Edinburgh; Churchill Livingstone.

Walsh, R., Budtz-Olsen, I., Leader, C. & Cummins, R. (1981). The menstrual cycle, personality and academic performance. *Archives of General Psychiatry*, **38**, 219–221.

Warner, P. & Bancroft, J. (1990). Factors related to self-reporting of the pre-menstrual syndrome. *British Journal of Psychiatry*, **157**, 249–260.

Weidegar, P. (1976). *Female Cycles.* London; The Women's Press.

Wilbur, J., Dan, A., Hedricks, C. & Holm, K. (1990). The relationship among menopausal status, menopausal symptoms, and physical activity in midlife women. *Family and Community Health*, **13**, 67–78.

Wilcoxen, L., Schrader, S. & Sherif, C. (1976). Daily self reports on activities, life events, moods, and somatic changes during the menstrual cycle. *Psychosomatic Medicine*, **38**, 399–417.

Williams, L. (1983). Beliefs and attitudes of young girls regarding menstruation. In S. Golub (ed) *Menarche.* Lexington, MA; Lexington Books.

Wilson, C.A. & Key, W.R. (1989). A survey of adolescent dysmenorrhea and premenstrual symptom frequency: A model program for prevention, detection, and treatment. *Journal of Adolescent Health Care*, **10**, 317–322.

Wilson, R.A. (1966). *Feminine Forever.* New York; Evans.

Wood, C. & Jakubowicz, D. (1980). The treatment of premenstrual symptoms with mefenbamic acid. *British Journal of Obstetrics and Gynaecology*, **87**, 627–30.

Woods, N., Dery, M. & Most, E. (1982). Recollections of menarche, current menstrual attitude and peri-menstrual symptoms. *Psychosomatic Medicine*, **44**, 285–97.

World Health Organisation (1981). Research on the menopause. Report of a WHO scientific group. *Technical Report Series*, **670**. Geneva; WHO.

ISSUES OF CONTROL AND HEALTH: THE ACTION IS IN THE INTERACTION

KENNETH A. WALLSTON* AND M. SHELTON SMITH

Butler (1976) delineates three "symptoms" of middle age. The first is counting the number of years left before death rather than counting the years since birth. The second involves looking at what one has done and evaluating accomplishments in relation to goals. The third is an awareness of the body and a monitoring of the body systems and states. As one ages and one's health status declines this third symptom plays an increasingly important role.

The middle-aged years are a time of "settling down" (Levinson, 1977). Middle-aged adults experience greater control over their lives and have stronger feelings of security and stability than at other developmental periods. During these years, individuals struggle with resolving the "crisis" between generativity versus stagnation (Erikson, 1968). Generativity is the ability to care for others and to help them accomplish their goals as well as to manage one's own life and to care for oneself. Stagnation is hanging on to the same goals established early in life regardless of the likelihood of achieving those goals, or using unhealthy or self-destructive methods for coping with disillusionment or failure.

Middle-aged is an ambiguous term. Various definitions exist as far as when someone should be considered middle-aged. Some theorists have marked the decades between 30 and 70 as the middle years (Kerckhoff, 1976). The US census more narrowly delimits the range to between 45 and 64 years of age. Chronological age is not the only determinant of when middle-age begins and ends. The perspectives of similarly-aged people vary as to whether they consider themselves middle-aged or not. The tasks one is attempting to accomplish and the characteristics of one's life also mark the middle years.

*Address all correspondence regarding this chapter to K.A. Wallston, School of Nursing, Vanderbilt University, Nashville, TN 37240 USA.

Generally, the developmental tasks of middle-age involve the establishment of oneself in one's career, the raising of children, caring for elderly parents, and, in a real sense, managing the world. This is usually the most productive period of one's life. Typically one is more in control over one's own life, as well as other people's lives, when one is middle-aged than at any other time. In addition to managing one's own life, the middle-aged individual is also a member of the primary group that is responsible for the major decisions and activities of society as a whole.

Of course, not all individuals in this period of life experience equivalent levels of control. Women in traditional domestic roles may begin to struggle with their own dependency on their husbands (Sheehy, 1976). Their crisis is less one of learning to care for other people and more of learning to care for oneself. People in lower socioeconomic status groups also do not feel as much in control over their destinies as those with more financial resources. At the same time when one is at the peak of productivity, one is also beginning to notice and deal with the decline of youth and vigorous health, both of which have implications for one's feelings of control over one's health status.

The effects of aging on health are relatively gradual and may not be noticed until much later. The first effects of aging may become evident during the early 40s – wrinkles, gray hairs, vision and hearing loss, weight gain. Certain effects of aging (e.g. weight gain; wrinkles) can also be delayed or diminished through regular exercise, a good diet, and avoiding tobacco. Health issues during this period are variable from individual to individual. Some may begin to experience the effects of cardiovascular disease or other chronic illnesses such as arthritis or diabetes. Even those who do not suffer from serious illness usually observe more of their contemporaries having health problems. The impact of declining health has differential effects on individuals depending upon a variety of factors, most of which interact with one another to produce varying outcomes.

In addition to health issues, there are many other stressors that go along with this highly significant period in life. The management of multiple roles, the responsibilities and obligations that accompany power, all produce stress as well as rewards. Middle age is the most complex period in the life-cycle. Personality characteristics, beliefs, values, attitudes, societal expectations, environmental factors, and role demands are only a few of the numerous factors that influence the behavior and psychological states of middle-aged adults. This chapter focuses on one of these factors: the extent to which an individual believes he or she is "in control" of some aspect of his/her health.

Elsewhere we have defined perceived control as "the belief that one can determine one's own internal states and behaviour, influence one's environment, and/or bring about desired outcomes" (Wallston, Wallston, Smith and Dobbins, 1987, p. 5). Perceived control is related to, but different from, desire for control – a motivational construct which also plays a role in determining behavior (R. Smith, Wallston, Wallston, Forsberg and King, 1984). Also, perceived control of health encompasses more than "health locus of control" (Wallston, 1992). Control beliefs, however, are only one of the possible factors that may predict behavior. Because behavior is multiply determined, it is unlikely that control beliefs alone would have a singular impact on a middle-aged adult's behavior. It is also the case that one's own behavior may be only a minor determinant of one's health status (Kaplan, 1984). Control beliefs are far more likely to interact with a myriad of other factors in predicting behavior and outcomes for this group than would be evident if only one looked for "main effects" of such beliefs.

For example, consider a middle aged male who has spent a lifetime experiencing many positive outcomes as a result of his behavior and who, therefore, has developed an "internal locus of control orientation" (i.e. the generalized belief that one's outcomes are the result of one's actions; Rotter, 1966). Suppose that one day he experiences chest pains and is hospitalized for "tests and observation" in an institution where all decisions are made for him by the staff. The experience of not having control in that setting may result in more negative outcomes for the person who expects control than for another person who has experienced little control up to that point. This latter patient might just as soon relinquish all control to the doctors and nurses. In other words, the patient's control beliefs (locus or desire) may interact with situational factors in predicting how the patient will adjust to the situation.

In applying Rotter's (1954) social learning theory to the prediction of health-related phenomena, Wallston and his colleagues have consistently stated that one's expectations about the outcomes of one's health behavior (typically assessed by a measure of health locus of control beliefs: Wallston, Wallston and DeVellis, 1978; Wallston, Wallston, Kaplan and Maides, 1976) are moderated by the value one places on being healthy and, perhaps, by other factors as well (see Wallston, 1991, or Wallston and Wallston, 1984, for explications of this theoretical proposition).

Theoretically, one's health behavior is only predictable by one's health locus of control beliefs if one values being healthy. Testing this theoretical proposition calls for, at minimum, examining the interaction between a measure of expectancies and a measure of values. For example, Kaplan and Cowles (1978) found that individuals who simultaneously held internally-oriented health locus of control beliefs (Wallston *et al.*, 1976) *and* who valued their health highly were the only subjects able to maintain reduced smoking levels post-treatment. Internally-oriented subjects who were lower in health value were able to reduce their smoking levels during the treatment phase, but relapsed during maintenance. (See Smith and Wallston, 1992, for a discussion of how to assess health values).

The remainder of this chapter consists of a potpourri of studies in which some measure of health-related control beliefs was examined in interaction with some other variable in order to explain some health-related phenomenon. Only some of these studies were conducted by Wallston and his students/colleagues, and only some employed one or other of the health locus of control scales developed by Wallston and his colleagues. All of these illustrations, however, involve people with either chronic illnesses or people who are receiving medical or surgical attention. In addition, the vast majority of subjects in these studies were middle-aged. Finally, they all have in common the fact that the most interesting findings were interactions rather than main effects. In effect, the action was in the interaction.

MEASURES OF CONTROL AND COPD PATIENTS

Chronic Obstructive Pulmonary Disease (COPD) is a set of conditions (such as chronic bronchitis, emphysema, and asthma) that are characterized by a persistent slowing of airflow while attempting to exhale air rapidly (Brashear, 1980). From both an economic and personal health standpoint, COPD is a serious, debilitating condition and a significant public health problem. The condition, however, is amenable to behavioral intervention, especially attempts at getting the patient to engage in appropriate physical conditioning exercises. If COPD patients can be motivated to carry out these exercises, they can improve their oxygen consumption and utilization, lower their heart rate, improve ventilation, and increase their tolerance for additional physical activity. The problem, however, is getting COPD patients to comply with a physical exercise regimen. Initially, in sedentary patients, physical activity may lead to serious shortness of breath. Experiencing shortness of breath is often frightening, causing the patient to avoid not only exercise but, also, many "essential" activities of daily living.

In the early 1980s, Bob Kaplan and Cathie Atkins, colleagues of the first author's out in San Diego, California, developed a number of cognitive-behavioral interventions to help COPD patients maintain a daily exercise program involving mostly walking. These interventions were based on Bandura's social learning theory (Bandura, 1977a), especially that aspect of his theory involving situationally-specific self-efficacy beliefs as mediators of behavior change (Bandura, 1977b; 1982). In order to test whether COPD patients' beliefs in their abilities to do the exercises did, in fact, contribute to their exercise compliance, Kaplan, Atkins, and their students (Kaplan, Atkins and Reinsch, 1984) administered a set of six self-efficacy scales. Within each scale, the patient was presented with a series of progressively more difficult performance requirements within a specified domain of activity. For example, the scale for walking included: walk one block (in approximately five minutes); walk two blocks (in 10 minutes); . . . walk three miles (in 90 minutes). Altogether, the walking efficacy scale consisted of nine items representing increasing gradients (in nonequal intervals) of difficulty. These self-efficacy scales (which we consider to be measures of perceived control of behavior; Wallston *et al.*, 1987) were administered at baseline – after the patient had been given a walking prescription – and at follow-up, three months later.

Kaplan *et al.* also administered the unidimensional HLC Scale to their subjects on the same occasions they had them fill out the behaviorally specific self-efficacy scales. Their reason for doing so was to show that measures based on Bandura's social learning theory were superior to one based on Rotter's social learning theory when it came to predicting health behaviors and outcomes. In their initial analyses, Kaplan and Atkins confirmed their (West Coast biased) expectations: for example, walking compliance over the three-month study period correlated .63 with self-efficacy for walking, but was essentially uncorrelated (r = −.08) with HLC scores. However, after a suggestion by the first author of this chapter, Kaplan and Atkins carried out additional analyses examining the hypothesis that HLC beliefs moderated the relationship between specific self-efficacy beliefs and health outcomes. Using a median split, they divided their sample into two groups: "HLC internals" and "HLC externals." Lo and behold, the correlations between self-efficacy for physical activity and the criterion variables were mostly positive and significant for the "HLC internals" and insignificant for the "HLC externals." In other words, only for those COPD patients who believed that their health was dependent on their actions did expectations of one's ability to carry out those actions predict health status. These findings, which are consistent with both Rotter's and Bandura's social learning theories, can be found in the article about these analyses published by Kaplan, Atkins and Reinsch (1984).

We turn next to a series of studies done by Glenn Affleck, Howard Tennen, and their colleagues at the University of Connecticut, with patients with rheumatoid arthritis. Rather than illustrating interactions among different measures of control beliefs, their work demonstrates how control beliefs interact with disease severity to predict psychological well-being.

ADAPTATION TO RHEUMATOID ARTHRITIS

Rheumatoid arthritis (RA) is a debilitating chronic illness characterized by severe pain, fatigue, disfiguration, and joint damage. It may occur at any age, but its onset is most prevalent during the late 30s through the early 50s. Although RA is incurable, it is not life-threatening; its prognosis is variable and most patients experience intermittent periods of disease flare and remission. In fact, living with the uncertainty of the disease, especially not knowing from day-to-day how one will feel, is a major stressor associated with this condition (Wiener, 1975). In illnesses such as RA, perceptions of control over the illness and its symptomatology are likely to play a significant role in patients' psychological well-being (Wallston, 1993).

Many investigators interested in psychological adaptation to RA have used the health locus of control scales as their sole means of assessing the control perceptions of RA patients. With few exceptions, these investigators contented themselves with simply correlating HLC or MHLC scores with outcome measures such as anxiety or depression. The group headed up by Glenn Affleck and Howard Tennen at the University of Connecticut, however, has not only approached measurement of control in a novel manner, they have also examined interactions of control perceptions and symptom severity as predictors of RA patients' mood disturbance.

Affleck, Tennen, Pfeiffer and Fifield (1987) interviewed a sample of 92 patients with RA (mean age = 50.4 years). In the context of that interview, they asked patients to rate the degree of personal control they felt they had over (1) day-to-day symptoms, (2) the future course of the disease, and (3) their medical care and treatment. Patients made these control appraisals on scales ranging from 0 to 10 (0 = "absolutely no control;" 10 = "extreme amount of control"). Their measure of disease severity was a composite index of physician-rated joint involvement, joint deformity, joint erosions, and global disease severity. As dependent variables, Affleck *et al.* (1987) assessed patients' mood (using the Profile of Mood States-B; Lorr and McNair, 1982) and global adjustment to their illness (by having rheumatologists and nurse practitioners treating these patients make ratings using the scale developed by Derogatis, 1975).

In two hierarchical multiple regression analyses in which background and illness-status variables were controlled, Affleck *et al.* (1987) found that RA patients' rating of the degree to which they had control over their treatment process was predictive of both positive mood and global adjustment. More importantly, with both dependent measures, there was a significant interaction between appraisals of personal control over the disease and disease severity. Perceiving personal control over the course of the disease was marginally associated with positive mood in patients with mild disease but was significantly associated with negative mood in patients with severe RA. Similarly, perceiving control over the course of the disease was only weakly associated with global adjustment in patients with mild and moderate disease severity, but was significantly related to less positive adjustment in those with relatively severe disease (Affleck *et al.*, 1987).

Recently, Tennen, Affleck, Urrows, Higgins and Mendola (1992) have reported on another set of interactions involving control beliefs and illness factors in RA patients. This more recent investigation followed 54 RA patients (mean age = 53 years) for 75 days, obtaining daily reports of pain intensity, mood, and activity limitations due to pain. Controlling for disease activity and dispositional optimism (Scheier and Carver, 1985), those who believed at the onset of the study that they had more control over their pain experienced less daily pain. However, with increased levels of pain, greater control was associated with less positive mood. On the other hand, perceived benefits of having chronic pain – a construct Tennen *et al.* (1992) equate with "secondary control" (cf Rothbaum, Weisz and Snyder, 1982) – interacted in a different manner with pain severity to predict activity limitations. Those RA patients who perceived greater benefits and then experienced severe pain reported fewer days on which their activities were limited by their pain. These extremely complex, but clinically important, findings would not have been discovered had not Tennen *et al.* examined their data for interaction effects.

DEPRESSION IN END-STAGE RENAL DISEASE

Another example of how control beliefs interact with situational variables to predict psychological state comes from a study conducted by Christensen, Turner, Smith, Holman and Gregory (1991). In their study of patients with end-stage renal disease, health locus of control beliefs (Wallston *et al.*, 1978) were examined in interaction with the experience of a failed renal transplant to predict depression.

Their study was based on Folkman's (1984) assertion that the benefits of a particular set of control beliefs are dependent on the situational context. Christensen *et al.* predicted that the negative effects of a transplant failure would be greater for those who had strong beliefs in the controllability of their illness, whether through their own efforts or those of their health care providers. It was also predicted that among those patients who had not experienced a transplant failure, those with stronger beliefs in control would have better psychological outcomes. Christensen *et al.* also predicted that disease severity would moderate the interaction described above, such that the more severe the disease the stronger the interaction.

The subjects for this study were 96 dialysis patients – 66 of whom had never had a transplant and consequently had never experienced a failure, and 30 who had had unsuccessful transplants. The measures given were the PHLC and IHLC subscales of the MHLC, the Sickness Impact Profile (SIP, Bergner, Bobbit, Carter and Gilson, 1981), and the Beck Depression Inventory (BDI, Beck, Ward, Mendelson, Mock and Erbaugh, 1961). (The BDI was administered without the somatic items due to the possible confound with symptoms of end-stage renal disease.) All measures were administered at one time point. Subjects were classified as high or low on internal and powerful other control beliefs based on a median split on each of the scales. Subjects were also classified as high or low in disease severity based on a median split on the SIP.

A separate 2 (Treatment Condition) × 2 (Control Beliefs) × (Disease Severity) ANCOVA was conducted for each dimension of control beliefs. The covariates were age and time since diagnosis, two variables that were significantly different between the treatment groups. For both analyses, the predicted three-way interactions were found to be significant: for IHLC × Disease Severity × Condition ($F(1,86) = 6.53$, $p < .05$); and for PHLC × Disease Severity × Condition ($F (1,86) = 4.71, p < .05$). The pattern of results were similar for both types of control beliefs. Within the low disease severity group, the two-way interactions between control beliefs and treatment conditions were not significant. However, the predicted interaction was found among the high disease severity group. In the failed transplant group, the high IHLC patients and high PHLC patients were significantly more depressed than the low IHLC and low PHLC patients, respectively. Among the patients who never had transplants, the opposite effects were found.

The implication of these results is that contextual variables are very important to consider in interaction with control beliefs when predicting the effects of an illness on psychological states. Beliefs in the controllability of health are more critical when those beliefs are challenged. When challenged, strong beliefs in control can actually be detrimental rather than beneficial. The experience of illness in and of itself challenges a belief in control over one's health.

Next we turn to the prediction of the "ultimate" dependent variable of interest to health psychologists: survival.

PREDICTING CANCER PATIENTS' LENGTH OF SURVIVAL

The study of the relationship between individual differences among cancer patients and how long they survive with the disease has generated an increasing amount of attention from health researchers. Investigations in this area are based on the clinical evidence that, despite similarity in histology and stage of cancer at diagnosis, cancers do not advance at the same rate across patients (Levy, 1983). Some patients die within a few weeks or months after diagnosis while others live long, nearly normal lives. The controversy over whether and to what extent we can use knowledge of individual differences to predict how long a patient will live after being diagnosed with cancer has led to much interdisciplinary attention and debate (e.g. Angell, 1985).

At the time the analysis to be described below was conducted, literature considering the effect of psychological variables on the course of cancer was replete with diverse and inconsistent findings. With the exception of a few studies (e.g. Bloom, 1982; Cassileth *et al.*, 1985; Funch and Marshall, 1983; Weisman and Worden, 1975), the majority of cancer survival investigations typically employed univariate analyses examining isolated main effects of the individual difference variables (e.g. Bieliauskas *et al.*, 1979; Derogatis, Abeloff and Melisaratos, 1979; Greer, Morris and Pettingale, 1979; Jamison, Burish and Wallston, 1987). We were aware of no studies that had examined interactions among psychological constructs.

While univariate analyses offer advantages of design simplicity and ease of interpretation, one major disadvantage is that examining one isolated factor at a time does not allow for the conjoint influences among the factors. It is, perhaps, too simplistic to believe that any one individual difference factor (or even a linear combination of these variables – such as was examined by Cassileth *et al.*, 1985) would predict an outcome as multidetermined as cancer survival. Thus, the analytical strategies employed in most past studies may have resulted in either losing or obscuring important information and may very well have contributed to the "discrepancies" in the literature.

This study, which was carried out by Maribeth Smith (no relation to the second author of this chapter), had as its primary goal the investigation of a multicomponent model of length of cancer patient survival time. The model consists of selected psychological variables (health locus of control beliefs and coping style) along with selected nonpsychological factors (i.e. age, sex, severity of type of cancer, and length of time since diagnosis). Smith was stimulated to look for interactions by Dinardo's (1972) finding (cited in Strickland, 1978) that the best adjustment for patients with spinal cord injuries were for those with both an internal locus of control orientation and a high degree of emotional repression. Those patients with an external locus who tended to be open about their negative emotional feelings had the poorest adjustment (Dinardo, 1972). It was hypothesized that interactions between health locus of control beliefs and coping style would be more predictive of survival from cancer than either construct alone, and that these interactions in combination with other individual differences would constitute a significant set of predictors.

The sample consisted of 56 terminal cancer patients, all of whom had received chemotherapy. Of the 56 subjects, 41 (73%) were female. The mean age of the sample at the time of testing was 51.3 years (s.d. = 11 years), and the average time from diagnosis to testing was 15.8 months (s.d. = 20 months). The following cancer types were represented in the sample: breast (39%), ovarian (21%), lung (21%), testicular (5%), melanoma, lymphoma, Hodgkins, colon, and leukemia. By the time of the analysis, all 56 patients had died of cancer.

All subjects had filled out a battery of psychological instruments as part of an earlier study of conditioned nausea and vomiting (conducted at Vanderbilt by Tom Burish and his associates, Burish *et al.*, 1984) in which they had participated. Inclusion criteria for Smith's sample were the availability of descriptive data (i.e. verification of date and cause of death; age; sex; cancer type; and date of diagnosis) and completion of the two psychological measures used in this analysis. Psychological testing occurred at various intervals from each patient's date of initial diagnosis. To control for these differences, the analysis included a measure of the number of months between diagnosis and time of testing (hereafter called "lead time").

Each patient completed the Multidimensional Health Locus of Control (MHLC) Scale (Wallston *et al.*, 1978) and the Situation-Response Inventory of General Trait Anxiousness (S-RI: Endler and Okada, 1974). The S-RI is a multidimensional measure of anxiety which assesses three response modes across five situations. For purposes of this study, the response mode of distress/avoidance in a new or strange situation was used as the indicator of coping style. Thus, the more a subject indicated he/she typically felt uneasy, tense or anxious when in a new or strange situation, the higher his/her distress and the greater the sensitizing coping style. Conversely, low scores on those items were indicative of avoidance or a repressive coping style.

For use in the analysis, the subscales of the MHLC (i.e. IHLC, PHLC, CHLC) and distress/avoidance scores were converted to standardized T-scores before multiplying each of the MHLC subscales by distress/avoidance to create six interaction terms. This procedure gave equal weighting to health locus of control and coping style in the resultant interactions. It also allowed separate interaction terms (e.g. IHLC × distress and IHLC × avoidance) to be included to examine the exact shape of the interaction among the constructs.

Because of the wide range of cancer types included in the sample, it was felt necessary to control for the influence of cancer severity on survival time. This was done using normative five-year survival rates (American Cancer Society, 1984). The five-year probability of surviving, based on the patient's cancer type, was subtracted from 1.00 to produce a relative severity rating. These severity ratings ranged from .18 (melanoma) to .88 (lung) with a mean of .49 (s.d. =.26).

Survival time, the dependent variable in this analysis, was operationalized as the number of months between psychological testing and death. Using a stepwise multiple regression analysis, survival time was regressed upon age, sex, cancer severity, lead time, the four psychological measures (IHLC, PHLC, CHLC, and distress/avoidance), and the six interaction terms (IHLC × distress, IHLC × avoidance, PHLC × distress, PHLC × avoidance, CHLC × distress, and CHLC × avoidance).

The regression analysis indicated that six predictors accounted for 28% of the variance (adjusted $R^2 = .176$) in cancer survival. This six predictor regression equation – consisting of CHLC × distress, sex, PHLC × distress, cancer severity, lead time, and IHLC × avoidance – was significantly different from 0.00, $\{F_{(6, 49)} = 2.96;$ $p < .02\}$, although, in the final model, no one predictor was significant by itself. CHLC × distress was the only predictor that ever contributed significantly to the equation, but it did so only on the first and second steps $\{F_{(1, 54)} = 8.94 \ p < 01;$ $F_{(1, 53)} = 5,15, \ p < .01\}$. None of the psychological measures taken by themselves (i.e. considered as main effects as opposed to interactions) entered the regression equation.

Maribeth Smith's (1985) results did not exactly fit the pattern Dinardo (1982) reported with spinal cord injured patients. Instead of the combination of internality and repression leading to the best outcome ("adjustment" in Dinardo's study, survival in Smith's), it appears that those with the *lowest* scores on IHLC × avoidance survived longer than those with the highest scores. On the other hand, the PHLC × distress interaction term appears to replicate Dinardo's finding that externals with a sensitizing coping style had the poorest outcome. It should be noted, however, that "adjustment" and length of survival time are quite different outcomes. In fact, the results of Derogatis *et al.* (1979) could indicate that those cancer patients who indicated the best "adjustment" (i.e. low levels of anxiety and depression) were those who died most quickly.

Given the complexity of an event such as dying from cancer and the controversy which has arisen over trying to predict the time of occurrence of that event from individual differences or psychological constructs, it is indeed remarkable that Smith was able to account for an adjusted 18% of the variance in cancer survival time. If she had done so merely through the use of predictors such as degree of disease severity and/or length of time since diagnosis, her findings would not be of much interest or importance to health psychologists. However, that was not the case in this study. In and of themselves, those nonpsychological individual difference factors were not significant predictors of survival. It was only when they were combined with measures of psychological constructs that the model became statistically significant and psychologically intriguing.

Taylor (1983) described a multicomponent adaptation process necessary for adequate coping with cancer. Her model consisted of a number of components, each of which was necessary, but none alone were sufficient. The fact that the only psychological terms that entered Smith's prediction equation were interactions rather than main effects may explain why other investigators (e.g. Cassileth *et al.*, 1985; Jamison, Burish and Wallston, 1987) failed to predict cancer survivorship from psychological measures. Up until Smith's (1985) study, few people reported looking for effects of interactions in predicting survival.

In the next section we review a series of three field experiments carried out by our research team at Vanderbilt under the auspices of a grant from the National Center for Health Services Research. In each of these three studies, we attempted to manipulate patient's perceived control over some aspect of their health-care situation. We also assessed how much control the patients said they wanted in those settings, so that we might examine the interactions between our control manipulations and the patients' control preferences. As will be seen, the action *was* in the interaction, but not in the form we originally thought it would be.

ENHANCING CONTROL IN HEALTH-CARE SETTINGS AS A FUNCTION OF INDIVIDUAL DIFFERENCES IN DESIRE FOR CONTROL

The major objective of this line of research was to enhance patients' sense of control by giving certain patients predictability information about and/or choice over selected aspects of their health-care regimen. We based this work on the findings of social psychologists who had demonstrated the positive health benefits of small-scale control-enhancing interventions such as (a) letting blood donors choose from which arm the blood should be drawn (Mills and Krantz, 1979); (b) giving nursing home residents a plant to take care of and letting them choose which night to attend a movie (Rodin and Langer, 1977); or (c) allowing nursing home residents to select the frequency and timing of a visit from a college student volunteer (Schulz, 1976).

In each of the three experiments we conducted, we measured, at the outset, how much control each patient wanted in the particular health care setting (see R. Smith, Wallston, Wallston, Forsberg and King, 1984). Our theoretical prediction was that the outcome variables (e.g. psychological well-being; compliance; etc.) would be determined by an interaction between this individual difference variable, desire for control (DFC), and the experimental conditions (in which we felt we would be differentially manipulating perceived control). When we first began these studies, we hypothesized that patients high in DFC would respond very favorably to our choice condition and negatively to being assigned to the condition where they were neither given choice nor enhanced predictability information. Conversely, we felt that those low in DFC would do all right if left alone, but might even become somewhat stressed if "forced" to make choices (i.e. exercise decisional control) or if presented with sensory and procedural information (i.e. heightened informational control). We soon learned how naive we were in making those predictions. We were correct in looking for an interaction, but the form of the interaction surprised us.

In the first experiment in this series (B. Wallston, Wallston, Smith *et al.*, 1987) the stressor was having to prepare for a barium enema on an outpatient basis. Having a barium enema is, in and of itself, a highly stressful experience for any patient. The unpleasantness of the situation, however, is compounded by having to follow a strict bowel cleansing regimen at home or at work for 24 to 48 hours prior to the radiological examination. (The standard regimen at that time involved a combination of a liquid diet, ingesting an evil tasting, caster-oil like preparation, and taking laxatives in order to insure that one's bowels and intestines would be empty before being given the barium enema.) Our proposed means of "improving" the situation was to develop two other alternative regimens, each of which had equal efficacy. One-third of our patient-subjects were allowed to choose from among the three regimens after we carefully described what each experience would involve. We hypothesized that patients randomly assigned to this "choice" condition would perceive the greatest amount of control and, subsequently, would have the most favorable outcomes (e.g. be less distressed and most likely to follow the regimen).

To complete the design of this randomized clinical trial, another third of the patients were given one of the regimens along with the complete description of what it would involve – including the sensations they would experience. These patients constituted the "predictability" condition. We were not sure how much perceived control to hypothesize for these subjects, since Schulz (1976) had found that his "predictability alone" subjects fared as well as those given choice. The remaining patients were given neither choice nor enhanced sensory information about the regimen assigned them. We hypothesized that these latter subjects would have the least perceived control.

In the second study (K. Wallston, Smith, King *et al.*, 1991), the stressor was receiving chemotherapy for cancer and its attendant side effects, especially nausea and vomiting. We used a two-group experimental design. Half of the patients were randomly assigned to the "choice" condition where they were given information about three distinctly different antiemetic treatments, each purportedly equivalent in reducing the noxious side effects of the chemotherapy treatments. The other group of cancer patients were assigned an antimetic treatment, rather than being given a choice, but were provided the same sensory and procedure information as those in the "choice" condition. (For ethical reasons, we did not feel comfortable in utilizing a no information "control" group in this study.) The patients, all of whom were just beginning chemotherapy or resuming chemotherapy after at least a year's time, were studied for four consecutive sessions.

In the final study in this series (R. Smith, Wallston, King and Zylstra, 1991), the health care stressor was the post-operative period in the hospital following major surgery. Patients were studied for five days post-surgery (or after being released from the surgical intensive care unit). Typically, patients feel dreadful for a day or two post surgery, then they begin to recover. By five to seven days post surgery, if complications have not occurred, they are usually well enough to be discharged. In the immediate post-operative period, when one is not feeling well, being "in control" is probably not highly salient for most patients. However, as they begin to recover, many patients become distressed at being in a situation characterized by some (e.g. Taylor, 1979) as lacking in opportunities for patients to have any control. We reasoned that this would especially be the case for those aspects of the patients' lives that they would normally control if they were at home instead of being in the hospital (such as if and when to take a bath or to receive visitors).

In the hypothesized high perceived control condition, one of our research nurses visited the patient-subject on four consecutive post-op days to offer a menu of choices in a number of areas: sleeping aids; bathing; diet; visitors; telephone calls. The patient was free to make as many, or few, choices off the "menu" as desired, and could change the selections on a daily basis. In contrast, those randomly assigned to the "predictability only" condition were not given choices but were, instead, given enhanced predictability information (e.g. told they would/would not receive a back rub that evening, or half bath in the morning). Finally, those assigned to the "standard operating procedure" SOP) condition received only the routine nursing care available to all patients on those post-surgical units.

In analyzing the data for Study One, while attempting to test the hypothesized interaction between DFC and the experimental conditions, we soon realized that we had many more "significant" findings if we did a three-way rather than a two-way split on DFC. This decision to trichotomize rather than dichotomize our individual difference variable proved fortuitous. By doing so, we established a pattern of findings which we replicated over the next two studies. If we had stuck by our initial decision to simply separate patients into high and low DFC (or if we had adopted a linear regression rather than an ANOVA approach to the analysis), we likely would have missed the most important findings. Briefly, what we found in all three of these studies, was that the only patients who profited by our "enhanced control" manipulation were those who were moderate in DFC. Contrary to prediction, those high in DFC who were given choices did poorly (e.g. became upset, were non-compliant), while those low in DFC who were given choices did fine, but not as well as those moderate in DFC.

What did we learn from these three studies? We learned that, for these particular settings, we could not give a sufficient amount of control to the high DFC patients to meet their needs. For patients with a high desire (or need) for control, the kinds of choices we were able to give were not enough to satisfy them. We may, in fact, have raised their expectations by dangling choices in front of them, and then dashed their hopes when the choices did not lead to the control they desired. Perhaps, certain patients can only feel in control by seizing it. Control which is "given" to them does not meet their needs. Additionally, the whole experience of being ill is characterized by uncontrollability. Individuals with a high need for control are placed in a particularly stressful situation; simply giving them limited choices over a treatment regimen may be irrelevant when they were unable to choose whether or not to be ill in the first place.

We also learned that health care providers won't do any harm by offering enhanced choices and/or information to patients who do not want control. Across all three studies, our low DFC patients did fine no matter which condition they were in. Because "being in control" was not a salient issue for them, they were not affected by whether or not they had choices or predictability information. In examining the demographic correlates of DFC, two variables – age and educational level – consistently showed negative relationships with DFC scores. When controlling for educational level, we still found significant age effects for DFC. Persons aged sixty or older professed less of a desire to control their health care setting than younger adults (R. Smith, Woodward, Wallston *et al.*, 1988). Given our finding that elderly patients are more apt to be lower in desire for control than younger patients, it is reassuring that those low in DFC were not adversely affected by our interventions.

Most importantly, we learned that providing opportunities for taking control had a positive benefit for at least some patients – those with moderate DFC. Although their perceived control scores were no different than any other subjects, the moderate DFC patients who were given choices did significantly better on many of the other dependent variables than other patients given choices or moderate DFC patients in other conditions.

SUMMARY IMPLICATIONS

We have just described seven different studies involving predominantly middle-aged subjects all of whom were experiencing health problems. In each of these studies, the investigators assessed some aspect of belief about control over some aspect of their health and analyzed the data for interactions among these health beliefs and some other aspect of the situation. In each of these analyses, it was the interaction effect which produced the most interesting findings, not the main effects. In other words, the action was in the interaction.

As we stated in the introduction to this chapter, the middle-aged years involve a number of complexities; any person who attempts to understand and/or predict the behavior or experiences of persons who are middle-aged must be open to an interactionist perspective. Control beliefs do play an important role in helping to explain/predict the behavior and/or experiences of individuals, but they do not do so alone. One of the most consistent findings across several of the studies we described was that strong beliefs in control over one's health do not necessarily lead to positive outcomes. This is particularly the case in situations which challenge one's beliefs in control, such as when one has a severe chronic illness. The more severe the disease, the more strongly one's control beliefs are confronted. As control beliefs are disconfirmed by disease progression, one's view of the world changes, and one becomes psychologically disturbed. For many persons in this situation, it might be psychologically "healthier" to desire and/or expect a lesser degree of control (cf. Burish, Carey, Wallston *et al.*, 1984).

For researchers, it is important not only to examine interactions, but also to recognize that the interactions among the variables might not always be linear. Also, in choosing which variables to examine in interaction with control beliefs, it is better to be guided by theory (or at least some well thought out conceptual framework) than to capitalize on chance by exploring all possible combinations of variables. As several of the studies we reviewed suggest, when looking at chronically ill populations it is a good idea to block on disease severity. Other situational characteristics, such as whether the patient has experiences that confirm or disconfirm controllability beliefs, may also be important moderators. A similar case could be made for other individual differences interacting with control beliefs, such as one's feelings of susceptibility (cf. Smith, 1988). Finally, it is quite possible that the interaction effects described in this chapter are limited to middle-age persons who are experiencing health difficulties; the presence, nature, and direction of interaction effects might be very different in healthy, younger populations.

REFERENCES

Affleck, G., Tennen, H., Pfeiffer, C. & Fifield, J. (1987). Appraisals of control and predictability in adapting to a chronic disease. *Journal of Personality and Social Psychology*, **53**, 273–279.

American Cancer Society (1984). *Cancer facts and figures.*

Angell, M. (1985). Editorial: Disease as a reflection of the psyche. *New England Journal of Medicine, 312, 1570–1572.*

Bandura, A. (1977a). *Social learning theory.* Englewood Cliffs, NJ: Prentice-Hall.

Bandura, A. (1977b). Self-efficacy: Toward a unifying theory of behavioral change. *Psychological Review, 84, 191–215.*

Bandura, A. (1982). Self-efficacy mechanisms in human agency. *American Psychologist, 37, 122–147.*

Beck, A.T., Ward, C.H., Mendelson, M., Mock, J. & Erbaugh, J. (1961). An inventory for measuring depression. *Archives of General Psychiatry, 4, 561–571.*

Bergner, R.N., Bobbit, R.A., Carter, W.B. & Gilson, B.S. (1981). The sickness impact profile: Development and final revision of a health status measure. *Medical Care, 191, 787–805.*

Bieliauskas, L., Shekelle, R., Garron, D., Maliza, C., Ostfeld, A., Paul, O. & Raynor, W. (1979). Psychological depression and cancer mortality. *Psychosomatic medicine, 41, 77–78.*

Bloom, J.R. (1982). Social support, accommodation to stress and adjustment to breast cancer. *Social Science and Medicine, 16, 1329–1338.*

Brashear, R.E. Chronic obstructive pulmonary disease (1980). In D. Simmons (Ed.). *Current pulmonology,* (Vol. 6). Boston: Houghton-Mifflin.

Burish, T.G., Carey, M.P., Wallston, K.A., Stein, M.J., Jamison, R.N. & Lyles, J.N. (1984). Health locus of control and chronic disease: An external orientation may be advantageous. *Journal of Social and Clinical Psychology, 2, 326–332.*

Butler, R.N. (1976). We should end commercialization in the care of older people in the United States: Some thoughts. *International Journal of Aging and Human Development, 7, 87–88.*

Cassileth, B.R., Lusk, E.J., Miller, D.S., Brown, L.L. & Miller, C. (1985). Psychosocial correlates of survival in advanced malignant disease? *New England Journal of Medicine, 312, 1551–1555.*

Christensen, A.J., Turner, C.W., Smith, T.W., Holman, J.M. & Gregory, M.C. (1991). Health locus of control and depression in end-stage renal disease. *Journal of Consulting and Clinical Psychology, 59, 419–424.*

Derogatis, L. (1975). *Global adjustment to illness scale.* Baltimore, MD: Clinical Biometrics Research Series.

Derogatis, L.R., Abeloff, M.D. & Melisaratos, N. (1979). Psychological coping mechanisms and survival time in metastatic breast cancer. *Journal of the American Medical Association, 242, 1504–1508.*

Dinardo, Q.E. (1972). Psychological adjustment to spinal cord injury. *Dissertation Abstracts International, 32, 4206B–4207B.*

Endler, N.S. & Okada, M. (1974). A multidimensional measure of generalized trait anxiety: The S-R inventory of general trait anxiousness. *Journal of Consulting and Clinical Psychology, 46, 319–329.*

Erikson, E.H. (1968). *Identity: Youth and crisis.* New York: Norton.

Folkman, S. (1984). Personal control and stress and coping processes: A theoretical analysis. *Journal of Personality and Social Psychology, 46, 839–852.*

Funch, D.P. & Marshall, J. (1983). The role of stress, social support and age in survival from breast cancer. *Journal of Psychosomatic Research, 27, 77–83.*

Greer, S., Morris, T. & Pettingale, K.W. (1979). Psychological response to breast cancer: Effect on outcome. *The Lancet, 2, 785–787.*

Jamison, R.M., Burish, T.G. & Wallston, K.A. (1987). Psychogenic factors in predicting survival of breast cancer patients. *Journal of Clinical Oncology, 5, 768–772.*

Kaplan, G.D. & Cowles, A. (1978). Health locus of control and health value in the prediction of smoking reduction. *Health Education Monographs, 6, 129–137.*

Kaplan, R.M. (1984). The connection between clinical health promotion and health status: A critical review. *American Psychologist, 39, 755–765.*

Kaplan, R.M., Atkins, C.J. & Reinsch, S. (1984). Specific efficacy expectations mediate exercise compliance in patients with COPD. *Health Psychology*, **3**, 223–242.

Kerchoff, R.K. (1976). Marriage and middle age. *The Family Coordinator*, **25**, 5–11.

Levinson, D. (1977). The mid-life transition: A period in adult psychosocial development. *Psychiatry*, **40**, 99–112.

Levy, S.M. (1983). Host differences in neoplastic risk: Behavioral and social contributors to the disease. *Health Psychology*, **2**, 21–44.

Lorr, M. & McNair, D. (1982). *Profile of mood states-B*. San Diego, CA: Educational and Industrial Testing Service.

Mills, R.T. & Krantz, D.S. (1979). Information, choice, and reactions to stress: A field experiment in a blood bank with laboratory analogue. *Journal of Personality and Social Psychology*, **37**, 608–620.

Rodin, J. & Langer, E.J. (1977). Long-term effects of a control-relevant intervention with the institutionalized aged. *Journal of Personality and Social Psychology*, **35**, 897–903.

Rothbaum, F., Weisz, J. & Snyder, S. (1982). Changing the world and changing the self: A two-process model of perceived control. *Journal of Personality and Social Psychology*, **42**, 5–37.

Rotter, J.B. (1954). *Social learning and clinical psychology*. Englewood Cliffs, NJ: Prentice-Hall.

Rotter, J.B. (1966). Generalized expectancies for internal versus external control of reinforcement. *Psychological Monographs*, **80**, No. 1, (Whole No. 609).

Scheier, M. & Carver, C. (1985). Optimism, coping, and health: Assessment and implications of generalized outcome expectancies. *Health Psychology*, **4**, 219–247.

Schulz, R. (1976). The effects of control and predictability on the physical and psychological well-being of the institutionalized aged. *Journal of Personality and Social Psychology*, **33**, 563–573.

Sheehy, G. (1976). *Passages: The predictable crises of adult life*. New York: E.P. Dutton & Company.

Smith, M. (1985). *Predicting cancer patient survival length*. Unpublished masters thesis. Vanderbilt University, Nashville, TN.

Smith, M.S. (1988). *Growing health nuts: Preventive health behavior of young adults as a function of perceived control, relative health value, and susceptibility beliefs*. Unpublished doctoral dissertation. Vanderbilt University, Nashville, TN.

Smith, M.S. & Wallston, K.A. (1992). How to measure the value of health. *Health Education Research, Theory & Practice*, **7**, 129–135.

Smith, R.A.P., King, J.E., Wallston, K.A. & Zylstra, M. (1991). *Individual differences in response to control interventions among surgical patients*. Unpublished manuscript. Vanderbilt University, Nashville, TN.

Smith, R.A., Wallston, B.S., Wallston, K.A., Forsberg, P.R. & King, J.E. (1984). Measuring desire for control of health care processes. *Journal of Personality and Social Psychology*, **47**, 415–426.

Smith, R.A.P., Woodward, N.J., Wallston, B.S., Wallston, K.A., Rye, P. & Zylstra, M. (1988). Health care implications of desire and expectancy for control in elderly adults. *Journal of Gerontology*, **43**, P1–P7.

Strickland, B.R. (1978). Internal-external expectancies and health related behaviors. *Journal of Consulting and Clinical Psychology*, **46**, 1192–1211.

Taylor, S.E. (1983). Adjustment to threatening events: A theory of cognitive adaptation. *American Psychologist*, **38**, 1161–1173.

Taylor, S.E. (1979). Hospital patient behavior: Reactance, helplessness or control? *Journal of Social Issues*, **35**, 156–184.

Tennen, H. Affleck, G., Urrows, S., Higgins, P. & Mendola, R. (1992). Perceiving control, construing benefits, and daily processes in rheumatoid arthritis. *Canadian Journal of Behavioral Sciences*, **24**, 186–203.

Wallston, B.S., Smith, R.A.P., Wallston, K.A., King, J.E., Rye, P.D. & Heim, C. (1987).

Choice and predictability in the preparation for barium enemas: A person-by-situation approach. *Research in Nursing and Health*, 10, 13–22.

Wallston, B.S. & Wallston, K.A. (1984). Social psychological models of health behavior: An examination and integration. In A. Baum, S. Taylor & J.E. Singer (Eds.), *Handbook of psychology and health*, Volume 4: Social aspects of health. Hillsdale, NJ: Erlbaum. 23–53.

Wallston, B.S., Wallston, K.A., Kaplan, G.D. & Maides, S.A. (1976). The development and validation of the health related locus of control (HLC) scale. *Journal of Consulting and Clinical Psychology*, 44, 580–585.

Wallston, K.A. (1991). The importance of placing measures of health locus of control beliefs in a theoretical context. *Health Education Research, Theory & Practice*, 6, 251–252.

Wallston, K.A. (1992). Hocus-Pocus, the focus isn't strictly on locus: Rotter's social learning theory modified for health. *Cognitive Therapy and Research*, 16, 183–199.

Wallston, K.A. (1993). Psychological control and its impact in the management of rheumatological disorders. In S. Newman & M. Shipley (Eds), *Psychological aspects of rheumatic disease. Baillière's Clinical Rheumatology 7:2*. London, England: Baillière Tindall.

Wallston, K.A., Smith, R.A. P., King, J.E., Smith, M.S., Rye, P.D. & Burish, T.G. (1991). Interaction of desire for control and choice of antiemetic treatment for cancer chemotherapy. *Western Journal of Nursing Research*, 13, 12–29.

Wallston, K.A., Wallston, B.S., Smith, S. & Dobbins, C.J. (1987). Perceived control and health. *Current Psychological Research and Reviews*, 6, 5–25.

Wallston, K.A., Wallston, B.S. & De Vellis, R. (1978). Development of the Multidimensional Health Locus of Control (MHLC) Scales. *Health Education Monographs*, 6, 160–170.

Weisman, A.D. & Worden, J.W. (1975). Psychosocial analysis of cancer deaths. *Omega*, 6, 61–75.

Wiener, C. (1975). The burden of rheumatoid arthritis: Tolerating the uncertainty. *Social Science and Medicine*, 9, 97–104.

SECTION V
Old Age

THE COSTS OF CARING FOR ELDERLY PEOPLE

SIOBHAN HART

INTRODUCTION

Ours is an ageing society. Improved standards of living and of health care provision in industrialized societies have resulted in an unprecedented growth in the number of older people, both in absolute numbers and as a proportion of the total population (Brody *et al.*, 1987; Office of Health Economics 1989). Currently about one person in six of the population of Britain is over retirement age (i.e. 60 or 65 years). By the year 2031, some one in five of the population of the UK will be over 65 years of age (Office of Health Economics, 1989). Of particular importance is the spectacular growth in the population aged 75 or more years, whose numbers are expected to increase by around 44 per cent in the next 40 years. Comparable demographic trends are apparent in other countries. These trends present a formidable challenge to the organization and provision of health care because of the high prevalence of disease amongst elderly people and the extent to which they draw upon health-care resources.

Increased longevity is not synonymous with increased health (Brody *et al.*, 1987; Office of Health Economics, 1989). The burden of illness borne by elderly people is primarily due to the high prevalence of chronic diseases, the majority suffering from at least one chronic condition and many from two or more. In economic terms, some 41 per cent of National Health Service expenditure in 1986/87 went on providing health care to people aged over 65 years, although they only constituted about one in six of the population (Office of Health Economics, 1989). However, the costs entailed in caring for elderly people extend far beyond those accounted for by funding of formal health and social care agencies. While elderly people do occupy many hospital beds and in various ways draw upon the services of formal health care staff, the vast majority remain resident in the community where the main providers of care are relatives and friends – the so-called informal or unpaid carers to whom attention is increasingly being directed. Although it has been recent UK government policy that, wherever possible, sick and disabled people should be cared for in the community rather than in institutions, the thrust towards community care received new impetus with the introduction of the White Paper "Caring for People: Community Care in the Next Decade and Beyond" (1989) and subsequently with the passing the National Health Service and Community Care Act (1990).

Such policies, together with the demographic trends outlined above, emphasise the importance of informal care. Indeed a recent survey (Opportunities for Women, 1990) found that many individuals in our society expect to care for an elderly relative at some time in their lives. This expectation was almost as prevalent among men as among women (72 and 76 per cent, respectively).

Some of the wider social and political implications of these shifts in patterns of care provision are considered by Jordan (1990) who notes that some individuals who carry out informal care may not consider their caring role to be anything more than an implicit responsibility of family membership. Whether such views change over time, or as a function of the costs entailed in caregiving, and whether they affect the emotional state of informal carers if and when they are forced to call upon the help of formal care staff, have yet to be assessed. However, one consequence is that surveys tapping the subjective judgements of informants concerning whether they are informal carers are likely to yield conservative estimates.

The potential consequences of the lack of any widely accepted definition of informal care were acknowledged by Green (1988). Nonetheless the Department of Health and Social Security survey on which she reported indicated that one adult in seven (14 per cent) of the population of Great Britain was providing informal care to a sick, handicapped or elderly person. The majority of carers were women but, allowing for the differential sex ratio in the general population, the proportion of men and women who were carers was remarkably similar (12 and 15 per cent, respectively). About half of the carers had dependants aged 75 or over, and 42 per cent were looking after a female dependant aged 75 or more years. The majority of these elderly dependants (73 per cent) were described as suffering from physical, as opposed to mental disabilities. However, since respondents' concepts of what constituted physical and mental illness were not explored, this categorization may not be entirely accurate. The majority of carers were aged between 45 and 64 years, although a sizeable proportion (13 per cent) were aged 65 or more years. The most common patterns of care provision were for a spouse living in the same household and for a parent living in a separate household. The largest single group of carers were those looking after parents. Broadly similar data for the United States were reported by Stone *et al.* (1987). Here too the majority of carers were women (72 per cent) but American carers tended to be older (36 per cent over the age of 65 years) and more lived permanently in the same household as the dependant (74 per cent versus 29 per cent in the United Kingdom).

MORBIDITY IN ELDERLY PEOPLE

Health problems in people older than 65 years are many and varied. They include cardiovascular and cerebrovascular diseases, malignant neoplasms of lung and breast, pneumonia, bronchitis and emphysema, diabetes mellitus, arthritis, depression, accidents involving motor vehicles and dementia (Brody *et al.*, 1987; Office of Health Economics, 1989). The characteristics of these conditions and the signs and symptoms that generate dependency are diverse and often evolving. Comparative research involving carers whose elderly dependants are affected by different conditions might highlight aspects of the caregiving role which have health consequences for carers. These might include social attitudes and expectations regarding the various conditions and therefore the perceived merit of caregivers' activities, the nature of the specific tasks performed for dependants, the time course over which care is provided and the differential outcomes of providing care for those afflicted by different conditions. However, such comparative research is for the most part lacking. Although some studies have included subjects caring for physically ill elderly people (e.g. Caradoc-Davies and Dixon, 1991; Carey *et al.*, 1991; Fitzgerald, 1989), most research on the various costs (emotional, physical, social and financial) and health outcomes of caregiving has been concerned with dementia.

The importance of dementia lies in the devastating effects it can have upon those afflicted, rendering them highly dependent upon others, its high prevalence amongst older people and, the major focus of this chapter, its effects upon the lives of immediate family and friends. Dementia attacks the very humanity of its victims. Most of the conditions that give rise to dementia, including Alzheimer's disease (the most common cause), are relentlessly progressive, are currently incurable and are likely to remain so for the forseeable future.

Although there are marked individual differences, the general picture is one of progressive cognitive decline. Mnestic and communicative difficulties, together with spatial and temporal disorientation, are compounded by diminishing capacity for self-care and emergence of aberrant behaviours such as verbal and physical aggression, shouting, repetitive questioning, wandering (sometimes at night when victims wake from sleep at unusual hours), incontinence and/or inappropriate toileting behaviours, disturbed eating habits and inappropriate sexual behaviour. Patients gradually lose their social and personal identities. Family and friends become strangers and the reciprocity that lies at the heart of human relationships is eroded. Unless the course of progression is interrupted by death, the final state for most victims of dementia is one of mutism and unresponsiveness, usually totally bedridden with double incontinence and marked physical deterioration. The average duration of survival following diagnosis of dementia is of the order of five to ten years, although it can be considerably shorter or longer.

Kay *et al.* (1964) estimated that dementia affected around 10 per cent of the population aged 65 or more years. More recent prevalence studies (see Kay, 1991) are in substantial agreement, allowing for differences in the samples employed, the criteria used to define dementia and the methods used to detect it (see Hart and Semple, 1990). Problems of definition and detection are particularly acute with respect to mild dementia as its boundaries with normal ageing remain poorly defined. The prevalence of dementia rises steeply with age so that it approximately doubles every five years after the age of 60. This pattern is particularly significant since the "old elderly" are the fastest growing group in society. The early epidemiological work of Kay *et al.* (1964) showed that even in the 1960s, before thrusts towards care in the community became such a prominent feature of public policy, more than 80 per cent of all victims of dementia were resident in the community and in about half of these the condition was judged to be severe.

THE IMPACT OF CAREGIVING

Caring for an individual with dementia can profoundly affect many aspects of the life and wellbeing of carers. The concept of "caregiver burden" represents an attempt to provide a global catch-all metric. High levels of burden have been reported in those caring for elderly people with dementia (e.g. Gilleard *et al.*, 1984a; Liptzin *et al.*, 1988; Pratt *et al.*, 1985, 1987; Scott *et al.*, 1986; Zarit *et al.*, 1980). However, the utility of the term burden is flawed by lack of conceptual clarity and by methodological inadeqacies in its measurement. Like the term "stress", caregiver burden has been used to refer to the "load", i.e. the additional tasks entailed in care provision and the limitations imposed by the caring role, and also to the perception of this role and its incumbent demands as oppressive (see Montgomery, 1989). Even if the term is restricted to the negative impact of being a carer, there remain conceptual and practical issues regarding the utility of a situation-specific concept. Montgomery (1989) provides a critical appraisal of the referent-specific notion of "caregiver burden" as opposed to more generic concepts and measures of stress or of well-being (George and Gwyther, 1986). Whatever the utility of caregiver burden and measures thereof in other contexts, it is not appropriate for the initial task of documenting the impact of caregiving since, by definition, non-caregivers cannot meaningfully be employed for comparative purposes.

Some investigators have focused more directly upon the health outcomes of adopting and maintaining a caregiving role. Most have been concerned with psychological morbidity. Feelings of depression, stress, low morale, poor self-esteem and reduced life satisfaction are commonly reported by caregivers (e.g. Anthony-Bergstone *et al.*, 1988; Chenoweth and Spencer, 1986; Drinka *et al.*, 1987; Dura *et al.*, 1990; Fiore *et al.*, 1983; Fitting *et al.*, 1986; Gallagher *et al.*, 1989; George and Gwyther, 1986; Gilleard *et al.*, 1984a; Haley *et al.*, 1987a; Kiecolt-Glaser *et al.*, 1987; Kinney and Stephens, 1989; Moritz *et al.*, 1989; Pruchno and Potashnik, 1989). While these results support the popular view that caring for an individual with dementia must be a negative experience, not all studies have revealed high levels of psychological distress amongst carers (e.g. Eagles *et al.*, 1987a, b). Indeed, some have highlighted the positive aspects of caregiving such as learning more about the care recipient, feelings of self-satisfaction and pride in one's ability to manage problems and deal with crises, a more balanced perspective regarding other life stresses and relief from worry concerning whether the dependant is being cared for properly (e.g. Kinney and Stephens, 1989; Motenko, 1989; see also Brody, 1985; Horowitz, 1985). Unfortunately, the generality of these studies is open to question. Diverse criteria have been used to identify carers (see Barer and Johnson, 1990). The samples employed are also unlikely to be representative since subjects are typically recruited from local branches of carers' associations, through formal social and health care agencies or in response to advertisements offering places in caregiver training programmes. Such people are likely to be distressed or to perceive a need for help. Carers who can cope adequately without recourse to additional support are likely to be underrepresented and likewise those who are overwhelmed by the demands of caring. Since most studies have not employed control groups, it is difficult to evaluate the reported levels of depressive and stress-related symptoms. Cut-off scores associated with standardized instruments may not be particularly useful when the carers studied are themselves elderly since older individuals tend to be under-represented, if indeed they are included, in standardization samples. Becker and Morrisey (1988), acknowledging the prevalence of depressive affect amongst carers, rightly distinguished between this and clinical depression and proposed that caring for victims of dementia was unlikely to precipitate clinical depression, except in predisposed individuals. Nevertheless, many carers fall far short of enjoying health in the positive sense of "a state of complete physical, mental and social well-being and not simply the absence of disease and infirmity" (World Health Organization, 1983).

In view of the literature (some referring to studies of elderly subjects) documenting strong positive relationships between physical and mental health (see Hart 1990; Pruchno *et al.*, 1990a), together with the fact that caregiving can entail onerous physical demands (Mace and Rabins, 1985) and the convergent data linking depression with impaired immune function (see O'Leary, 1990), there are grounds for enquiring about the physical health status of carers. To date comparatively few studies have done so. Some data from self-report questionnaires and interviews (e.g. Chenoweth and Spencer, 1986; Haley *et al.*, 1987a; Pruchno and Potashnik, 1989) would be consistent with the notion that the physical health of carers is impaired in that they report higher rates of anaemia, arthritis, back pain, cancers, cardiovascular disorders and diabetes than non-caregiving peers or than would be expected from population norms. Indeed Pruchno and Potashnik (1989) reported that only 24.1 per cent of their caregiving subjects rated their own health as better than that of their dependants. There has long been controversy concerning the direction of causality in the covariation of physical and mental health status and Pruchno *et al.*, (1990a) rightly appreciated the potential afforded by those caring for patients with dementia to address this unresolved question. They applied mathamatical modelling techniques to longitidinal data from carers which included single-item subjective self-ratings of health and of burden, respectively, the Center for Epidemologic Studies Depression Index and a measure of the functional capacity of dependants. It was concluded that psychological distress predicted physical health problems and therefore that depression increased the susceptibility of carers to poor physical health, rather than vice-versa, possibly through failure to attend to their own needs. However, their methodology was not sufficiently rigorous to allow these conclusions to be more than tentative. Indeed many of the methodological criticisms levelled against studies of psychological morbidity amongst carers are equally applicable to most investigations into physical health status (e.g. methods of recruiting subjects and absence of appropriate control groups). Moreover, not all studies suggest a decline in the physical health of carers. For example, those who took part in George and Gwyther's (1986) study did not differ from comparison samples in the number of consultations with physicians during the previous six months nor in how they rated their own physical health although there were marked differences between the samples on the mental health indicators employed. Discrepancies between self-ratings of physical and mental health respectively, pointing to greater morbidity on the latter, were also reported by Kiecolt-Glaser *et al.*, (1987).

In all investigations requiring subjects to rate their own health, questions arise regarding the accuracy with which they can do so. Although correlations between subjective and objective assessments of the physical health of elderly subjects are indeed significant, they are generally modest so that subjective ratings are likely to be of limited utility as outcome measures or in decisions regarding individuals (see Hart, 1990).

An obvious solution would be to employ more direct and objective physiological indicators of physical health status but this has rarely been done. A notable exception is the investigation of Kiecolt-Glaser *et al.* (1987), based upon the considerable body of evidence that stressful events are associated with adverse effects on immune function (see O'Leary, 1990). They found that carers were compromised relative to matched control subjects on a number of immunological indices and that the observed immunosuppression could not be accounted for by differences in nutrition or by differential engagement in health-related behaviours such as consumption of caffeine, alcohol or nicotine. The authors considered their results to be particularly significant since their subjects appeared to be less distressed and had greater financial resources than is typical of carers in many other reports. If immunosuppression is indeed a consequence of caregiving, this might be particularly sinister for elderly carers given the decline in immunologic competence that occurs with ageing processes *per se* (see O'Leary, 1990) together with evidence that poor immunocompetence is associated with increased mortality in elderly people (Roberts-Thomson *et al.*, 1974).

Pomara *et al.* (1989) also produced direct evidence of an effect of caring upon caregiver physiology. Investigating the neurochemical changes associated with Alzheimer's disease, they compared levels of the inhibitory neurotransmitter GABA in the cerebrospinal fluid (CSF) of patients with that of control subjects and made the serendipitous discovery that the CSF GABA levels in the control group were bimodally distributed, being significantly higher in those control subjects who were caregivers (spouses of the patients included in the study) than in the non-caregiving control subjects. No significant differences were found between carers and non-caregiving control subjects with respect to biochemical markers of other neuro-transmitter systems examined. Pomara *et al.* speculated that these results might reflect an adaptive physiological response to the stresses of caring and cited data suggesting that acute stress can produce increased activity in GABAergic systems.

The time and energy demands of caregiving, and the possibility that dependants' behaviour might be deemed socially unacceptable, could restrict the opportunities or readiness of carers to interact with others and/or participate in social activities – an important buffer between stress and adverse outcomes (Cohen and Wills, 1985). Social costs of caregiving have indeed been noted by many investigators (e.g. Cantor, 1983; Chenoweth and Spencer, 1986; Deimling and Bass, 1986; George and Gwyther, 1986; Gilhooly, 1984; Haley *et al.*, 1987a; Miller and Montgomery, 1990). However there is considerable variation in the nature and extent of social engagement among carers and in their experience of the caregiving role as a cause of social limitations. The level of dependency of the person cared for cannot alone account for the time and energy invested in caring, nor for carers' perception of their role as costly in social terms (Miller and Montgomery, 1990). Male carers, even when they satisfy criteria for designation as the primary caregiver, are less likely to provide intensive personal care (Green, 1988) and are more willing than female carers to leave dependants alone in order to pursue other activities (Miller, 1987). Role conflict is one potential adverse consequence of elder care responsibilities and is particularly likely to affect women who remain the major providers of informal care to elderly dependants and shoulder the major responsibility for child care (Brody, 1981). Such conflict will be exacerbated as female participation in the labour force increases. Interest in the interaction between family and work roles is growing (Brody, 1987; Creedon, 1991; Kola and Dunkle, 1988), but it remains unclear what effect the re-entry of women into the work force will have on family care of the elderly and vice versa. Irrespective of how potential conflicts are resolved, social costs seem inevitable and could, at one extreme, amount to decreasing availability of informal caregivers in the face of increasing numbers of elderly people in need of care. If, however, role conflict is diminished by relinquishing the work role, as many have done (see Creedon 1991), adverse economic consequences are likely to be compounded by social costs insofar as work outside the home offers opportunities for social fulfilment in addition to providing financial remuneration (Opportunities for Women, 1990; Stoller and Pugliesi, 1989).

Providing care for others can make significant demands upon the financial resources of carers, especially in the absence of extensive state-funded health care. Although seldom invoked, a number of states in the USA have passed so-called "relatives' responsibility laws" whereby not only spouses, but also children and more distant kin, are financially liable for the costs incurred by elderly relatives in nursing homes (see Gilhooly, 1986a). These costs can be considerable and can rapidly lead to impoverishment (Creedon, 1991). In view of the financial implications, together with other adverse consequences (see Cahill and Rosenman, 1991), many investigators have sought to determine what factors lead to institutionalization, often with a view to combatting these (e.g. Cahill and Rosenman, 1991; Chenoweth and Spencer, 1986; Colerick and George, 1986; Gilhooly, 1986b; Montgomery *et al.*, 1985; Morycz, 1985; Pruchno *et al.*, 1990b; Wilder *et al.*, 1983; Zarit *et al.*, 1986). It is clear from such research that the level of the dependant's disability is a less important determinant of institutionalization than are factors such as the kinship bond and quality of the relationship between carer and dependant and characteristics of the caregiver such as their acceptance of the caregiving role, perceived capacity to cope with its demands and their physical wellbeing.

Caring for a chronically incapacitated individual within the community can also impose a heavy financial strain upon carers who may be forced to cease full-time employment or forego further training and/or promotion which would entail increased responsibility or time commitment. The loss of income and/or career prospects, together with conflicting demands of employment and caregiving, is a source of considerable stress and frustration to many carers (Opportunities for Women, 1990). Moreover reduced efficiency in the workplace, and likewise partial or complete withdrawal from the workforce, can prove financially burdensome for employers (see Creedon, 1991).

FACTORS DETERMINING THE IMPACT AND OUTCOMES OF CAREGIVING

Clearly the costs of caregiving are multiple and diverse. Understanding the factors which determine the impact of caregiving upon carers is important for inter-related theoretical and practical reasons. These include accounting for the variability of carers' responses to the challenges of caregiving, identifying carers at risk of adverse outcomes, designing intervention strategies to ameliorate the costs of caring and elucidating further the way(s) in which environmental and behavioural factors relate to mental and physical illness. While the concept of caregiver burden does have some relevance in the context of research drawing comparisons between carers, its utility may still be limited by methodological inadequacies inherent in many purported indices of burden (e.g. Kosberg and Cairl, 1986; Morycz, 1985; Robinson, 1983; Zarit *et al.*, 1980). For example, the tendency to use unidirectional phrasing of questions renders response bias highly probable (see Dillehay and Sandys, 1990) and the practice of summating responses to obtain global scores may obscure domain-specific patterns of caregiving impact.

There is little evidence that caregiver burden or wellbeing is significantly affected by the severity of cognitive impairment in patients with dementia (e.g. George and Gwyther, 1986; Gilhooly, 1984; Haley *et al.*, 1987b; Montgomery *et al.*, 1985; Scott *et al.*, 1986; Wilder *et al.*, 1983; Zarit *et al.*, 1980, 1986), although some studies have suggested a link (Deimling and Bass, 1986; Eagles *et al.*, 1987a, b; Moritz *et al.*, 1989), and only equivocal evidence regarding the contribution of dependants' ability to attend to basic self care needs (e.g. Deimling and Bass, 1986; Fitting *et al.*, 1986; Gilhooly, 1984; Gilleard *et al.*, 1982; Haley *et al.*, 1987b; Pagel *et al.*, 1985; Zarit *et al.*, 1980). There is better evidence that carers are affected adversely by aberrant behaviours on the part of dependants (e.g. Coppel *et al.*, 1985; Deimling and Bass, 1986; Eagles *et al.*, 1987b; George and Gwyther, 1986; Gilleard *et al.*, 1982, 1984a; Kiecolt-Glaser *et al.*, 1987; Pruchno and Resch, 1989a) but this too remains inconclusive (Haley *et al.*, 1987b; Zarit *et al.*, 1980). Little comparative research has been carried out, and while some reports suggest that caring for victims of dementia affects carers more adversely than providing care for other dependent groups (Birkel, 1987; Scharlach, 1989; Whittick, 1988) not all results concur with this (Drinka *et al.*, 1987; Liptzin *et al.*, 1988).

Although some investigators have reported that younger carers are more adversely affected (e.g. Barusch and Spaid, 1989; Gilleard *et al.*, 1984b; Fitting *et al.*, 1986; Haley *et al.*, 1987b) others have documented increased vulnerability in older carers on some outcome measures (Fiore *et al.*, 1986) or have failed to find a relationship between caregiver age and impact of the role (Gilhooly, 1984; Gilleard *et al.*, 1984a; Pagel and Becker, 1987; Pratt *et al.*, 1985). Some data (Cantor, 1983; George and Gwyther, 1986) suggest that the adverse effects of caregiving are more marked for spouses than for children, but others have not found a significant kinship effect (e.g. Eagles *et al.*, 1987b; Gilleard *et al.*, 1984a; Quayhagen and Quayhagen, 1988; Zarit *et al.*, 1980). Since age and kinship are likely to be confounded it may be difficult to determine the contribution of each, and both are likely to be further confounded by living arrangements.

Despite equivocal results regarding gender differences in caregiver burden (Fitting *et al.*, 1986; Zarit *et al.*, 1986), female carers consistently report higher levels of depressive symptomatology (e.g. Anthony-Bergstone *et al.*, 1988; Cantor, 1983; Fitting *et al.*, 1986; Horowitz, 1985; Moritz *et al.*, 1989; Pruchno and Resch, 1989b), but the baseline rate of depression is higher amongst women in general (Boyd and Weissman, 1982). Pruchno and Resch, (1989b) found that self-ratings of physical health were lower in women caregivers. Many explanations have been tendered to account for the apparent gender difference in the impact of caregiving. Although traditionally ascribed to women, the role can be a source of conflict, as, for example, in daughters who may face competing demands from partners, children and/or work. Male carers are more likely to receive support from health and social services and, as already noted, differ from women in the types of care they provide (see Morris *et al.*, 1991).

Gilhooly (1984) found that the quality of the relationship between carer and dependant prior to the development of dementia did not correlate significantly with the mental health or morale of carers. However Gilleard *et al.* (1984b) and L. Morris *et al.*, (1988) found that a positive prior relationship ameliorated the negative impact of caregiving.

Investigations into how support from relatives and friends affects carers' wellbeing have yielded contradictory results. There are reports that carers who receive more informal social support feel less burdened (George and Gwyther, 1986; Scott *et al.*, 1986; Zarit *et al.*, 1980) or depressed (Pagel and Becker, 1987), rate their health as better (Haley *et al.*, 1987b) and make fewer demands upon formal services such as intermittent respite care, day care and care provided in the home (Caserta *et al.*, 1987). However others (e.g. Fiore *et al.*, 1986; Gilhooly, 1984; Gilleard *et al.*, 1984a; Pratt *et al.*, 1985) have found that informal support does not enhance caregiver wellbeing and may indeed have negative effects (Pagel *et al.*, 1987). For various reasons carers may under-report the extent and utility of the support they receive from others (see Pruchno, 1990). Spouse caregivers may conceal from their children the full extent of their plight so as to protect the dignity of their life-long partner but at the same time attribute their own coping difficulties to a real or perceived lack of support from others. Children may under-rate the needs of a parent who is a spouse caregiver because they need to maintain their image of parents as powerful figures or they may withhold support supposedly to avoid infringing the independence and autonomy of the carer. Theories and methodologies for explicating family dynamics (Bentovim *et al.*, 1987) could fruitfully be applied to caregiving families.

The many inconsistencies in the literature are a consequence of the multiplicity of outcome measures employed and inadequate recognition of the heterogeneity of caregivers or of the complex and interactive nature of the variables which may influence outcome. While many investigators have made passing reference to the wider literature on cognitive models of stress or of depression, few have used such frameworks to guide their own research on determinants of the impact of caring, or have recognized the potential afforded by caregiving to test and refine such models. The limited amount of relevant research has highlighted the importance of carers' perceptions of the demands of caregiving and the coping responses they adopt.

Consistent with the reformulated learned helplessness model of depression (Abramson *et al.*, 1978), psychological distress amongst carers is associated with negative causal attributions that are global and stable: distressed carers perceive their caregiving role as infringing upon many aspects of their lives and believe that it will continue to do so (Coppel *et al.*, 1985; Cohen and Eisdorfer, 1988; Morris *et al.*, 1989). However the data provide only equivocal evidence regarding the need for causal attributions to be internal. Cohen and Eisdorfer (1988) found that depressed and non-depressed caregivers did not differ in their ratings of internal versus external locus of control although Pagel *et al.* (1985) reported that those who felt responsible for their dependant's behaviour were more depressed. Consistent with the views expounded by Wortman and Dintzer (1978) psychological distress in carers relates to how they perceive their own ability to cope with the challenges of caregiving and their sense of control over their own emotional responses to these challenges (Coppel *et al.*, 1985; Morris *et al.*, 1989; Pagel *et al.*, 1985).

Some research has focused upon the coping strategies adopted by carers. Seeking dementia-related information emerges as a strategy that is common and widely rated as being effective (Elias *et al.*, 1987; Scott *et al.*, 1987), although there are circumstances in which it may not prove beneficial (see Hart, 1990). Stephens *et al.* (1988) found that carers who reappraised events so as to derive inspiration and/or personal growth experienced greater positive affect. However, escape-avoidance strategies were associated with higher levels of dysphoria, consistent with the view that avoidance/denial strategies may only be effective in response to acute stressors and are maladaptive in chronic situations (see also Barusch, 1988; Elias *et al.*, 1987). Barusch (1988) highlighted the importance of a varied repertoire of coping skills and strategies to address the diverse problems associated with caregiving. These results, plus the finding that carers often preferred to manage without assistance from others, have important implications for the design of support programmes and the manner in which these are offered. Killeen (1990) found that carers typically employed both problem-focused and emotion-focused strategies (Lazarus and Folkman, 1984). Use of the latter was positively related to perceived burden and to reported duration of caregiving.

Most research on caregiving has involved measurements at a single point in time. However, the relationship between carers and their dependants is interactive and evolving. Since dementia is generally progressive, the challenges confronting carers will change and so too the strategies which will be most appropriate and the resources necessary to cope. Moreover, because of the extended period over which care is provided, blurring of cause and effect seem inevitable. Unfortunately there have been few longitudinal studies. Nevertheless, some scenarios have been outlined regarding possible changes in caregiver wellbeing during long-term provision of care (see Townsend *et al.*, 1989). The "wear and tear" hypothesis posits that carers will be gradually overwhelmed by an accumulation of stressors. Alternatively they may learn more efficient ways of coping so that their own wellbeing does not decline in step with disease progression, and indeed may even improve over time – the "adaptation" hypothesis. Implicit in each hypothesis is the notion that increases in disease severity will inevitably entail greater objective demands, but many of the behavioural disturbances that carers find most taxing (e.g. wandering, repetitive questioning and sleep disturbances) actually decrease in the later stages of dementia (Haley and Pardo, 1989).

Cross-sectional data (e.g. Gilhooly, 1984; Novak and Guest, 1989; Townsend *et al.*, 1989) and longitudinal data (Townsend *et al.*, 1989; Zarit *et al.*, 1986) favour the adaptation hypothesis. However these studies may be confounded by selective attrition which removes carers who do not adapt from the subject pool. Moreover longitudinal investigations will need to extend over a more prolonged time course than hitherto (14 months and 2 years, respectively) in order to determine how the wellbeing of carers changes over the course of caregiving which may extend over many years and require carers to respond to demands that change in nature and magnitude over its duration. Such investigations will have important practical implications for healthcare professionals in that the types of intervention programmes that will be appropriate for any given carer may vary over time.

INTERVENTION PROGRAMMES

There is an abundant literature on intervention programmes aimed at ameliorating the impact of caring for dependants with dementia. Unfortunately many reports contain little more than programme outlines with little or no attempt at evaluation of efficacy. Even when programmes have been evaluated there is all too often inadequate description of participants and an absence of theoretical foundation, thereby neglecting explanatory, but more importantly heuristic, potential. Most programmes include some or all of the following: an information package aimed at increasing awareness about the nature of dementia and/or the availability of support from voluntary and statutory bodies; training in methods to reduce stress; advice on behavioural management and problem solving techniques (e.g. Chiverton and Caine, 1989; Gendron *et al.*, 1986; Glosser and Wexler, 1985; Goodman and Pynoos, 1990; Kahan *et al.*, 1985; Mohide *et al.*, 1990; Pinkston and Linsk, 1984; Robinson, 1988; Russell *et al.*, 1989; Sutcliffe and Larner, 1988). Both group and individual modalities of presentation have been employed.

Although the results of intervention studies have generally been reported as positive in terms of enhancing caregivers' perceived well-being, capacity to cope and/or postponing institutionalization of dependants, there remain important questions regarding how best to maximize the benefits and minimize the potential pitfalls of interventions through selection or design of programmes and modules that are best suited to the needs and coping styles of individual carers. Recent empirical comparisons of different methods of delivering support to carers represent a welcome step forward (Toseland *et al.*, 1989, 1990; Zarit *et al.*, 1987). However it must be emphasised that positive group results can hide harmful effects upon individuals (see Hepburn and Wasow, 1986). There is a compelling need to determine the characteristics of subjects who do or do not respond favourably to particular types of intervention or components thereof.

Despite the substantial public resources involved, few investigations have assessed the impact of more "traditional" formal support services such as home-help provision, meals-on-wheels, attendance at day centres or day hospitals and short-term respite from the caregiving role. Gilleard *et al.* (1984a) failed to demonstrate a significant association between availability of support (either formal or informal) and caregivers' psychological wellbeing but, in a separate study on the impact of psychiatric day hospital care, Gilleard *et al.*, (1984c) found that carers typically perceived such care as beneficial for themselves although of little benefit to their dependants. Gilhooly (1984) found that while some aspects of formal care (such as frequency of home-help attendance and visits from a community nurse) bore a positive relationship to caregiver morale, others (availability of day hospital care and meals-on-wheels) bore no relationship to this. Although the intervention programme reported by Lawton *et al.* (1989) served to delay institutionalization of dependants it did not ameliorate burden or produce a significant improvement in carers' mental health. There is a clear need for further research which takes account of the quantity and quality of the formal care that is made available and how it can be delivered in a flexible manner to meet the changing needs of individual carers. Personal experience leads me to believe that the efficacy of intermittent admissions of dependants to provide respite for carers can be enhanced by appropriate counselling to counter the feelings of guilt and inadequacy that are often

associated with relinquishing, even temporarily, the caregiving role. Such psychological intervention increases the probability that carers will be able to exploit the
period of separation so as to replenish their physical and psychological resources. This
is particularly important since the changes in surroundings and routine experienced by
dependants may cause them to be more confused upon returning home.

In much of the literature on caregiving it is clear that the health status of carers has
only been of interest to researchers and clinicians insofar as it bears upon the welfare
and ultimate fate of care recipients. Further evidence of this limited perspective lies in
the paucity of studies which have investigated carers following the permanent
institutionalization of their former dependants. The few studies that have been carried
out suggest that carers continue to suffer considerable distress (Cahill and Rosenman,
1991; Colerick and George, 1986).

Many have commented upon the essential widowhood and living bereavement
endured by the carers of severely demented patients as they attempt to cope with "... a
death that never ends, and a mourning process that can never properly take place
because the dead personality lingers in a surviving body" (Levine *et al.*, 1984).
Surprisingly little attention has been directed to the fate of carers following death of
their dependants. Guilt is a common component of the process of grieving, but in the
case of bereaved carers this may be fuelled by uncertainty surrounding the manner in
which they have coped, or failed to cope, with the burden arising out of a disease
incurred by their loved ones. Bass and Bowman (1990) found a direct relationship
between caregiving strain and the severity of bereavement responses, illustrating the
need for continuing support for carers after the death of their dependants. For many
carers caregiving has been the dominant focus of their lives for a number of years and
has necessitated radical changes in their life styles. Relinquishing the role of caregiver
may require considerable adaptation from individuals whose coping resources have
already been severely taxed.

CONCLUDING REMARKS

There is no evidence to support the myth that the willingness of individuals to provide
care for elderly relatives has declined (Brody, 1981). Indeed Brody (1985) rightly
emphasises that some people need to be helped to reduce the amount of care they
provide (see also Hart, 1991). The significance of informal care has been increased by
demographic trends, social changes such as increased re-entry of women into the
workforce and by government policies promoting care in the community. There has
been much research into the effects of informal caregiving, particularly in relation to
victims of dementia whose multiple and changing needs are such as to require
continuous care, epitomized in the phrase "the 36 hour day" (Mace and Rabins, 1985).

Methodological difficulties notwithstanding, the cumulative data available suggest
a strong association between caregiving and adverse health outcomes. However the
multiplicity and complexity of the factors bearing upon the effects of caregiving calls
for research that is conceptually and methodologically more sophisticated than has
typically been attempted to date. There is a particular need for longitudinal research to
disentangle the interactions of cause and effect and to document the long-term
outcomes for carers after they have relinquished the caregiving role (recognizing that

there may be a time lag in the manifestation of some effects). Future research on those caring for patients with dementia should take greater account of the specific conditions giving rise to this syndrome since the demands made upon carers are likely to be different, at least in the earlier stages (Hepburn and Gates, 1988). It is also important that the database be extended to include those caring for victims of other debilitating conditions which do not involve mental impairment.

The costs entailed in caring for elderly people are indeed significant but this reality does not justify ageist stereotypes which construe all people deemed old by the social criterion of chronological age as mere parasites upon the rest of society. Many care providers are themselves elderly. However the increased susceptibility to disease and infirmity inherent in the process of ageing will complicate further the already difficult task of elucidating causal relationships regarding adverse outcomes associated with caregiving. Likewise this enhanced vulnerability, together with the heterogeneity of those encompassed within the gross and global socially-defined category of "the elderly" will make demonstration of the efficacy of intervention programmes more difficult.

The heterogeneity of carers, the challenges they face and the resources they mobilize amount to a rich natural laboratory for exploration of the relationship(s) between psychosocial, cognitive, behavioural and physiological factors on the one hand and health and wellbeing on the other, as well as affording a medium through which psychological models and theories can be evaluated and refined. However, despite the plethora of research on caregiving and interventions to ameliorate its adverse effects, few investigators have demonstrated adequate appreciation of these possibilities. For the most part the aim of preventing illness in carers appears to have been a secondary goal with little interest in promoting their health and wellbeing for its own sake. Despite the emphasis on choice in recent reorganizations of health care delivery, the thrust towards care in the community has in effect reduced the availability of choice for carers since there are fewer alternative facilities available and the expectation is that elderly people, like others in need of care, will remain in the community, preferably in domestic settings. Such policies, with their questionable assumption that community care will always be in the best interests of dependants, may unwittingly infringe the rights of family members to not adopt or to relinquish the caregiver role and thereby distort their sense of personal versus external control in decisions to care or abandon caring for a dependant. They may even promote elder abuse. There are already many, hopefully influential, advocates proclaiming the needs and rights of carers to attention and consideration in their own right (e.g. Richardson *et al.*, 1989). Most research to date has been concerned with the adverse effects of caregiving, but it is important to note that detailed investigation of that sizeable portion of carers who report little or no burden might yield valuable information concerning effective coping styles and/or strategies, although longitudinal research will be required before it can be concluded unequivocally that they have indeed emerged unscathed from the caregiving experience.

REFERENCES

Abramson, L.Y., Seligman, M.E.P. & Teasdale, J.D. (1978). Learned helplessness in humans: critique and reformulation. *Journal of Abnormal Psychology*, **87**, 49–74.

Anthony-Bergstone, C.R., Zarit, S.H. & Gatz, M. (1988). Symptoms of psychological distress among caregivers of dementia patients. *Psychology and Aging*, **3**, 245–248.

Barer, B.M. & Johnson, C.L. (1990). A critique of the caregiving literature. *Gerontologist*, **30**, 26–29.

Barusch, A.S. (1988). Problems and coping strategies of elderly spouse caregivers. *Gerontologist*, **28**, 677–685.

Barusch, A.S. & Spaid, W.M. (1989). Gender differences in caregiving: why do wives report greater burden? *Gerontologist*, **29**, 667–676.

Bass, D.M. & Bowman, K. (1990). The transition from caregiving to bereavement: the relationship of care-related strain and adjustment to death. *Gerontologist*, **30**, 35–42.

Becker, J. & Morrissey, E. (1988). Difficulties in assessing depressive-like reactions to chronic severe external stress as exemplified by spouse caregivers of Alzheimer patients. *Psychology and Aging*, **3**, 300–306.

Bentovim, A., Barnes, G.G. & Cooklin, A. (1987). *Family Therapy: Complementary Frameworks of Theory and Practice*. London: Academic Press.

Birkel, R.C. (1987). Toward a social ecology of the home-care household. *Psychology and Aging*, **2**, 294–301.

Boyd, J.H. & Weissman, M.M. (1982). Epidemiology. In *Handbook of Affective Disorders*. E.S. Paykel (ed). New York: Guilford.

Brody, E.M. (1981). "Women in the middle" and family help to older people. *Gerontologist*, **21**, 471–480.

Brody, E.M. (1985). Parent care as a normative family stress. *Gerontologist*, **25**, 19–29.

Brody, E.M. (1987). Work status and parent care: a comparison of four groups of women. *Gerontologist*, **27**, 201–208.

Brody, J.A., Brock, D.B. & Williams, T.F. (1987). Trends in the health of the elderly population. *Annual Review of Public Health*, **8**, 211–234.

Cahill, S. & Rosenman, L. (1989). Caregiver considerations in institutionalizing dementia patients. In D. O'Neill (ed) *Carers, Professionals and Alzheimer's Disease*. London: John Libbey.

Cantor, M.H. (1983). Strain among caregivers: a study of experience in the United States. *Gerontologist*, **23**, 597–604.

Caradoc-Davies, T.H. & Dixon, G.S. (1991). Stress in caregivers of elderly patients: the effect of an admission to a rehabilitation unit. *New Zealand Medical Journal*, **104**, 226–228.

Carey, P.J., Oberst, M.T., McCubbin, M.A. & Hughes, S.H. (1991). Appraisal and caregiving burden in family members caring for patients receiving chemotherapy. *Oncology Nursing Forum*, **18**, 1341–1348.

Caserta, M.S., Lund, D.A., Wright, S.D. & Redburn, D.E. (1987). Caregivers of dementia patients: the utilization of community services. *Gerontologist*, **27**, 209–214.

Chenoweth, B. & Spencer, B. (1986). Dementia: the experience of family caregivers. *Gerontologist*, **26**, 267–272.

Chiverton, P. & Caine, E.D. (1989). Education to assist spouses in coping with Alzheimer's disease: a controlled study. *Journal of the American Geriatrics Society*, **37**, 593–598.

Cohen, D. & Eisdorfer, C. (1988). Depression in family members caring for a relative with Alzheimer's disease. *Journal of the American Geriatrics Society*, **36**, 885–889.

Cohen, S. & Wills, T.A. (1985). Stress, social support, and the buffering hypothesis. *Psychological Bulletin*, **98**, 310–357.

Colerick, E.J. & George, L.K. (1986). Predictors of institutionalization among caregivers of patients with Alzheimer's disease. *Journal of the American Geriatrics Society*, **34**, 493–498.

Coppel, D.B., Burton, C., Becker, J. & Fiore, J. (1985). Relationships of cognitions associated with coping reactions to depression in spousal caregivers of Alzheimer's disease patients. *Cognitive Therapy and Research*, **9**, 253–266.

Creedon, M.A. (1991). Economic consequences of Alzheimer's disease. In D. O'Neill (ed) *Carers, Professionals and Alzheimer's Disease.* London: John Libbey.

Deimling, G.T. & Bass, D.M. (1986). Symptoms of mental impairment among elderly adults and their effects on family caregivers. *Journal of Gerontology*, **41**, 778–784.

Dillehay, R.C. & Sandys, M.R. (1990). Caregivers for Alzheimer's patients: what we are learning from research. *International Journal of Aging and Human Development*, **30**, 263–285.

Drinka, T.J.K., Smith, J.C. & Drinka, P.J. (1987). Correlates of depression and burden for informal caregivers of patients in a geriatrics referral clinic. *Journal of the American Geriatrics Society*, **35**, 522–525.

Dura, J.R., Haywood-Niler, E. & Kiecolt-Glaser, J.K. (1990). Spousal caregivers of persons with Alzheimer's and Parkinson's disease dementia: a preliminary comparison. *Gerontologist*, **30**, 332–336.

Eagles, J.M., Beattie, J.A.G., Blackwood, G.W., Restall, D.B. & Ashcroft, G.W. (1987a). The mental health of elderly couples. I. The effects of a cognitively impaired spouse. *British Journal of Psychiatry*, **150**, 299–303.

Eagles, J.M., Craig, A., Rawlinson, F., Restall, D.B., Beattie, J.A.G. & Besson, J.A.O. (1987b). The psychological well-being of supporters of the demented elderly. *British Journal of Psychiatry*, **150**, 293–298.

Elias, J.W., Hutton, J.T., Bratt, A.H., Miller, B.A. & Weinstein, L.A. (1987). Caretaker coping and Alzheimer's patient decline. *Texas Medicine*, **83**, 46–47.

Fiore, J., Becker, J. & Coppel, D.B. (1983). Social network interactions: a buffer or a stress? *American Journal of Community Psychology*, **11**, 423–439.

Fiore, J., Coppel, D.B., Becker, J. & Cox, G.B. (1986). Social support as a multifaceted concept. *American Journal of Community Pscyhology*, **14**, 93–111.

Fitting, M., Rabins, P., Lucas, M.J. & Eastham, J. (1986). Caregivers for dementia patients: a comparison of husbands and wives. *Gerontologist*, **26**, 248–252.

Fitzgerald, G. (1989). Effects of caregiving on caregiver spouses of stroke victims. *AXON*, **10**, 85–88.

Gallagher, D., Rose, J., Rivera, P., Lovett, S. & Thompson, L.W. (1989). Prevalence of depression in family caregivers. *Gerontologist*, **29**, 449–456.

Gendron, C.E., Poitras, L.R., Engels, M.L., Dastoor, D.P., Sirota, S.E., Barza, S.L., Davis, J.C. & Levine, N.B. (1986) Skills training with supporters of the demented. *Journal of the American Geriatrics Society*, **34**, 875–880.

George, L.K. & Gwyther, L.P. (1986). Caregiver well-being: a multidimensional examination of family caregivers of demented adults. *Gerontologist*, **26**, 253–259.

Gilhooly, M.L.M. (1984). The impact of caregiving on caregivers: factors associated with the psychological well-being of people supporting a dementing relative in the community. *British Journal of Medical Psychology*, **57**, 35–44.

Gilhooly, M.L.M. (1986a). Legal and ethical issues in the management of the dementing elderly. In M.L.M. Gilhooly, S.H. Zarit and J.E. Birren (eds). *The Dementias: Policy and Management.* Englewood Cliffs N.J.: Prentice-Hall.

Gilhooly, M.L.M. (1986b). Senile dementia: factors associated with caregivers' preference for institutional care. *British Journal of Medical Psychology*, **59**, 165–171.

Gilleard, C.J., Belford, H., Gilleard, E., Whittick, J.E. & Gledhill, K. (1984a). Emotional distress among the supporters of the elderly mentally infirm. *British Journal of Psychiatry*, **145**, 172–177.

Gilleard, C.J., Boyd, W.D. & Watt, G. (1982). Problems in caring for the elderly mentally infirm at home. *Archives of Gerontology and Geriatrics,* 1, 151–158.

Gilleard, C.J., Gilleard, E., Gledhill, K. & Whittick, J. (1984b). Caring for the elderly mentally infirm at home: a survey of the supporters. *Journal of Epidemiology and Community Health,* 38, 319–325.

Gilleard, C.J., Gilleard, E. & Whittick, J. (1984c). Impact of psychogeriatric day hospital care on the patient's family. *British Journal of Psychiatry,* 145, 487–492.

Glosser, G. & Wexler, D. (1985). Participants' evaluation of educational/support groups for families of patients with Alzheimer's disease and other dementias. *Gerontologist,* 25, 232–236.

Goodman, C.C. & Pynoos, J. (1990). A model telephone information and support programme for caregivers of Alzheimer's patients. *Gerontologist,* 30, 399–404.

Green, H. (1988). *Informal Carers: General Household Survey 1985,* Supplement A. London: HMSO.

Haley, W.E., Levine, E.G., Brown, S.L., Berry, J.W. & Hughes, G.H. (1987a). Psychological, social, and health consequences of caring for a relative with senile dementia. *Journal of the American Geriatrics Society,* 35, 405–411.

Haley, W.E., Levine, E.G., Brown, S.L. & Bartolucci, A.A. (1987b). Stress, appraisal, coping and social support as predictors of adaptational outcome among dementia caregivers. *Psychology and Aging,* 2, 323–330.

Haley, W.E. & Pardo, K.M. (1989). Relationship of severity of dementia to caregiving stressors. *Psychology and Aging,* 4, 389–392.

Hart, S. (1990). Psychology and the health of elderly people. In P. Bennett, J. Weinman and P. Spurgeon (eds). *Current Developments in Health Psychology.* London: Harwood.

Hart, S. (1991). Non-drug therapy in dementing illness. In D. O'Neill (ed). *Carers, Professionals and Alzheimer's Disease.* London: John Libbey.

Hart, S. & Semple, J.M. (1990). *Neuropsychology and the Dementias.* Hove: Lawrence Erlbaum Associates.

Hepburn, K. & Wasow, M. (1986). Support groups for family caregivers of dementia victims: questions, directions, and future research. In N.S. Abramson, J.K. Quam & M. Wasow (eds) *The Elderly and Chronic Mental Illness. New Directions for Mental Health Services No. 29.* San Francisco: Josse-Bass.

Hepburn, K.W. & Gates, B.A. (1988). Family caregivers for non-Alzheimer's dementia patients. *Clinics in Geriatric Medicine,* 4, 925–940.

Horowitz, A. (1985). Family caregiving to the frail elderly. *Annual Preview of Gerontology and Geriatrics,* 5, 194–246.

Jordan, B. (1990). *Value for caring: recognizing unpaid carers.* London: King Edward's Hospital Fund for London.

Kahan, J., Kemp, B., Staples, F.R. & Brummel-Smith, K. (1985). Decreasing the burden in families caring for a relative with a dementing illness: a controlled study. *Journal of the American Geriatrics Society,* 33, 664–670.

Kay, D.W.K. (1991). The epidemiology of dementia: a review of recent work. *Reviews in Clinical Gerontology,* 1, 55–66.

Kay, D.W.K., Beamish, P. & Roth, M. (1964). Old age mental disorders in Newcastle-upon-Tyne. Part 1: A study of prevalence. *British Journal of Psychiatry,* 110, 146–158.

Kiecolt-Glaser, J.K., Glaser, R., Shuttleworth, E.C., Dyer, C.S., Ogrocki, P. & Speicher, C.E. (1987). Chronic stress and immunity in family caregivers of Alzheimer's disease victims. *Psychosomatic Medicine,* 49, 523–535.

Killeen, M. (1990). The influence of stress and coping on family caregivers' perceptions of health. *International Journal of Aging and Human Development,* 30, 197–211.

Kinney, J.M. & Stephens, M.A.P. (1989). Hassles and uplifts of giving care to a family member with dementia. *Psychology and Aging,* 4, 402–408.

Kola, L.A. & Dunkle, R.E. (1988). Eldercare in the workplace. *Social Casework: The Journal of Contemporary Social Work,* November, pp. 569–574.

Kosberg, J.I. & Cairl, R.E. (1986). The Cost of Care Index: a case management tool for screening informal care providers. *Gerontologist,* **26,** 273–278.

Lawton, M.P., Brody, E.M. & Saperstein, A.R. (1989). A controlled study of respite service for caregivers of Alzheimer's patients. *Gerontologist,* **29,** 8–16.

Lazarus, R.S. & Folkman, S. (1984). *Stress, Appraisal and Coping.* New York: Springer Publishing Company.

Levine, N.B., Gendron, C.E., Dastoor, D.P., Poitras, L.R., Sirota, S.E., Barza, S.L. & Davis, J.C. (1984). Existential issues in the management of the demented elderly patient. *American Journal of Psychotherapy,* **38,** 215–223.

Liptzin, B., Grob, M.C. & Eisen, S.V. (1988). Family burden of demented and depressed elderly psychiatric inpatients. *Gerontologist,* **28,** 397–401.

Mace, N.L. & Rabins, P.V. (1985). *The 36-Hour Day.* London: Hodder and Stoughton.

Miller, B. (1987). Gender and control among spouses of the cognitively impaired: a research note. *Gerontologist,* **27,** 447–453.

Miller, B. & Montgomery, A. (1990). Family caregivers and limitations in social activities. *Research on Aging,* **12,** 72–93.

Mohide, E.A., Pringle, B.M., Streiner, D.L., Gilbert, J.R., Muir, G., & Tew, M. (1990). A randomized trial of family caregiver support in the home management of dementia. *Journal of the American Geriatrics Society,* **38,** 446–454.

Montgomery, R.J.V. (1989). Investigating caregiver burden. In K.S. Markides and C.L. Cooper (eds) *Aging, Stress and Health.* Chichester: John Wiley and Sons.

Montgomery, R.J.V., Gonyea, J.G. & Hooyman, N.R. (1985). Caregiving and the experience of subjective and objective burden. *Family Relations,* **34,** 19–26.

Moritz, D.J., Kasl, S.V. & Berkman, L.F. (1989). The health impact of living with a cognitively impaired elderly spouse: depressive symptoms and social functioning. *Journal of Gerontology,* **44,** S17–S27.

Morris, L.W., Morris, R.G. & Britton, P.G. (1988). The relationship between marital intimacy and perceived strain and depression in spouse caregivers of dementia sufferers. *British Journal of Medical Psychology,* **61,** 231–236.

Morris, L.W., Morris, R.G. & Britton, P.G. (1989). Cognitive style and perceived control in spouse caregivers of dementia sufferers. *British Journal of Medical Psychology,* **62,** 173–179.

Morris, R.G., Woods, R.T., Davies, K.S. & Morris, L.W. (1991). Gender differences in carers of dementia suffers. *British Journal of Psychiatry,* **158** (Supplement 10) 69–74.

Morycz, R.K. (1985). Caregiving strain and the desire to institutionalize family members with Alzheimer's disease: possible predictors and model development. *Research on Aging,* **7,** 329–361.

Motenko, A.K. (1989). The frustrations, gratifications, and well-being of dementia caregivers. *Gerontologist,* **29,** 166–172.

Novak, M. & Guest, C. (1989). Caregiver response to Alzheimer's disease. *International Journal of Aging and Human Development,* **28,** 67–79.

Office of Health Economics (1989). *Compendium of Health Statistics.* Seventh Edition. London: OHE.

O'Leary, A. (1990). Stress, emotion, and human immune function. *Psychological Bulletin,* **108,** 363–382.

Opportunities for Women (1990). *Carers at Work.* London: Opportunities for Women.

Pagel, M. & Becker, J. (1987). Depressive thinking and depression: relations with personality and social resources. *Journal of Personality and Social Psychology,* **52,** 1043–1052.

Pagel, M.D., Becker, J., & Coppel, D.B. (1985). Loss of control, self-blame and depression: an investigation of spouse caregivers of Alzheimer's disease patients. *Journal of Abnormal Psychology,* **94,** 169–182.

Pagel, M.D., Erdly, W.W. & Becker, J. (1987). Social networks: we get by with (and in spite of) a little help from our friends. *Journal of Personality and Social Psychology,* **53,** 793–804.

Pinkston, E.M. & Linsk, N.L. (1984). Behavioural family intervention with the impaired elderly. *Gerontologist,* **24,** 576–583.

Pomara, N., Deptula, D., Galloway, M.P., LeWitt, P.A. & Stanley, M. (1989). CSF GABA in caregiver spouses of Alzheimer patients. *American Journal of Psychiatry,* **146,** 787–788.

Pratt, C.C., Schmall, V.L., Wright, S. and Cleland, M. (1985). Burden and coping strategies of caregivers to Alzheimer's patients. *Family Relations,* **34,** 27–33.

Pratt, C., Wright, S., & Schmall, V. (1987). Burden, coping and health status: a comparison of family caregivers to community dwelling and institutionalized Alzheimer's patients. *Journal of Gerontological Social Work,* **10,** 99–112.

Pruchno, R.A. (1990). The effects of help patterns on the mental health of spouse caregivers. *Research on Aging,* **12,** 57–71.

Pruchno, R.A., Kleban, M.H., Michaels, J.E. & Dempsey, N.P. (1990a). Mental and physical health of caregiving spouses: development of a causal model. *Journal of Gerontology,* **45,** 192–199.

Pruchno, R.A., Michaels, J.E. & Potashnik, S.L. (1990b). Predictors of institutionalization among Alzheimer disease victims with caregiving spouses. *Journal of Gerontology,* **45,** S259–S266.

Pruchno, R.A. & Potashnik, S.L. (1989). Caregiving spouses: physical and mental health in perspective. *Journal of the American Geriatrics Society,* **37,** 697–705.

Pruchno, R.A. & Resch, N.L. (1989a). Aberrant behaviours and Alzheimer's disease: mental health effects on spouse caregivers. *Journal of Gerontology,* S177–S182.

Pruchno, R.A. & Resch, N.L. (1989b). Husbands and wives as caregivers: antecedents of depression and burden. *Gerontologist,* **29,** 159–165.

Quayhagen, M.P. & Quayhagen, M. (1988). Alzheimer's stress: coping with the caregiving role. *Gerontologist,* **28,** 391–396.

Richardson, A., Unell, J. & Aston, B. (1989). *A New Deal for Carers.* London: King's Fund Informational Support Unit.

Roberts-Thomson, I.C., Whittingham, S., Young-Chaiyud, U. & MacKay, I.R. (1974). Ageing, immune response and mortality. *Lancet,* **ii,** 368–370.

Robinson, B.C. (1983). Validation of a Caregiver Strain Index. *Journal of Gerontology,* **38,** 344–348.

Robinson, K.M. (1988). A social skills training programme for adult caregivers. *Advances in Nursing Science,* **10,** 59–72.

Russell, V., Procter, L. & Moniz, E. (1989). The influence of a relative support group on carers' emotional distress. *Journal of Advanced Nursing,* **14,** 863–867.

Scharlach, A.E. (1989). A comparison of employed caregivers of cognitively impaired and physically impaired elderly persons. *Research on Aging,* **11,** 225–243.

Scott, J.P., McKenzie, P.N., Slack, D. & Hutton, J.T. (1987). The role of coping behaviours for primary caregivers of Alzheimer's patients. *Texas Medicine,* **83,** 48–50.

Scott, J.P., Roberto, K.A. & Hutton, J.T. (1986). Families of Alzheimer's victims: family support to the caregivers. *Journal of the American Geriatrics Society,* **34,** 348–354.

Stephens, M.A., Norris, V.K., Kinney, J.M., Ritchie, S.W. & Grotz, R.C. (1988). Stressful situations in caregiving: relations between caregiver coping and well-being. *Psychology and Aging,* **3,** 208–209.

Stoller, E. & Pugliesi, K. (1989). Other roles of caregivers: competing responsibilities on supporting resources *Journal of Gerontology,* **44,** S231–S238.

Stone, R., Cafferata. G.L. & Sangl, J. (1987). Caregivers of the frail elderly: a national profile. *Gerontologist, 27*, 616–626.

Sutcliffe, C. & Larner, S. (1988). Counselling carers of the elderly at home: a preliminary study. *British Journal of Clinical Psychology, 27*, 177–178.

Toseland, R.W., Rossiter, C.M. & Labrecque, M.S. (1989). The effectiveness of three group intervention strategies to support family caregivers. *American Journal of Orthopsychiatry, 59*, 420–429.

Toseland, R.W., Rossiter, C.M., Peak, T. & Smith, G.C. (1990). Comparative effectiveness of individual and group interventions to support family caregivers. *Social Work, 35*, 209–217.

Toseland, R.W. & Smith, G.C. (1990). Effectiveness of individual counselling by professional and peer helpers for family caregivers of the elderly. *Psychology and Aging, 5*, 256–263.

Townsend, A., Noelker, L., Deimling, G. & Bass, D. (1989). Longitudinal impact of interhousehold caregiving on adult children's mental health. *Psychology and Aging, 4*, 393–401.

Whittick, J.E. (1988). Dementia and mental handicap: emotional distress in carers. *British Journal of Clinical Psychology, 27*, 167–172.

Wilder, D.E., Teresi, J.A. & Bennett, R.G. (1983). Family burden and dementia. In R. Mayeux and W.G. Rosen (eds) *The Dementias*. New York: Raven Press.

World Health Organization (1983). *International Classification of Impairments, Disabilities and Handicaps*. Geneva: World Health Organization.

Wortman, C.B., & Dintzer, L. (1978). Is an attributional analysis of the learned helplessness phenomenon viable? A critique of the Abramson-Seligman-Teasdale reformulation. *Journal of Abnormal Psychology, 87*, 75–90.

Zarit, S.H., Anthony, C.R. & Boutselis, M. (1987). Interventions with caregivers of dementia patients: a comparison of two approaches. *Psychology and Aging, 2*, 225–232.

Zarit, S.H., Reever, K.E. & Bach-Peterson, J. (1980). Relatives of the impaired elderly: correlates of feelings of burden. *Gerontologist, 20*, 649–655.

Zarit, S.H., Todd, P.A. & Zarit, J.M. (1986). Subjective burden of husbands and wives as caregivers: a longitudinal study. *Gerontologist, 26*, 260–266.

SOCIAL SUPPORT, SOCIAL CONTROL, AND HEALTH AMONG THE ELDERLY

MEGAN A. LEWIS, KAREN S. ROOK AND RALF SCHWARZER

Few adults manage to avoid experiencing health problems as they grow old, yet the health status of older adults need not be viewed in an excessively bleak light. Much variability exists among the elderly, and some older adults continue to function at levels that are similar to or even surpass earlier levels of physical functioning. For example, many older men and women compete in marathons or participate in Senior Olympics. Nevertheless, the health status of older adults does differ in several important respects from that of young and middle-aged adults. Older adults have more chronic conditions, such as heart disease, arthritis, and hearing impairments (Vital and Health Statistics, 1989). Rates of arthritis, for example, are 2–3 times higher among the elderly than among younger age groups (Vital and Health Statistics, 1989). In addition, older adults are more likely to suffer from multiple chronic conditions simultaneously (National Center for Health Statistics, 1987). Acute conditions, such as the common cold or influenza, occur less often among the elderly, but they are more debilitating and require more care when they affect an older person (Verbrugge, 1983). Older adults experience more activity restrictions as a result of health problems, and spend more days in bed because of illness (Verbrugge, 1983). Thus, without exaggerating the extent of infirmity among the elderly, it is clear that contending with illness and disability represents a common experience in the lives of many older adults.

This observation invites attention to two basic questions: What factors might help to prevent illness and disability in late life? What factors might help older adults to manage the illnesses and disabilities that do develop? With respect to prevention, it is widely acknowledged that many health problems can be traced to unsound health behaviors such as smoking, eating foods high in fat, or leading a sedentary lifestyle (Hamburg, Elliot and Parron, 1982). Moreover, many of the health problems from which older adults suffer have their behavioral roots in young and middle adulthood (Verbrugge, 1983). For example, most people start smoking in the young adult years, and smoking is the major cause of death and disability in later years (Hamburg, Elliot and Parron, 1982). Similarly, vulnerability to bone fractures among the elderly may be traced not only to inactivity in late life but also to inadequate development of bone mass early in life and to bone loss induced by menopausal changes in midlife (Riggs and Melton, 1988). Thus, the prevention of disability in old age requires efforts to reduce unsound health practices (e.g. smoking or excessive drinking) and to promote sound health practices (e.g. exercise or regular self-exams) among young and middle aged-adults. This does not mean that preventive health practices become irrelevant by late life. Some preventive practices retain their importance throughout adulthood and old age, such as obtaining regular preventive exams (e.g. mammograms or blood pressure tests), and other practices have special significance in old age, such as obtaining innoculations for influenza. The cumulative effect of efforts to promote sound health practices throughout the life course should be a reduction in chronic health problems among the elderly, or a "compression of morbidity" to fewer years of a person's life (Fries and Crapo, 1981).

Until this goal of preventing or postponing chronic illness has been achieved, however, some degree of disability will remain a fact of life for most older adults. Indeed, Verbrugge (1990) has argued that the legacy of increasing life expectancy is that people now spend more years living with multiple chronic conditions and disability (see also Schneider and Brody, 1983). She contends that most research captures only the tip of the "iceberg of disability" experienced in the daily lives of individuals coping with chronic conditions. Additionally, as an increasing number of older individuals live longer with one or more chronic conditions, the "iceberg" will continue to grow. Thus, it becomes important to consider what factors might help older adults more effectively manage, or live with, their disability. Some conditions require older adults to adhere to complex medical regimens or to participate in rehabilitation programs. For example, recovery from a heart attack requires people to initiate and maintain dietary changes, to participate in cardiac rehabilitation involving varying degrees of physical activity, and to maintain regular use of prescription medications (Santinga, 1987). Older adults vary in how successfully they comply with such treatment regimens, and psychosocial factors undoubtedly affect their rates of compliance. Other chronic conditions, such as arthritis, do not require adherence to a complex treatment regimen but do impose limitations on older adults' functioning. Some older adults simply succumb to such limitations, whereas others circumvent these limitations, and continue to lead active and satisfying lives. Psychosocial factors may play an important role in determining how well older adults adapt to living with disability.

The goal of this chapter is to consider how *social relationships* may affect patterns of illness and disability in late life, both by helping to prevent or delay the onset of chronic conditions and by helping older people to manage chronic conditions once they occur. We begin by briefly discussing epidemiological evidence that provides a rationale for focusing on social relationships in the context of physical health. This evidence indicates that people with greater social network involvement generally live longer than do people with more limited social network involvement. We then consider evidence that addresses how specific relationships with spouses, children, friends, and others may affect health outcomes. The next section considers the mechanisms by which social relationships may function to promote behaviors that prevent disability in old age or that help older adults to manage disabling conditions. Our discussion emphasizes two complementary aspects of social relationships – social support and social control. We use the term social support to refer to various forms of assistance and comfort provided by network members in times of need. Social control, in contrast, refers to actions by network members that are designed to influence or regulate behavior. Others' efforts to provide support can reduce the health-damaging consequences of life stress, can sustain self-initiated efforts to improve one's health practices, and can buoy one's spirits in the face of disabling health conditions. Others' efforts to exercise control can deter one from engaging in health-compromising behaviors such as smoking or excessive alcohol consumption, and can prompt one to engage in health-enhancing behaviors such as maintaining a regular exercise regimen or adhering to prescribed medications. We consider how social support and social control may influence health behaviors prior to the onset of health problems. We also consider how social support and social control may influence health behaviors and functioning after the onset of health problems. We conclude by identifying issues and questions for future research.

A comprehensive review of the numerous possible links between health status in late life and social relationships is beyond the scope of the present chapter. This chapter accordingly seeks to illustrate a subset of these links, emphasizing two key elements of social relationships – social support and social control – and emphasizing links of a behavioral rather than psychobiological nature. Other authors have provided excellent treatments of older adults' social networks (e.g. Antonucci, 1990), and the psychophysiological and immunological consequences of interpersonal loss or tensions (Kiecolt-Glaser and Glaser, 1988). In addition, other authors have addressed the illness behaviors of older adults (Krause, 1990), the utilization of health services by older adults (Wolinsky, 1990), and the general correlates of preventive health behaviors in late life (Rakowski *et al.*, 1987; Hickey, Rakowski and Julius, 1988). We do not wish to duplicate this work; rather, we wish to suggest a framework for thinking about how social relationships may affect health-related behavior and functioning before and after the onset of disability in late life. Additionally, we seek to illustrate how the questions subsumed by this framework have been (or could be) approached by researchers. The chapter is necessarily speculative in some places. We extrapolate periodically from research on young and middle-aged adults, because only a limited number of studies have focused specifically on social support and social control in relation to older adults' health behaviors and functioning. Finally, in referring to "the elderly" in this chapter, we do not mean to minimize the considerable heterogeneity that exists among older adults (Berkman, 1988). Hopefully, future research will provide a basis for refinement of current ideas about the links between older adults' social relationships and health, giving appropriate attention to gender, socioeconomic status, ethnicity, and other important differentiating factors.

EMPIRICAL EVIDENCE OF A LINK BETWEEN SOCIAL RELATIONSHIPS AND HEALTH

Evidence that links social relationships to important health outcomes comes from several sources. In an early and highly influential review of epidemiological research with humans and experimental studies with animals, Cassel (1976) concluded that social factors such as isolation and integration affect a wide range of health problems. His paper helped to call attention to the importance of social network factors as determinants of physical health outcomes. Many subsequent studies have supported his conclusion (see reviews by Berkman, 1984; Cohen, 1988; House, Landis and Umberson, 1988; House, Umberson and Landis, 1988; Schwarzer and Leppin, 1991).

A widely cited study by Berkman and Syme (1979) yielded strong evidence of a link between social integration and mortality. Over a 9-year period, the researchers investigated the social ties, health practices, and health status of a sample of 2,229 men and 2,496 women living in the United States. They found that people with more extensive social ties (e.g. those who were married or who belonged to community organizations) were less likely to die than were people with less extensive ties. This association was found to be independent of the respondent's health status at baseline measurement, the respondent's use of health services, and an overall index of health-risk behaviors (e.g. cigarette smoking, excessive drinking). Each type of social tie examined – marriage, contacts with friends and relatives, church membership, and informal and formal group associations – significantly predicted the risk of mortality, as did a composite measure of social integration that combined these various social ties. Additionally, more intimate social ties, such as bonds with a spouse or with family and friends, were more powerful predictors of mortality risk than were less intimate ties, such as group associations.

A further analysis of this data set was conducted by Seeman *et al.* (1987) to determine whether a comparable link between social integration and mortality exists for older people. Berkman and Syme (1979) included in their analyses only individuals aged 30–69 at baseline measurement, whereas Seeman *et al.* (1987) included people aged 38–94 at baseline measurement. In addition, Seeman *et al.* (1987) examined mortality records over a 17-year period, rather than a 9-year period. These analyses replicated the pattern obtained by Berkman and Syme (1979) for the composite measure of social integration but yielded somewhat different patterns for the measures of specific social ties. Relationships with friends and relatives (excluding the spouse) were found to be more important in predicting mortality risk for older adults than for middle-aged adults. Marital relationships, in contrast, were more important for middle-aged adults than for older adults (Seeman *et al.*, 1987). Seeman *et al.* (1987) speculated that friends and relatives assume greater importance in old age because so many older adults become widowed.

A prospective study by Blazer (1982) also demonstrated the importance of social relationships to older adults' health. In a sample of 331 older adults, Blazer (1982) examined social roles and attachments (e.g. marital status, number of children), perceived social support, and frequency of social interaction in relation to mortality risk 30 months later. Older adults with lower scores on these aspects of social network involvement were found to be at significantly greater risk of mortality, relative to older adults with moderate-to-high scores on these network indicators. This association remained significant even when statistical controls were included for potentially confounded variables, such as socioeconomic status, stressful life events, health practices, and health status at initial assessment.

Convergent evidence of the importance of social ties for physical health comes from research designed to address the question of whether it is beneficial to occupy certain social roles, such as the role of spouse or parent. For example, Gove (1973) compared mortality rates from the National Center for Health Statistics for married, single, widowed, and divorced individuals. He found that mortality risk was lower among married individuals than among individuals with all other marital statuses. In addition, mortality risk was greater for unmarried men than for unmarried women. Gove's (1973) analyses revealed further that, among the unmarried, mortality risk was greater for causes of death in which behavior or psychological states played a role, such as cirrhosis of the liver, lung cancer, or suicide. Fewer mortality differences between married and unmarried people were observed when the cause of death could not be attributed to lifestyle factors, such as leukemia. Thus, part of the health benefit that marriage confers relates to health practices and risk behaviors.

In analyses of several national health surveys in the United States, Verbrugge (1979) similarly found evidence that marital status was linked to patterns of morbidity. Divorced and separated people were found to have the worst health status, with higher rates of acute as well as chronic conditions, and higher rates of disability. Widowed people and single people, respectively, had the next worst health status, with married people enjoying the best health status. Such results are consistent with studies of health risk-taking, which have found divorced individuals to engage in riskier behavior than other individuals (Umberson, 1987). Later work by Verbrugge (1983, 1985, 1989) and other investigators (Wingard, 1982; Nathanson, 1984) reached similar conclusions regarding the association between marital status and morbidity and mortality.

Parental status has also been examined in relation to physical health outcomes. This work indicates that overall mortality risk is lower for people who are married and have children, especially when the children are young enough to be living at home (Korbin and Hendershot, 1977; Wingard, 1982; Umberson, 1987). Parenthood also appears to constrain health risk-taking, with parents engaging in fewer health-compromising behaviors, such as excessive drinking or smoking, than non-parents (Umberson, 1987).

The health implications of living with others versus living alone have been studied as well. Among unmarried people those who live alone have been found to engage in more health-compromising behaviors, such as drug and alcohol use, than those who live with others (Hughes and Gove, 1981; Dean, 1989). Interestingly, unmarried people who live alone fare nearly as well, and sometimes better than, unmarried people who live with others on measures of mental health (Hughes and Gove, 1981). These patterns have emerged in general population studies; more equivocal evidence has emerged in studies of older adults. Lawton, Moss and Kleban (1984) found in three large probability samples that, compared to older individuals who lived with others, those who lived alone had better functional health but lower psychological well-being. Those who lived alone apparently suffered from fewer disabilities than did those who lived with others. Yet Cafferata (1987) found in data from the National Medical Care Expenditure Survey that older adults who lived with others reported fewer physician visits than did those who lived alone. Thus, the health implications for older adults of living alone versus living with others remain somewhat uncertain, particularly since health may represent both a cause and a consequence of living arrangements in late life.

Overall, findings from these different lines of research converge in suggesting that social relationships often influence health behaviors and important health outcomes. Well-controlled prospective studies indicate that people who have limited connections to others experience increased risk of morbidity and mortality. This increased risk of mortality cannot easily be discounted as a mere artifact of other factors, such as socioeconomic status, use of health services, or initial health status. Moreover, evidence suggests that at least part of the health benefit conferred by social relationships can be attributed to the role these relationships play in fostering sound health practices and deterring unsound practices (e.g. Cwikel *et al.*, 1988; Umberson, 1987). The next section seeks to elaborate on this mediating role.

IMPLICATIONS OF SOCIAL SUPPORT AND SOCIAL CONTROL FOR HEALTH PROBLEMS IN LATE LIFE

Competing ideas been offered to explain how social networks may influence health across the life span. Many researchers emphasize the role of social support provided through informal social networks in mitigating the health-damaging consequences of life stress (see reviews by Cohen and Wills, 1985; Kessler and McLeod, 1985; Vaux, 1988). Other researchers emphasize the role of controlling or regulatory actions by social network members in promoting sound health practices and deterring unsound practices (e.g. Hughes and Gove, 1981; Umberson, 1987). This section contrasts these two perspectives, considering how social support and social control may influence health status in late life by helping to prevent the onset of chronic conditions and by helping older adults to manage chronic conditions that do develop. We also recognize that the efforts of social network members to provide social support or to exercise social control do not always succeed and sometimes even backfire, aggravating rather than alleviating any existing problems (Wortman and Lehman, 1985; Coyne, Wortman and Lehman, 1988). We illustrate several such paradoxical effects in this section.

The Social Support Perspective

Many social scientists assume that the health benefits afforded by social integration are attributable to the positive, affirming, supportive aspects of relationships with others (e.g. Sarason *et al.*, 1987). In this tradition of research, social relationships are thought to influence health by providing needed resources that help to alleviate the potentially deleterious effects of stressful circumstances. These resources can take many forms, such as talking with the person, providing concrete aid, or helping the person appraise a stressful situation as less threatening (House, 1981). The empirical and theoretical work that has focused on understanding social support processes generally has emphasized this stress-buffering aspect of social ties. Some theorists have argued that social ties offer important health benefits, regardless of the stress a person may experience. This work has been guided by the view that a sense of being loved, esteemed, and cared for is the mechanism by which social relationships enhance health (Sarason *et al.*, 1987).

  Much recent research on the association between older adults' social involvement and their physical or emotional health reflects an interest in understanding how relationships buffer older adults from the adverse effects of stress (e.g. see reviews by Schulz and Rau, 1985; Antonucci, 1985, 1990). Studies investigating caregiver stress, or events such as widowhood or retirement, have probed the role that socially supportive relationships play in facilitating adaptation to such circumstances (e.g. Lopata, 1979; Wan, 1982; Haley *et al.*, 1987). Research has also begun to focus on the role that social support may play in facilitating recovery from illness, and compliance with medical regimens (e.g. Revenson, Wollman and Felton, 1983). The following discussion focuses on the role that social support may play in preventing the development of chronic conditions through its effect on health practices. In addition, we consider how socially supportive relationships may influence adaptation to chronic conditions once they have occurred by promoting compliance with prescribed medical regimens, and influencing patients' perceptions of health. Lastly, we consider paradoxical psychological reactions that may accompany the receipt of social support in later years.

The role of social support prior to the onset of chronic conditions
It has been well-established that people initiate high-risk health behaviors as a means of coping with life stress and resulting emotional strain. For example, drinking alcohol, smoking cigarettes, or using drugs can represent efforts to cope with stress and to regulate negative emotional states (Wills and Shiffman, 1985). Grunberg and Baum (1985) found that smokers who were experiencing stressful circumstances, reported increased rates of smoking and also reported fewer stress-related negative emotions. To the extent that social support helps to reduce emotional strain in the face of life stress, people may be less likely to turn to substance use and other unhealthy behaviors for relief (Wills, 1990).

Bereavement is a common stressful event in late life that sometimes results in coping behaviors that jeopardize health. Widowed individuals report greater use of alcohol, tobacco, and tranquilizers, compared with matched, nonwidowed controls, and this difference persists for as long as 13 months after the death of the spouse (Gass, 1989). In addition, such coping strategies have been found to be correlated with feelings of grief and depression (Gallagher, Thompson and Peterson, 1982). Men may be particularly likely to rely on alcohol use as a coping mechanism following the death of a spouse, as evidenced by higher rates of mortality from cirrhosis of the liver among widowers than among widows (Stroebe and Stroebe, 1983). Although few studies have focused specifically on the coping responses of older bereaved adults (Wortman and Silver, 1990), it is plausible that social support could reduce widowed individuals' reliance on unhealthy coping behaviors, thereby helping to prevent or delay the development of debilitating conditions, such as cirrhosis of the liver or heart and lung diseases.

Another way in which social support may help to prevent the development of chronic conditions in late life is by helping people to sustain self-initiated changes in their health behaviors (e.g. Zimmerman and Conner, 1989). Reviews provide a mixed assessment of the effectiveness of social support in helping to sustain self-initiated behavioral risk reduction (Baranowski and Nader, 1985), but it does appear that social support can help to sustain efforts to quit smoking. Several studies indicate that partner support can be especially helpful during initial behavior change and early in the maintenance of abstinence (Mermelstein, Lichtenstein and McIntyre, 1983; Coppotelli and Orleans, 1985; Morgan, Ashenberg and Fisher, 1988). Cohen *et al.* (1988) concluded from a review of social support interventions incorporated in smoking cessation studies that social support is most effective in the earlier stages of quitting and in helping people cope with the potentially stressful physical and emotional discomfort associated with quitting. During later stages of maintenance social support becomes less important.

Additionally, studies have begun to identify the specific kinds of behaviors that are most effective in supporting abstinence from smoking. Helpful behaviors include being understanding, listening, and helping the ex-smoker cope in positive ways, and avoiding interpersonal conflicts or stressful circumstances (Coppotelli and Orleans, 1985). Furthermore, the ratio of a spouse's supportive behaviors to unsupportive behaviors is more effective in predicting smokers who will remain abstinent than the receipt of supportive spousal behaviors alone (Cohen and Lichtenstein, 1990). Findings such as these demonstrate the value of examining supportive behaviors in the context of other interpersonal behaviors in investigating how social relationships influence health behavior changes.

In sum, research has demonstrated at least two ways in which social support may be helpful in delaying the onset of chronic conditions in late life. Supportive relationships may influence health-related behaviors prior to the development of chronic conditions by decreasing the likelihood that people who are experiencing life stress will engage in maladaptive coping behaviors. In addition, social support can more directly influence health-related behaviors prior to the development of chronic conditions by facilitating behavioral risk reduction and encouraging health-promoting behaviors.

The role of social support after the onset of chronic conditions
Even if chronic health conditions develop in later years social support may prove to be of value in helping people adapt to the challenges posed by chronic conditions. Supportive relationships have the potential to help people comply with prescribed behavioral and medical recommendations (DiMatteo and Hays, 1981). In addition, supportive relationships encourage more positive perceptions of health and functional abilities among those with chronic conditions. Positive perceptions of health are associated with important health outcomes ranging from better daily functioning to mortality risk (Idler and Kasl, 1991). The following discussion addresses how these social support processes may help older adults to manage chronic conditions and disability in later years.

Several reviews have examined the role social support plays in the process of adapting to chronic conditions. These reviews provide a mixed assessment of the role that social support may play in enhancing compliance with medical recommendations (DiMatteo and Hays, 1981; Levy, 1983; Wortman and Conway, 1985; Felton, 1990). Social support sometimes has no effect on patient compliance with medical regimens (e.g. Kaplan and Hartwell, 1987), and at other times has a detrimental effect (e.g. Carpenter and Davis, 1976). It does appear, however, that support facilitates recovery from coronary heart disease. For example, in patients with coronary heart disease, social support has been associated with appropriate medication use (Doherty *et al.*, 1983), and with maintenance of desirable weight and reduced smoking (Finnegan and Suler, 1985). Social support has also been shown to facilitate recovery by buffering the negative effects of stress (Fontana *et al.*, 1989). Results such as these have led to the conclusion that social support can be an influential factor in the course of recovery from coronary heart disease (Davidson and Shumaker, 1987). Recent reviews, however, caution that many studies that have linked social support with favorable health-related outcomes in cardiac patients have included only men, and that a complete understanding of how social support effects compliance in late life will not be complete until more representative samples are included in future studies (Shumaker and Hill, 1991).

In spite of these positive results investigators have begun to explore why social support sometimes has detrimental effects on patient compliance (for example see, Kaplan and Hartwell, 1987), and at other times has no effect at all (for example see, Carpenter and Davis, 1976). In explaining inconsistent results, investigators have pointed to both poor conceptualization and operationalization of support and compliance measures, and to the lack of attention to contextual aspects of relationships as factors that impede this area of research (Levy, 1983; Wortman and Conway, 1985).

Greater attention to the operationalization of both compliance and support measures would help sort out conflicting results in this area of research. Clinical outcomes such as blood pressure or cholesterol have been used as the sole indicators of compliance in some studies. Yet such clinical indicators may deteriorate or improve for reasons unrelated to actual compliance (Levy, 1983). Regarding social support, authors have suggested that specific types of support be distinguished in studies to determine which kinds of support benefit versus irritate individuals who are adapting to chronic health conditions (Wortman and Conway, 1985). For example, in a study of women breast cancer patients who had undergone surgery, emotional and instrumental support were associated with enhanced psychological adjustment after surgery, while financial support was related to physical recovery (Funch and Mettlin, 1982). In addition, the importance of support may vary at different points in the process of recovery (Fontana *et al.*, 1989). Thus, investigators need to give thought to the time frame in which supportive exchanges may benefit older adults who are adapting to chronic health conditions.

Considering both the support provider's and recipient's perspectives on support exchanges may also help us understand conflicting results in this area (Wortman and Conway, 1985). Recent work with rheumatoid arthritis patients illustrates this point. Melamed and Brenner (1990) found that when rating the supportiveness of their spouse's behaviors, 74% of patients rated the statement: "Asked me how he or she could help," as an *unsupportive* behavior. Of all the behaviors that these patients rated as unsupportive, only "Expressed irritation" was endorsed equally frequently (Melamed and Brenner, 1990). Thus, support providers' good intentions alone do not guarantee a positive outcome; some well intended actions only serve to aggravate the support recipient. Other studies with cancer patients indicate that the perception of support gestures as helpful or unhelpful depends not only on the type of support, but also the source of support (Dakof and Taylor, 1990).

Another way in which support may influence health and well-being after the onset of chronic conditions in late life is by encouraging positive evaluations of health and functioning. For example, patients with kidney disease who have supportive family ties exhibit higher morale and better social functioning during hemodialysis than do patients with fewer supportive ties (Dimond, 1979). Demonstration of such links would be important because current perceptions of health status have been shown to predict later morality risk, independent of physical health problems, disability, or behavioral risk factors for disease (Idler and Kasl, 1991). Emerging evidence suggests that social support is associated with positive perceptions of health status in late life (Siegler and Costa, 1985). For example, in one study of older adults, several types of supportive exchanges with network members were related to positive changes in indices of physical health, including self-perceptions of health status (Cutrona, Russell and Rose, 1986). Similarly, "emotional bondedness" with a confidant or close friend was found to be associated significantly with positive ratings of health in another elderly sample (Snow and Crapo, 1982).

Social support may enhance self-ratings of health in later years, in part, by alleviating psychological distress and depression. Research indicates that distress and depression are associated with lower self-rated health status (Tessler and Mechanic, 1978; Blazer and Houpt, 1979). Compared to nonbereaved control groups, bereaved older adults have been found to endorse lower self-ratings of health status (Thompson *et al.*, 1984), and it is well-known that the bereaved suffer from higher rates of depression. Stoller (1984) used path analysis to delineate the relationship between social network influences and health status among community residing older adults. She found that social isolation contributed to depressive symptoms, which in turn resulted in lower ratings of health status. Furthermore, depressive symptoms were more strongly related to lower self-rated health than were functional and medical impairment measures. Such findings suggest that psychological states can play an important role in self-rated health status.

Empirical studies connecting social processes with perceptions of health are not consistent, however. Some studies have found perceptions of health to be unrelated to psychosocial processes (Idler and Kasl, 1991; Kunter, 1987). Drawing distinctions among different types of support may aid in understanding equivocal results in this area of research. For example, Seeman, Seeman and Sayles (1985) found that social ties characterized as providing tangible forms of support were associated with better perceptions of health. Social ties characterized as providing consultation and advice, however, were not associated with better perceptions of health in their study. These authors noted that the relationship between social ties and ratings of health are modest, but that modest results should not be looked upon with disappointment. Such findings may realistically reflect the nature of the association between social ties and physical health outcomes.

Paradoxical effects of social support processes
In the preceding discussion we have outlined several ways in which social support processes can enhance health-related practices or perceptions prior to and after the onset of chronic conditions in late life. Research with older adults indicates, however, that social exchanges with network members do not uniformly result in positive outcomes (e.g. Fiore, Becker and Coppel, 1983; Pagel, Erdly and Becker, 1987; Rook, 1984, 1990a; Stephens *et al.*, 1987). Well-intentioned gestures of support can backfire. Family members can inadvertently reinforce sick-role behavior (e.g. DiMatteo and Hays, 1981), can support some parts of a patient's prescribed treatment regimen while undermining other parts (Kaplan and Toshima, 1990), and can provoke frustration and erode independence by being overly protective (Coyne, Wortman and Lehman, 1988). Such miscarried help can undermine emotional health, and impede adaptation to chronic conditions (DiMatteo and Hays, 1981; Bohm and Rodin, 1985; Burish and Bradley, 1983). Metabolic control of diabetes, for example, requires family members to support (or at least not to interfere with) a patient's efforts to make changes in diet, weight, and medication use. Yet research indicates that family support is not uniformly targeted to these different components of the treatment regimens, and does not uniformly promote regimen adherence; indeed, social support has been found to be associated with worse diabetic control in some studies (Kaplan and Toshima, 1990).

Mixed effects of social network support have been documented in geriatric stroke patients (Stephens *et al.*, 1987; Norris, Stephens and Kinney, 1990). For example, Norris, Stephens and Kinney (1990) assessed social supports, social problems, and adaptation to disability in a study of older adults who were disabled by a stroke. These investigators found that patients who reported problems in obtaining aid and assistance from family members also experienced greater dependence in terms of activities of daily living after hospitalization. This potential for social exchanges to hinder positive adjustment to chronic illness has also been documented in rheumatoid arthritis patients (Manne and Zautra, 1989), and in severely disabled cancer patients (Revenson, Wollman and Felton, 1983). Such results demonstrate the importance of examining both the potentially negative and positive effects of social ties on behavioral and psychological dimensions of adaptation to chronic conditions. Hopefully, such research will lead to development of theoretical models that will allow us to predict beneficial versus detrimental health outcomes of social network ties.

The Social Control Perspective

Most psychological work linking social relationships to health has focused on the stress-buffering, psychologically affirming aspect of social support, but a complete understanding of the processes by which social relationships influence health requires attention to an additional aspect of social relationships, namely social control. Just as social support contributes to health by alleviating stress, social control can contribute to health by constraining risky, health-damaging behaviors or promoting self-care behaviors. Social control has been defined as "the mechanism by which social relationships affect health behaviors" (Umberson, 1987, p. 309), and "the controlling or regulating quality of social relationships, which depending on the behaviors controlled or regulated, may be either health promoting or health damaging" (House, Umberson, Landis, 1988 p. 302). A similar definition to that of House, Umberson and Landis (1988) has been proposed by Rook and Pietromonaco (1987), who view the regulatory, restraining function of the social bond as social control.

Social control theorists have conceptualized the health benefits of social relation-ships as occurring through two basic mechanisms. Social control affects health behaviors and well-being *indirectly* when a person has internalized a feeling of responsibility, or has a significant role obligation to others, and adheres to norms that accompany such social roles as being married or being a parent. According to social control theorists, people who have responsibilities or obligations to others lead more orderly, regular, and less risky lives than do people who lack such obligations or responsibilities (Umberson, 1987). For example, someone who has the primary care-taking responsibility for a disabled spouse may be less likely to drink excessively or otherwise take risks. In addition, he or she may be more likely to engage in appropriate self-care (e.g. sleeping regularly) as a result of a perceived obligation to continue functioning effectively as a caregiver.

Social control also effects health behaviors *directly* through the efforts of social network members to prompt a person to engage in preventive health actions, to discourage risky or deviant behavior, or to prompt compliance with prescribed medical regimens. For example, a spouse who intervenes to stop his or her partner's excessive drinking would be making an attempt to exercise direct social control (Durkheim, 1897/1951; Hughes and Gove, 1981; Rook and Pietromonaco, 1987; Umberson, 1987; House, Umberson and Landis, 1988). Early theoretical formulations and studies of social control focused on health-related behaviors that were clearly deviant and risky such as alcoholism or attempted suicide (Durkheim, 1897/1951). More recent work has emphasized less risky self-care behaviors in addition to deviant or risky actions (Hughes and Gove, 1981; Umberson, 1987; Rook, Thuras and Lewis, 1990).

Sociological investigations typically have operationalized social control in terms of marital status, living arrangement, and parenthood. That is, individuals who are married, have children, and/or who live with others are assumed to experience greater social control than their counterparts who are unmarried, childless, and/or who live alone. The studies reviewed earlier of the health-enhancing effects of marriage, parenthood or living with others are viewed by social control theorists as evidence that social control influences health-related outcomes. Few of these studies have assessed social control attempts directly, but instead have treated marital status or parental status as proxies for the interpersonal processes implied by the social control construct. More recent work has attempted to include more explicit assessment of social control phenomena that occur in the context of social networks (Rook, Thuras and Lewis, 1990; Umberson and Greer, 1990).

The following discussion considers the role of social control processes in enhancing health behaviors prior to and after the onset of chronic conditions in late life. In addition, we consider potentially paradoxical effects of social control. This discussion is necessarily speculative in describing how both direct and indirect forms of social control experienced by older adults may influence their health behaviors and health outcomes.

The role of social control prior to the onset of chronic conditions
Both direct forms of social control (i.e. interpersonal influence and regulation) and indirect forms of social control (i.e. role obligations) can influence health-related behaviors prior to the development of chronic conditions. Network members can use direct forms of social control to deter an individual from personally desired but health-compromising behaviors, such as smoking or excessive drinking. In addition, network members can use persuasion to promote good self-care behaviors or preventive health behaviors that an older person might otherwise resist, such as exercise. The following discussion concerns these direct forms of social control as well as the potential impact of role obligations on health-related behaviors prior to the development of chronic conditions in late life.

Evidence indicates that the experience of direct forms of social control is not uncommon among older adults. In a sample of community residing older adults, almost 80% reported that network members had prompted them to engage in positive health behaviors, and almost 78% reported that others had tried to deter them from engaging in unhealthful behaviors. Network members who were most frequently named as engaging in such forms of social control were adult children and friends (Rook, Thuras and Lewis, 1990). Consistent with this, Dillard (1989) found that a common influence goal in close personal relationships is changing and influencing another's health-related behaviors. The behaviors that were targeted most frequently in this sample of college students were health-risk behaviors such as drinking, using drugs, or smoking. Thus, although the available evidence is limited, it suggests that direct social control attempts aimed at changing or regulating health-related behavior are relatively common in interpersonal relationships.

Utilizing panel data from a representative national sample, Umberson and Greer (1990) conducted analyses that provide interesting descriptive and some predictive data on direct social control attempts and the impact of role obligations on health risk-taking. These investigators were interested in how being the target of direct social control attempts by others may vary by gender and by marital status. In addition, these researchers tested the hypothesis that direct social control would be related to lower levels of health risk-taking. Men reported experiencing more direct social control from network members than did women, and married people reported experiencing more direct social control than did unmarried people. In addition, a significant interaction between marital status and gender emerged revealing that married men and unmarried women reported experiencing more direct social control than other groups. Contrary to expectation, these authors found that more frequent social control attempts were associated with an increase rather than a decrease in health risk-taking.

Umberson and Greer (1990) also investigated whether transition from marriage into divorce or widowhood would be accompanied by an increase in health risk-taking. As reviewed previously, statuses such as marriage, parenthood, and living with other people are associated with less health risk-behavior (Verbrugge, 1979; Hughes and Gove, 1981; Umberson, 1987). Social control theorists postulate that the obligations and responsibilities that accompany such roles serve to constrain health-risk taking (Hughes and Gove, 1981). Thus, the transition to a single status (widowed or divorced) from being married would be expected to be accompanied by an increase in detrimental health behaviors. Indeed, Umberson and Greer (1990) did find that transition to a single status was associated with the practice of unhealthy behaviors. For example, men who became divorced or widowed between the two panel measurements smoked more cigarettes and drank more alcohol than did men who remained married. Women who became widowed or divorced lost more weight, and slept less than did women who remained married during that same time period (Umberson and Greer, 1990). Because these authors used marital status as a proxy for direct social control attempts, however, it could also be argued that the observed increase in negative health behaviors was due not to the lack of restraining role obligations, but to the stress that accompanies divorce and widowhood (Bloom, Asher and White, 1978). Future research should examine how transition from one marital status to another is related to direct social control attempts and to health risk-behaviors. Additionally, future work in this area should distinguish between health risk-taking, self-care, and preventive behaviors in an attempt to determine whether social control processes have similar or dissimilar effects on these classes of behaviors.

The role of social control after the onset of chronic conditions
Indirect and direct forms of social control can influence health-related behavior after the onset of chronic conditions in several ways. Members of one's social network can cajole or coerce an individual to comply with prescribed medical regimens. For example, network members may coerce a person who has cancer to quit smoking. Additionally, social role obligations in late life, if they are not too taxing, may facilitate self-care and adaptive functioning. Despite the potential importance of social control processes after the onset of late-life chronic conditions, the available evidence on these processes is sparse. The few empirical studies that have examined social control have not distinguished between the effects of social control prior to versus after the onset of chronic conditions. Also, studies that have examined social role obligations in late life have not necessarily involved social control as the explanatory mechanism. Therefore, the following discussion extrapolates from relevant studies that have been conducted with elderly samples, even if they were not designed to investigate social control phenomena.

One way in which social control may influence health-related behaviors in late life is through responsibilities and obligations that accompany many social roles. There is some indication that social role obligations facilitate treatment outcomes. For example, in a sample of alcoholics being treated for their drinking problems, those who had stable marriage and/or work situations at the beginning of treatment evidenced better treatment outcomes (Bromet and Moos, 1977). Unfortunately, there has been little methodologically sound research that has investigated how older adults' social roles influence their health-related behavior and physical health outcomes (Rodin, Cashman and Desiderato, 1987). An exception in this regard is research on caregiving, which documents the toll taken on older adults by burdensome caregiving demands (e.g. Haley, *et al.*, 1987). Researchers have argued, however, that providing meaningful social roles for the elderly would be an appropriate intervention to combat social isolation, and to facilitate positive adaptation in old age (Heller *et al.*, 1991). Future research needs to examine in a more rigorous fashion how the provision of social roles, such as volunteer or paid work, or opportunities to provide companionship to others, influences both physical and psychological well-being among older adults.

Rook, Thuras and Lewis (1990) examined the effect of direct and indirect mechanisms of social control among community residing older adults. This study tested the hypothesis, derived from the work of Hughes and Gove (1981), that social control discourages risky health practices. The risky health practices included in this study were alcohol and cigarette consumption, medication misuse, an overall index of fifteen health risk-behaviors, and an index of medication misuse. Analyses revealed that smoking rates were lower if participants in the study had someone who depended on them regularly (social role obligations). In addition, medication misuse was positively associated with network members' attempts to deter unwise health practices. Such a finding could mean that social control attempts backfire, serving to increase rather than decrease medication misuse. It is also plausible that medication misuse elicits social control from network members. These data revealed no significant associations between social control (direct or indirect) and alcohol consumption or the overall index of health risk-taking. Thus, initial evidence indicates that for older adults, social control is not consistently related to health risk-taking, rather, its effects depend on the type of health behavior under investigation.

It is premature, however, to conclude that direct social control is unrelated to health practices in late life. Future studies in this area would do well to strengthen measures of direct social control and to distinguish among self-care behaviors, compliance-related health activities, and health risk-taking behaviors. In addition, future work would also benefit from distinguishing among various sources of social control. For example, are social control attempts less effective with chronic risky behaviors (e.g. life-long smoking) than with "everyday" self-care behaviors (e.g. sound nutritional practices). In addition, do older adults who have more serious or debilitating chronic conditions receive more social control from network members? Similarly, is social control from certain network members (e.g. friends versus family members) more effective in constraining detrimental health behaviors? Addressing questions such as these would extend preliminary studies that have tried to link direct social control with health practices in late life.

Paradoxical effects of social control processes
In the previous section we have highlighted the hypothesized benefits of social control processes in late life. There is reason to suspect, however, that social control sometimes promotes maladaptive behaviors. Others can cajole or pressure us into

unhealthy actions, such as eating or drinking or abandoning adherence to a prescribed treatment regimen. Such processes have been studied most extensively among adolescents (see review by Wills, 1990), but they may occur in middle and late adulthood as well. For example, Rook, Thuras and Lewis (1990) found that 19% of the older adults in their study reported that network members had tried to influence them to engage in unhealthy and unwanted behaviors. Such results suggest that "peer pressure" still operates in late adulthood, although this form of social control is rarely studied in late life.

Social control may also have paradoxical effects by engendering psychological and behavioral reactance (Brehm and Brehm, 1981). Psychological reactance theory outlines several propositions about what people do when pressured to act in certain ways. When a person's behavioral "freedom" is threatened s(he) may feel motivated to resist or oppose the demand, in an attempt to reassert personal control (Brehm and Brehm, 1981). Network members who try to dissuade older adults from engaging in unhealthy but personally enjoyed behaviors (e.g. eating high fat diets or smoking) may provoke psychological reactance, thereby increasing the older adults' commitment to the unhealthy behavior.

Social control theorists (e.g. Hughes and Gove, 1981) explicitly acknowledge the potential for social bonds to provoke psychological distress while simultaneously seeking to promote sound health practices. This dual nature of social control – arousing psychological distress while discouraging unhealthy behaviors – was examined by Hughes and Gove (1981). These researchers found that people who lived alone (and who presumably had little exposure to controlling actions by others) engaged in more health-compromising behaviors, such as drinking and using sleeping pills, but also reported better psychological functioning than did those who lived with others. Hughes and Gove (1981) reasoned that "constraint may be the source of considerable frustration; at the same time it tends to reduce the probability of problematic or maladaptive behaviors" (p. 71). This hypothesis was examined in a study of older adults by Rook, Thuras and Lewis (1990). These investigators found, however, that attempts by network members to exercise health-related social control were associated with better, not worse, psychological functioning. In addition, attempts by network members to influence the elderly participants to take health-risks were associated with lower self-esteem. How older adults respond psychologically to others' efforts to exercise social control (positive and negative control) deserves further attention. Further work is also needed that can clarify causal associations among social control, behavioral outcomes, and psychological reactions.

CONCLUSION

Although many adults live with chronic conditions in their later years (Vital and Health Statistics, 1989), it has been argued that the practice of sound health behaviors can delay morbidity in later years, and reduce the number of chronic health problems in late life (Fries and Crapo, 1981). This chapter has examined how social relationships may help to delay the onset of chronic conditions in late life. We also considered how social relationships may help older adults to manage chronic conditions and disability. Social support and social control were emphasized as two key elements of social relationships that may influence health-related behaviors and perceptions. Social support may help to delay the onset of chronic conditions by decreasing the likelihood that unhealthy behaviors will be initiated in response to stressful circumstances, and by supporting self-initiated behavioral risk reduction. Social control can help to constrain health risk-taking, and to increase the likelihood that important self-care behaviors are practiced. If chronic conditions develop in late life, social support can help encourage compliance with prescribed medical recommendations and can enhance positive perceptions of health, which are associated with lower mortality risk. Social control processes similarly can help to insure compliance with prescribed medical regimens, and can facilitate self-care and adaptive functioning. In addition, we have considered potentially negative psychological and behavioral outcomes that, at times, accompany the provision of social support and exposure to social control.

Although we have considered social support and social control as independent processes, future work should consider the interactive effects of supportive or controlling transactions in older adults' relationships. Many close relationships undoubtedly provide social support some of the time, and exercise social control at other times. By examining social control processes in the context of supportive relationships, we can extend our understanding of how social relationships function to enhance health-related behaviors. Social control attempts may be more palatable (and therefore, more effective) when they are made by network members who also provide valued forms of social support in other contexts (Rook, 1990b). For example, an elderly widower may be more likely to comply with his daughter's efforts to persuade him to stop smoking when the daughter has a track record of providing support than when she lacks such a record. Much more remains to be learned about the interdependent effects of social support and social control.

Future work in this area should address the possible negative or unexpected side-effects of both social support and social control processes. Research has indicated that miscarried social support can have detrimental effects (Kaplan and Toshima, 1990; Coyne, Wortman and Lehman, 1988; Wortman and Lehman, 1985), and that social control attempts can backfire or provoke psychological distress (Hughes and Gove, 1981). More systematic evaluation of the causes and consequences of positive and negative interactions in the context of the health problems or health-related behaviors will aid in understanding how social relationships influence health and well-being in late life.

REFERENCES

Antonucci, T.C. (1985). Personal characteristics, social support, and social behavior. In *Handbook of Aging and the Social Sciences*, edited by R.H. Binstock & E. Shanas, pp. 94–128. New York: Van Nostrand-Reinhold.

Antonucci, T.C. (1990). Social supports and social relationships. In *Handbook of Aging and the Social Sciences*, edited by R.H. Binstock & L.K. George, pp. 205–226. San Diego: Academic Press, Inc.

Baranowski, T. & Nader, P.R. (1985). Family involvement in health behavior change programs. In *Health, Illness, and Families: A Lifespan Perspective*, edited by D.C. Turk & R.D. Kerns, pp. 81–107. New York: John Wiley & Sons.

Berkman, L.F. (1984). Assessing the physical health effects of social networks and social support. *Annual Review of Public Health*, 5, 413–432.

Berkman, L.F. (1988). The changing and heterogeneous nature of aging and longevity: A social and biomedical perspective. In *Annual Review of Gerontology and Geriatrics*, edited by G.L. Maddox & M.P. Lawton, pp. 37–68. New York: Springer Publishing Co.

Berkman, L.F. & Syme, L.S. (1979). Social networks, host resistance, and mortality: A nine-year follow-up study of Alameda County Residents. *American Journal of Epidemiology*, 109, 186–204.

Blazer, D.G. (1982). Social support and mortality in an elderly community population. *American Journal of Epidemiology*, 115, 684–694.

Blazer, D.G. & Houpt, J.L. (1979). Perception of poor health in the healthy older adult. *Journal of the American Geriatrics Society*, 27, 330–334.

Bloom, B., Asher, S.J. & White, S.W. (1978). Marital disruption as a stressor: A review and analysis. *Psychological Bulletin*, 85, 867–894.

Bohm, L.C. & Rodin, J. (1985). Aging and the family. In *Health, Illness, and Families: A Lifespan Perspective*, edited by D.C. Turk & R.D. Kerns, pp. 279–310. New York: John Wiley & Sons.

Brehm, S.S. & Brehm, J.W. (1981). *Psychological Reactance*. New York: Academic Press.

Bromet, E. & Moos, R.H. (1977). Environmental resources and the post-treatment functioning of alcoholic patients. *Journal of Health and Social Behavior*, 18, 326–338.

Burish, T.G. & Bradley, L.A. (1983). Coping with chronic disease: Definitions and issues. In *Coping with Chronic Disease*, edited by T.G. Burish and L.A. Bradley, pp. 3–12. New York: Academic Press.

Cafferata, G.L. (1987). Marital status, living arrangements, and the use of health services by elderly persons. *Journal of Gerontology*, 42, 613–618.

Carpenter, J.O. & Davis, L.J. (1976). Medical recommendations – Followed or ignored? Factors influencing compliance in arthritis. *Archives of Physical Medicine and Rehabilitation*, 57, 241–246.

Cassel, J. (1976). The contribution of the social environment to host resistance. *American Journal of Epidemiology*, 104, 107–123.

Cohen, S. (1988). Psychosocial models of the role of social support in the etiology of physical disease. *Health Psychology*, 7, 269–297.

Cohen, S. & Lichtenstein, E. (1990). Partner behaviors that support quitting smoking. *Journal of Consulting and Clinical Psychology*, 58, 304–309.

Cohen, S., Lichtenstein, E., Mermelstein, R., Kingsolver, K., Baer, J.S. & Kamarck, T.W. (1988). Social support interventions for smoking cessation. In *Marshaling Social Support: Formats, Processes, and Effects*, edited by B.H. Gottlieb, pp. 211–240. Newbury Park: Sage Publications.

Cohen, S. & Wills, T.A. (1985). Stress, social support, and the buffering hypothesis. *Psychological Bulletin*, 98, 310–357.

Coppotelli, H.C. & Orleans, C.T. (1985). Partner support and other determinants of smoking cessation maintenance among women. *Journal of Consulting and Clinical Psychology*, 53, 455–460.

Coyne, J.C., Wortman, C.B. & Lehman, D.R. (1988). The other side of support: Emotional over-involvement and miscarried helping. In *Social Support: Formats, Processes, and Effects*, edited by B.H. Gottlieb, pp. 305–330. Beverly Hills, CA: Sage.

Cutrona, C., Russell, D. & Rose, J. (1986). Social support and adaptation to stress by the elderly. *Journal of Psychology and Aging*, 1, 47–54.

Cwikel, J.M.G., Dielman, T.E., Kirscht, J.P. & Israel, B.A. (1988). Mechanisms of psychosocial effects on health: The role of social integration coping style, and health behavior. *Health Education Quarterly*, 15, 151–173.

Dakof, G.A. & Taylor, S.E. (1990). Victims' perceptions of social support: What is helpful from whom? *Journal of Personality and Social Psychology*, 58, 80–89.

Davidson, D.M. & Shumaker, S.A. (1987). Social support and cardiovascular disease. *Arteriosclerosis*, 7, 101–104.

Dean, K. (1989). Self-care components of lifestyles: The importance of gender, attitudes and the social situation. *Social Science and Medicine*, 29, 137–152.

DiMatteo, M.R. & Hays, R. (1981). Social support and serious illness. In *Social Networks and Social Support*, edited by B.H. Gottlieb, pp. 117–147. Beverly Hills: Sage Publications.

Dillard, J.P. (1989). Types of influence goals in personal relationships. *Journal of Social and Personal Relationships*, 6, 293–308.

Dimond, M. (1979). Social support and adaptation to chronic illness: The case of maintenance hemodialysis. *Research in Nursing and Health*, 2, 101–108.

Doherty, W.J., Schrott, H.G., Metcalf, L. & Iasiello-Vailas, L. (1983). Effect of spouse support and health beliefs on medication adherence. *The Journal of Family Practice*, 17, 837–841.

Durkheim, E. (1897/1951). *Suicide: A Study in Sociology*. Translated by J. Spaulding & G. Simpson. New York: Free Press.

Felton B.J. (1990). Coping and social support in older people's experiences of chronic illness. In *Stress and Coping in Later-Life Families*, edited by M.A.P. Stephens, J.H. Crowther, S.E. Hobfoll & D.L. Tennenbaum, pp. 153–171. New York: Hemisphere Publishing, Corp.

Finnegan, D.L. & Suler, J.R. (1985). Psychological factors associated with maintenance of improved health behaviors in postcoronary patients. *The Journal of Psychology*, 119, 87–94.

Fiore, J., Becker, J. & Coppel, D. (1983). Social network interactions: A buffer or a stress? *American Journal of Community Psychology*, 11, 423–439.

Fontana, A.F., Kerns, R.D., Rosenberg, R.L. & Colonese, K.L. (1989). Support, stress, and recovery from coronary heart disease: A longitudinal causal model. *Health Psychology*, 8, 175–193.

Fries, J.F. & Crapo, J.M. (1981). *Vitality and Aging*. San Francisco: W.H. Freeman & Co.

Funch, D.P. Mettlin, C. (1982). The role of support in relation to recovery from breast surgery. *Social Science and Medicine*, 16, 91–98.

Gallagher, D.E., Thompson, L.W. & Peterson, J.A. (1982). Psychosocial factors affecting adaptation to bereavement in the elderly. *International Journal of Aging and Human Development*, 14, 79–95.

Gass, K.A. (1989). Appraisal, coping and resources: Markers associated with the health of aged widows and widowers. In *Older Bereaved Spouses*, edited by D.A. Lund, pp. 95–110. New York: Hemisphere Publishing, Corp.

Gove, W.R. (1973). Sex, marital status, and mortality. *American Journal of Sociology*, 79, 45–67.

Grunberg, N.E. & Baum, A. (1985). Biological commonalities of stress and substance abuse. In *Coping and Substance Abuse*, edited by S. Shiffman & T.A. Wills, pp. 25–62. New York: Academic Press, Inc.

Haley, W.E., Levine, E.G., Brown, S.L. & Bartolucci, A.A. (1987). Stress, appraisal, coping, and social support as predictors of adaptational outcomes among dementia caregivers. *Psychology and Aging*, 2, 323–330.

Hamburg, D.A., Elliot, G.R. & Parron, D.L. (1982). *Health and Behavior*, pp. 3–24. Washington, D.C.: National Academy Press.

Heller, K., Thompson, M.G., Vlachos-Weber, I., Steffen, A.M. & Trueba, P.E. (1991). Support interventions for older adults: Confidante relationships, perceived family support, and meaningful role activity. *American Journal of Community Psychology*, 19, 139–148.

Hickey, T., Rakowski, W. & Julius, M. (1988). Preventive health practices among older men and women. *Research on Aging*, 10, 315–328.

House, J.S. (1981). *Work Stress and Social Support*. Reading, MA: Addison-Wesley.

House, J.S., Landis, K.R. & Umberson, D. (1988). Social relationships and health. *Science*, 241, 540–545.

House, J.S., Umberson, D. & Landis, K.R. (1988). Structures and processes of social support. *Annual Review of Sociology*, 14, 293–318.

Hughes, M. & Gove, W.R. (1981). Living alone, social integration, and mental health. *American Journal of Sociology*, 87, 48–74.

Idler, E.L. & Kasl, S. (1991). Health perceptions and survival: Do global evaluations of health status really predict mortality? *Journal of Gerontology: Social Sciences*, **46**, S55-65.

Kaplan, R.M. & Hartwell, S.L. (1987). Differential effects of social support and social network on physiological and social outcomes in men and women with Type II Diabetes Mellitus. *Health Psychology*, **6**, 387-398.

Kaplan, R.M. & Toshima, M.T. (1990). The functional effects of social relationships on chronic illness and disability. In *Social Support: An Interactional View*, edited by B.R. Sarason, I.G. Sarason & G. Pierce, pp. 427-453. New York: Wiley.

Kessler, R.C. & McLeod, J.A. (1985). Social support and mental health in community psychology. In *Social Support and Health*, edited by S. Cohen & L. Syme, pp. 219-240. Orlando, FL: Academic Press.

Kiecolt-Glaser, J.K. & Glaser, R. (1988). Psychological influences on immunity: Implications for AIDS. *American Psychologist*, **43**, 892-898.

Korbin, F.E. & Hendershot, G.E. (1977). Do family ties reduce mortality? Evidence from the United States, 1966-1968. *Journal of Marriage and the Family*, **39**, 737-745.

Krause, N. (1990). Illness behavior in late life. In *Handbook of Aging and the Social Sciences*, edited by R.H. Binstock & L.K. George, pp. 227-244. San Diego: Academic Press, Inc.

Kunter, N.G. (1987). Social ties, social support, and perceived health status among chronically disabled people. *Social Science and Medicine*, **25**, 29-34.

Lawton, M.P., Moss, M. & Kleban, M.H. (1984). Marital status, living arrangement, and the well-being of older people. *Research on Aging*, **6**, 323-345.

Levy, R.L. (1983). Social support and compliance: A selective review and critique of treatment integrity and outcome measurement. *Social Science and Medicine*, **17**, 1329-1338.

Lopata, H.Z. (1979). *Women as Widows: Support Systems*. New York: Elsever.

Manne, S.L. & Zautra, A.J. (1989). Spouse criticism and support: Their association with coping and psychological adjustment among women with rheumatoid arthritis. *Journal of Personality and Social Psychology*, **56**, 608-617.

Melamed, B.C. & Brenner, G.F. (1990). Social support and chronic medical stress: An interaction-based approach. *Journal of Social and Clinical Psychology*, **9**, 104-117.

Mermelstein, R., Lichtenstein, E. & McIntyre, K. (1983). Partner smoking and relapse in smoking-cessation programs. *Journal of Clinical and Consulting Psychology*, **51**, 465-466.

Morgan, G.E., Ashenberg, Z.S. & Fisher, E.B. (1988). Abstinence from smoking and the social environment. *Journal of Consulting and Clinical Psychology*, **56**, 298-301.

Nathanson, C.A. (1984). Sex differences in mortality. *Annual Review of Sociology*, **10**, 191-213.

National Center for Health Statistics (1987). *Current Estimates from the National Health Interview Survey: U.S. 1986*, DHHS Publication No. (PHS)82-1569. Hyattsville, MD: U.S. Dept. of Health & Human Services.

Norris, V.K., Stephens, M.A.P. & Kinney, J.M. (1990). The impact of family interactions on recovery from stroke: Help or hinderance? *The Gerontologist*, **30**, 535-542.

Pagel, M.D., Erdly, W.W. & Becker, J. (1987). Social networks: We get by with (and in spite of) a little help from our friends. *Journal of Personality and Social Psychology*, **53**, 793-804.

Rakowski, W., Julius, M., Hickey, T. & Halter, J.B. (1987). Correlates of preventive health behavior in late life. *Research on Aging*, **9**, 331-355.

Revenson, T.A., Wollman, C.A. & Felton, B.J. (1983). Social supports as stress buffers for adult cancer patients. *Psychosomatic Medicine*, **45**, 321-331.

Riggs, B.L. & Melton, L.J. III (1988). Osteoporosis and age-related fracture syndromes. In *Research and the Aging Population*, edited by D. Evered & J. Whelan, pp. 129-142. Chichester, U.K.: Wiley.

Rodin, J., Cashman, C. & Desiderato, L. (1987). Intervention and aging: Enrichment and prevention. In *Perspectives in Behavioral Medicine: The Aging Dimension*, edited by M.W. Riley, J.D. Matarazzo & A. Baum, pp. 149-172. Hillsdale, NJ: Lawrence Erlbaum Associates, Pub.

Rook, K.S. (1984). The negative side of social interaction. *Journal of Personality and Social Psychology*, **46**, 1097-1108.

Rook, K.S. (1990a). Stressful aspects of older adults' social relationships: Current theory and research. In *Stress and Coping in Later-Life Families*, edited by M.A.P. Stephens, J.H. Crowther, S.E. Hobfoll & D.L. Tennenbaum, pp. 173-192. New York: Hemisphere Publishing, Corp.

Rook, K.S. (1990b). Social networks as a source of social control in older adults' lives. In *Communication, Health, and the Elderly*, edited by H. Giles, N. Coupland & J. Wiemann, pp. 45-63. Manchester, England: University of Manchester Press.

Rook, K.S. & Pietromonaco, P. (1987). Close relationships: Ties that heal or ties that bind? In *Advances in Personal Relationships, Vol. 1*, edited by W.H. Jones & D. Perlman, pp. 1-35. Greenwich, CT: JAI Press.

Rook, K.S. Thuras, P.D. & Lewis, M.A. (1990). Social control, health risk-taking, and psychological distress among the elderly. *Psychology and Aging*, **5**, 327-334.

Santinga, J.T. (1987). Cardiovascular disease. In *Handbook of Clinical Gerontology*, edited by L.L. Carstensen & B.A. Edelstein, pp. 132-143. New York: Pergamon Press.

Sarason, B.R., Shearin, E.N., Pierce, G.R. & Sarason, I.G. (1987). Interrelations of social support measures: Theoretical and practical implications. *Journal of Personality and Social Psychology*, **50**, 845-855.

Schneider, E.L. & Brody, J.A. (1983). Aging, natural death, and the compression of morbidity: Another view. *New England Journal of Medicine*, **309**, 854-856.

Schulz, R. & Rau, M.T. (1985). Social support through the life course. In *Social Support and Health*, edited by S. Cohen & S.L. Syme, pp. 129-149. Orlando, FL: Academic Press.

Schwarzer, R. & Leppin, A. (1991). Social support, and health: A theoretical and empirical overview. *Journal of Social and Personal Relationships*, **8**, 99-127.

Seeman, T.E., Kaplan, G.A., Knudsen, L., Cohen, R. & Guralnik, J. (1987). Social network ties and mortality among the elderly in the Alameda County Study. *American Journal of Epidemiology*, **126**, 714-723.

Seeman, M., Seeman, T. & Sayles, M. (1985). Social networks and health status: A longitudinal analysis. *Social Psychology Quarterly*, **48**, 237-248.

Shumaker, S.A. & Hill, D.R. (1991). Gender differences in social support and physical health. *Health Psychology*, **10**, 102-111.

Siegler, I.C. & Costa, P.T. (1985). Health behavior relationships. In *Handbook of the Psychology of Aging*, edited by J.E. Birren & K.W. Schaie, pp. 144-166. New York: Van Nostrand Reinhold Co.

Snow, R. & Crapo, L. (1982). Emotional bondedness, subjective well-being, and health in elderly medical patients. *Journal of Gerontology*, **37**, 609-615.

Stephens, M.A.P., Kinney, J.M., Norris, V.K. & Ritchie, S.W. (1987). Social networks as assets and liabilities in recovery from stroke by geriatric patients. *Psychology and Aging*, **2**, 125-129.

Stoller, E. (1984). Self-assessments of health by the elderly: The impact of informal assistance. *Journal of Health and Social Behavior*, **25**, 260-270.

Stroebe, M.S. & Stroebe, W. (1983). Who suffers more? Sex differences in health risks of the widowed. *Psychological Bulletin*, **93**, 279-301.

Tessler, R. & Mechanic, D. (1978). Psychological distress and perceived health status. *Journal of Health and Social Behavior*, **19**, 254-262.

Thompson, L.W., Breckenridge, J.N. Gallagher, D. & Peterson, J. (1984). Effects of bereavement on self-perceptions of physical health in elderly widows and widowers. *Journal of Gerontology*, **39**, 309-314.

Umberson, D. (1987). Family status and health behaviors: Social control as a dimension of social integration. *Journal of Health and Social Behavior*, **28**, 306-319.

Umberson, D. & Greer, M. (1990). Social relationships and health behaviors: The wellness regulation model. Paper presented at the annual American Sociological Meeting.

Vaux, A. (1988). *Social Support: Theory, Research, and Intervention.* New York: Praeger.

Verbrugge, L.M. (1979). Marital status and health. *Journal of Marriage and the Family*, 41, 267–285.

Verbrugge, L.M. (1983). Women and men: Mortality and health of older people. In *Aging in Society: Selected Reviews of Recent Research*, edited by M.W. Riley, B.B. Hess & K. Bond, pp. 139–174. Hillsdale, NJ: Lawrence Erlbaum Associates.

Verbrugge, L.M. (1985). Gender and health: An update on hypotheses and evidence. *Journal of Health and Social Behavior*, 26, 156–182.

Verbrugge, L.M. (1989). The twain meet: Empirical explanations of sex differences in health and mortality. *Journal of Health and Social Behavior*, 30, 282–304.

Verbrugge, L.M. (1990). The iceberg of diability. In *The Legacy of Longevity*, edited by S.M. Stahl, pp. 55–75. Newbury Park: Sage Publications.

Vital and Health Statistics (1989). *Current estimates from the national health interview survey, 1988.* DHHS Publication No. (PHS) 89–1501. Hyattsville, Maryland: U.S. Dept. of Health & Human Services.

Wan, T.T. (1982). *Stressful Life Events, Social Support Networks and Gerontological Health.* Lexington, MA: Lexington.

Wills, T.A. (1990). Multiple networks and substance use. *Journal of Social and Clinical Psychology*, 9, 78–90.

Wills, T.A. & Shiffman, S. (1985). Coping and substance use: A conceptual framework. In *Coping and Substance Abuse*, edited by S. Shiffman & T.A. Wills, pp. 3–24. New York: Academic Press, Inc.

Wingard, D.L. (1982). The sex differential in mortality rates. *American Journal of Epidemiology*, 115, 205–216.

Wolinsky, F.D. (1990). *Health and Health Behavior Among Elderly Americans.* New York: Springer Publishing Co.

Wortman, C.B. & Conway, T.L. (1985). The role of social support in adaptation and recovery from physical illness. In *Social Support and Health*, edited by S. Cohen & S.L. Syme, pp. 281–302. New York: Academic Press, Inc.

Wortman, C.B. & Lehman, D.R. (1985). Reactions to victims of life crises: Support attempts that fail. In *Social Support: Theory, Research, and Applications*, edited by I.G. Sarason & B.R. Sarason, pp. 463–489. Dordrecht, The Netherlands: Martinus Nijhoff.

Wortman, C.B. & Silver, R.C. (1990). Successful mastery of bereavement and widowhood: A life-course perspective. In *Successful Aging: Perspectives from the Behavioral Sciences*, edited by P.B. Baltes & M.M. Baltes, pp. 225–264. New York: Cambridge University Press.

Zimmerman, R.S. & Connor, C. (1989). Health promotion in context: The effects of significant others on health behavior change. *Health Education Quarterly*, 16, 57–75.

INDEX